THE
WHOLE
LIFE
PROSTATE
BOOK

**Everything That
Every Man—
at Every Age—
Needs to Know
About Maintaining
Optimal Prostate
Health**

H. BALLENTINE CARTER, MD
AND GERALD SECOR COUZENS

FREE PRESS
NEW YORK • LONDON • TORONTO • SYDNEY • NEW DELHI

*f*P

FREE PRESS

A Division of Simon & Schuster, Inc.
1230 Avenue of the Americas
New York, NY 10020

First Free Press hardcover edition June 2012

FREE PRESS and colophon are trademarks of Simon & Schuster, Inc.

For information about special discounts for bulk purchases,
please contact Simon & Schuster Special Sales at
1-866-506-1949 or business@simonandschuster.com.

The Simon & Schuster Speakers Bureau can bring authors to your live event.
For more information or to book an event, contact the Simon & Schuster Speakers
Bureau at 1-866-248-3049 or visit our Web site at www.simonspeakers.com.

Designed by Mspace/Maura Fadden Rosenthal

Illustrations by Rob Duckwall

Manufactured in the United States of America

1   3   5   7   9   10   8   6   4   2

Library of Congress Cataloging-in-Publication Data

Carter, H. Ballentine.
The whole life prostate book : everything that every man—at every age—
needs to know about maintaining optimal prostate health / H. Ballentine
Carter and Gerald Secor Couzens.—1st Free Press hardcover ed.
    p.   cm.
1. Prostate—Diseases—Popular works.   I. Couzens, Gerald Secor.   II. Title.
RC899.C34   2012
616.6'5—dc23
2012001415

ISBN 978-1-4516-2121-1
ISBN 978-1-4516-2123-5 (ebook)

To my wife

For her everlasting support.

—HBC

For Elisa and Gerald

Thanks for all the hard work.

This wouldn't have happened without you.

—GSC

CONTENTS

CONTENTS

NUMBER ONE,
IGNORE THE HYPE AND GET THE FACTS

Google the word *prostate*, and in 0.25 seconds you'll get more than eighty-two million Web hits bombarding you with information—much of it completely misleading. Sadly, there is a blinding storm of prostate-related content on the Internet, offering you everything from the latest intel on nondrug treatments for an enlarged prostate, to erectile dysfunction solutions too numerous to mention—and many others too dangerous to try.

For example, you might learn about robotic surgery for prostate cancer, cancer "eradication" with radiation, cryotherapy that will freeze the tumor, and ultrasound that will heat it. Or you could be impressed that the machine used to deliver proton beam radiation therapy for prostate cancer is housed in a facility the size of a football field, and although complete treatment costs $50,000, there is no scientific evidence to demonstrate that it's superior to any other form of prostate cancer treatment. Yet another online search might lead you to the Web site for a well-known maker of pomegranate juice, which claims that its product lowers the risk of both prostate cancer and erection problems. Naturally it neglects to mention that the US Federal Trade Commission (FTC), the federal agency responsible for preventing fraud, deception, and unfair business practices in the marketplace, has charged the company with making false statements.

Unsubstantiated claims abound and, unfortunately, there is no real way for men to know what Web-derived information is solid and what is potentially harmful. The deck is stacked against you. As a layperson, getting the right information online is not easy, and what's worse is that all of your sifting and digging can make it even more difficult to know which questions to ask your doctor.

With so many treatment options available with just a click of a mouse—surgical and nonsurgical, real and fabricated—it's nearly impossible for an average man to make the right choice and get the right advice. Your questions tend to take on lives of their own, multiplying exponentially.

- If I have lower urinary tract symptoms, do I actually need treatment right now?

- If I have prostate enlargement causing urinary symptoms, should I believe all the hype about the herbal supplements used to manage this condition?

- If I have prostate cancer, is treatment necessary immediately? How can I determine if I am a candidate for active surveillance? And how do I get a doctor to work with me?

- Do drugs work well for prostatitis? Are muscle spasms the reason for my chronic pelvic pain?

- How do I decide if getting a PSA test—short for prostate-specific antigen blood test—is right for me? At what age should I start? When do I stop?

- Should I have my prostate removed surgically if cancer is present? What is the best way to do it, and who should do it?

You will find no shortage of answers on the Internet, but be careful not to take them as fact. The most accurate information you are likely to find are the Google directions to get to the doctor's office.

It's not just the Internet that's to blame. Men today are ambushed by articles recommending over-the-counter supplements to maintain prostate health, infomercials touting prescription drugs that supposedly prevent or treat prostate enlargement, and billboards advertising "newer," more precise surgical and radiation treatments for prostate cancer. Yet much of what is being marketed is not backed by any evidence of effectiveness. Oftentimes these treatments are misdirected at the prostate when, in fact, the prostate is not the culprit behind the symptoms. Furthermore, many of these therapies are unnecessarily aggressive and invasive.

Why?

Despite great advances in medical research, our health care system today is driven by incentives that reward treating disease with medication, surgery, and radiation rather than preventing or managing it carefully before it actually strikes. Then there is the relative ease of approving, and promoting as "better," the newest drug or device that claims to improve health—even when there is no proof that new is actually better.

When it comes to maintaining male health and prostate health, there is no universal prescription. There are individual health histories and emerging data from ongoing studies to consider. And when it comes to prostate cancer, the stakes are higher and the need for answers is even more crucial.

Here are some facts to bear in mind:

- As many as two million men this year are going to seek medical attention for chronic pelvic pain syndrome, an ailment that has wrecked their quality of life. Obtaining a proper diagnosis and effective treatment will be very difficult, since most doctors rely on antibiotics to treat a problem that is not caused by an infection!

- Most men who live past the age of eighty will have prostate cancer that began decades earlier. Many will be diagnosed and opt for treatment, but a large proportion of those patients will not have needed it.

- More than half of males aged forty and above will have some degree of discomfort with lower urinary tract symptoms, acronymed LUTS, some triggered by their prostate. Deciding on what therapy to pursue will baffle most men.

According to a recent survey of men forty-five and older, 70 percent of them knew nothing about their prostate or about prostate cancer, the number two cause of cancer deaths in men, after lung cancer. I would like to see that percentage reduced significantly and to address all of the misinformation and misconceptions that abound.

Although we men now face many hurdles, I can show you how to maintain optimal health and avoid becoming a prostate patient—and how to make wise choices should you ever get diagnosed with a prostate disease.

LET ME BE YOUR GUIDE

"I can't sit through a meeting without having to excuse myself and scoot to the bathroom. Do I need one of the drugs I saw advertised on TV to eliminate these bathroom breaks?"

"I'm up two to three times every night going to the bathroom. Is this just normal aging?"

"I have been to countless doctors who have prescribed various treatments for my prostatitis, but it hasn't gotten better. It's been two years. What can I do?"

"I'm considering a laser procedure on my prostate so I don't have to urinate so much, especially at night. Is that my best option?"

"My erections are not as strong as they used to be, and I don't have as much interest in sex as I used to. Is this expected when you're older?"

"I'm scared out of my wits. I was just told that I have prostate cancer. Should I have my prostate removed next week like the doctor advised? What about proton beam therapy or high-intensity focused ultrasound?"

I am constantly asked questions such as these during medical consultations with patients of all ages. Answering them as honestly and as factually as possible is what being a good doctor is all about. For the last thirty years of my life, I have been dedicated to the study of urology and the prostate gland in particular. My ongoing interest in prostate research and treatment has taken me all over the world as a surgeon, scientist, teacher, and lecturer, and has stirred in me a deep and enduring kinship with men of every age, race, creed, and nationality.

I have had the incredible good fortune of spending my entire professional life at Johns Hopkins Hospital, which *U.S. News and World Report* has ranked the number one hospital in the United States for a record twenty-one years in a row—and number one in urology for that same time span. Johns Hopkins has given me the opportunity, the resources, and the support needed to invest myself fully in what has become my life's mission: leading men to a better understanding of male health and the symptoms and diseases associated with the prostate, and helping them maintain a healthy lifestyle in order to prevent the development of prostate disease with age. As I tell my patients, the prostate and overall male health are closely linked. The lifestyle that promotes male health also promotes prostate health. Conversely, adopting unhealthy habits increases the odds of disorders that are often associated with prostate disease, such as urinary symptoms and erectile dysfunction (ED).

Still, the fact is that for years most men—regardless of their individual symptoms—have been unequivocally led to believe that their prostates are to blame, instead of being encouraged to pay closer attention to their daily lifestyles. Granted, prostate disorders are common, but they are frequently misdiagnosed and often treated unnecessarily. Even with prostate cancer, which is diagnosed in over two hundred thousand men yearly, management is more often guided by the unfounded beliefs and personal fears of doctors and patients alike, which lead to needlessly invasive treatments.

Way back at the beginning of my career, the diagnoses and treatments for prostate-related diseases were handled much differently than they are today. Men who showed up at the doctor's office with significant complaints of urination difficulties or urinary retention (the inability to urinate) often underwent a surgical procedure called a TURP to remove prostate tissue. That's shorthand for transurethral resection of the prostate. In the 1980s, TURP was the second most commonly performed operation in the Medicare population. Today there is a better understanding of the causes of urination complaints, which are often unrelated to prostate disease. We have various medical therapies for these symptoms, and there has been a tremendous reduction in the need for surgery. Now there's even evidence that some urination problems can be prevented altogether.

Three decades ago, men also came to see the doctor with far more advanced prostate cancers—for which treatment was futile. In most of these cases, the disease had already spread beyond the prostate gland. Today, thanks to the PSA, or the prostate-specific antigen test, the majority of men are diagnosed with early stage prostate cancer and can be treated effectively with options that carry a lower risk of side effects. There's also growing evidence that a healthy lifestyle can prevent the development of prostate cancer as well as prevent or slow down the progression of prostate cancer that has already been diagnosed.

I will get to all of that later, but I bring it up because I have been the beneficiary of these advances, having spent my career at Johns Hopkins, where many discoveries about age-induced prostate disease have taken place. Perhaps, in some small way, I have contributed to these efforts.

When I first began practicing medicine in the 1980s, my goal was simple: make sick people well. And that's what I did as often as possible, utilizing medications in some cases, but more often than not, surgical procedures. However, as time went by, I began to realize that much pain and suffering could be avoided—if not eliminated—if only my patients were able to head off a problem before it developed, and that included preventing prostate disease.

Gradually, my medical approach changed, and prevention and careful management became its key component. The more men I saw suffering from prostate disease, the more I began to wonder why these men were ending up in my examining room in the first place and what I could do to prevent them from having to come back. I began to focus on the important roles of a physician, such as educating patients about their health and helping them reduce the development of disease.

It was then that I decided to look for every opportunity to teach men how to take better care of themselves, especially their prostates. No patient could leave my office without my telling him about the preventive aspects of a healthful diet and physical activity, both of which could help turn the tide of overall declining male health that has become epidemic in our society. Soon after, I saw firsthand how this approach could help restore the bounce in a man's step and the zest for life that many hadn't felt in twenty years.

I soon came to spend part of my time teaching and lecturing about the prostate to students at the Johns Hopkins School of Medicine, fellow doctors, and men's groups around the country, raising consciousness, increasing awareness, urging them to be proactive rather than reactive. This book is an extension of that important work.

Five years ago, this book could not have been written. The science and evidence on which it is based just weren't there. Back then, the focus was on diagnosis, when a low-risk prostate condition was already established, and then bringing out the big guns—surgery, most often—to bring relief or cure. The important connections between a healthful diet, weight loss, and regular exercise and their impact on the prostate had not been determined.

But now there is a better understanding of the link between lifestyle choices and disease development in the prostate. I now recommend a healthful lifestyle for patients as part of a prevention and treatment program for the often interrelated male health disorders that include lower urinary tract symptoms unrelated to the prostate, erectile dysfunction, prostate enlargement that causes urination symptoms, chronic pelvic pain syndrome, and newly diagnosed prostate cancer. By using this approach, many men see improvements in their quality of life without the need for any invasive treatments.

The content of this book comes from my firsthand experiences counseling anxious men with newly diagnosed prostate cancer. So many of these men had already experienced such a major decline in their overall health due to unwise lifestyle choices that prostate cancer was not the biggest threat to their lives—yet prostate cancer was their only concern. While counseling them about how we manage prostate cancer, I took the opportunity to point out shortcomings in their lifestyle choices and the potential for preventing further illness and prostate cancer progression with relatively simple behavioral changes.

Because I had a captive, frightened audience, perhaps my words were taken more seriously. But my message got through. I saw unexpected changes in my patients' health, including weight reduction and less need for drugs to lower blood pressure, glucose, and cholesterol. Reduced urinary symptoms and improved erectile function became the norm for many, along with an overall improved outlook on life.

I soon began to wonder why men wait for the proverbial anvil to drop—whether a heart attack or a prostate cancer diagnosis—before making important changes to improve their health. Thus began my efforts to educate and promote the healthy lifestyle that can prevent the deterioration in male health with age.

The theme of this book is educating yourself, changing your habits, and doing so with measures within your means. In the pages that follow, you will find information on modifying your lifestyle, including facts about food and exercise to help maintain not only the health of your prostate but also your general health while improving the quality of your life.

Since male health disorders such as benign prostatic enlargement, lower urinary tract symptoms, overactive bladder, prostatitis, chronic pelvic pain syndrome, and prostate cancer are managed in a variety of ways, I will analyze for you the strengths and weaknesses of the reasonable management options—as well as describe others that you should ignore entirely, even though they may be touted as "revolutionary breakthroughs."

A few examples follow:

- Mark C., a worried patient, recently informed me that he no longer wanted to have his PSA level tested. He'd based his decision on a front-page story in the *New York Times* reporting that men didn't need to get the PSA test anymore to detect prostate cancer early. "That is certainly something to think about," I told Mark, but I then had to spend the next twenty minutes of our visit explaining why the PSA test could save his life—based on his age (fifty-five), race (African American), and family history (an older brother had died of prostate cancer).

- In 2009 many national TV news programs carried stories claiming that the drug Avodart (generic name, dutasteride) and Proscar (generic name, finasteride) could be used to prevent prostate cancer. Ordinarily, these drugs are used to manage bothersome lower urinary tract symptoms. I immediately alerted my office manager to expect a steady stream of phone calls from patients wanting to know how to get this medication and when they should start taking it. I ended up speaking with many men over the next days and explaining to each that, contrary to the news report, these drugs, which are called 5-alpha reductase inhibitors, do not prevent prostate cancer; in fact, research showed that for some patients, they could *increase* their risk of developing a more aggressive form of prostate cancer. This advice was later validated in 2011, when the US Food and Drug Administration (FDA), which is responsible for protecting the public health by assuring the safety, effectiveness, and security of drugs, vaccines, medical devices, and our nation's food supply, voted not to approve the use of these drugs for the prevention of prostate cancer.

- An enlarged prostate can cause urination difficulties, and deciding on which management option to choose—surveillance, medication, in-office heat therapies, or surgery—takes careful thought and discussion. This can be a difficult process when a patient already has a preconceived notion of what he wants to do because of advertisements and Internet searches that often confuse the issues.

I bring this up because it took most of my afternoon meeting with Ron W. to convince him that the GreenLight laser surgery he had heard advertised on the radio was *not* the procedure that would work best for his lower urinary tract symptoms. Actually, weight loss and better food and beverage choices were a more logical first step. Six months later, after adopting an exercise program and losing weight, he returned and was more interested in talking to me about sailing than he was about his prostate! His urinary complaints were virtually forgotten without a single drug or surgical procedure.

- Supplements are popular with many of my patients. Richard M. recently emailed me saying that he had read on the Internet that selenium supplements are good for prostate health. Selenium is a mineral that many researchers had thought could play a key role in preventing prostate cancer. "How much should I start taking?" he wrote. This information was misleading and could prove harmful, and then I explained at great length just why that was so.

- Men fear a diagnosis of prostate cancer, especially when it has struck close to home. After a recent talk that I gave about prostate cancer to a local support group, a man asked me about his cancer susceptibility. "My father and brother had prostate cancer before age fifty-five," he said. "I am fifty years old. Does that mean I will get it too?" I explained that the odds of being diagnosed were higher for him than someone without a family history, but I then outlined basic ways that could help him effectively sidestep his genetic destiny through regular PSA screening and some dietary and exercise suggestions.

- Charles B. had been to several other urologists before meeting with me and had been misdiagnosed and treated for prostatitis for many years with various drugs. He had chronic pelvic pain from pelvic muscle spasm, and he could visibly describe the associated discomfort and the life stress that triggered it. After examining him and ruling out other causes for his discomfort, I gave Charles the contact information for a physical therapist who would work with him on a program for relieving his muscle spasm.

- I often see patients for second opinions about prostate cancer, and many men travel great distances. Liam M. had flown in from Ireland, and he was distraught. "My doctor says I have prostate cancer and need to have surgery. But I am sixty-five and recently married to a beautiful, loving thirty-eight-year-old woman," he said. "I know the possible side effects of surgery can include erection problems, so I am reluctant to undergo surgery. What if I chose to join your active surveillance program instead?"

In lieu of surgery or radiation therapy for men with very low- and low-risk prostate cancer, we started an active surveillance program more than sixteen years ago in which we monitored men with twice-yearly PSA tests and annual biopsy. I explained to Liam that if he met the criteria that I was going to describe, he just might be a perfect candidate. I then spent the rest of our session reviewing his medical records, explaining how the odds were overwhelming that something else would take his life rather than prostate cancer (even without treatment), and detailing the specific tests he would undergo every six months if he decided to join the program. Liam was eligible, and he did join our active surveillance program at Johns Hopkins. Five years later, he continues to enjoy a high quality of life that includes normal sexual function.

THE OVERDIAGNOSIS AND OVERTREATMENT OF PROSTATE CANCER

Although I have performed more than three thousand radical prostatectomy surgeries to remove cancerous prostates, I have since come to believe that prostate cancer is not only overdiagnosed but also overtreated in the United States. Let me explain.

Because we have been screening for prostate cancer in the United States with the PSA test since the late 1980s, one in six men are now diagnosed with prostate cancer. However, many of the cancers that are being uncovered would never cause any harm to a man during his lifetime, even without treatment. Some prominent prostate cancer experts are now terming this overdiagnosis of prostate cancer and calling for an end to mass PSA screening.

I don't agree with this assessment. The PSA screening dilemma will be covered in depth in chapter 10, where I offer the pros and cons in this contentious debate as well as explain the incredible benefit I believe there is in smart use of the PSA test, as opposed to mass screening with a one-size-fits-all approach. Together with colleagues at the Baltimore Longitudinal Study of Aging, I promoted this concept when PSA was first introduced as a screening test, arguing that not every man needs annual testing, that a baseline PSA can determine the optimal frequency of PSA testing, and that older men with low PSA levels during life can safely discontinue testing.

Unfortunately, prostate cancers are viewed too often as all being the same disease with the same threat for every individual, leading to unnecessary treatments in many men. This approach is grounded in the dread associated with the word *cancer*. A lack of information and fear too often result in men being treated unnecessarily and forced to accept the associated side effects of treatment that can diminish their quality of life.

Understanding the significance of overdiagnosis and overtreatment of prostate cancer, sixteen years ago I helped create and continue to direct the groundbreaking Johns Hopkins active surveillance program, which was the first of its kind to use the same strict criteria to enroll men and follow them carefully with regular testing twice a year. Almost one thousand men diagnosed with low-grade prostate cancer have enrolled, choosing for now to avoid surgery or radiation therapy and taking the alternate approach of having their cancer monitored carefully.

THE NEW PARADIGM

Historically, the prostate was something that concerned only older men. But in the current era of preventive medicine, I believe that educating the younger man about his prostate and associated male health is paramount. Young men will become older men. Hopefully, after a lifetime of awareness, education, and a variety of proactive steps that I prescribe— which call for diet and exercise modifications—they will be in a position to prevent or minimize the declines in male health that include the development of prostate disease.

This is a book for every man, at every important stage in his life. He can use it in the early part of his life, when he is in his twenties and thirties and needs to become informed about male health before it deteriorates—preventing that from happening through lifestyle choices like diet and exercise. It is also his definitive navigational guide to get him through the minefield of prostate-related medical issues that can arise in his forties, fifties, and beyond.

I see this as a book that a man uses to develop his prostate-healthy lifestyle of eating and exercise to prevent the common decline in male health that occurs with age caused by urinary symptoms, erectile dysfunction, and prostate diseases. Having the wrong information during this crucial period can not only affect quality of life but also take away life. My hope is that this book will help you—and all men—live longer, happier, and healthier.

NOW IT'S UP TO YOU

What you are about to read is a book that is the culmination of my life's endeavor to learn about male health and prostate disease. The information I'm providing comes from a combination of scientific opinions and studies from hospitals and university research labs around the world.

One final thought before we get under way. Since most male health problems—including those of the prostate—are so slow to develop, time is on your side. Use it wisely to make careful, well-informed decisions about prevention and management if a prostate disorder should develop. In the long run, this deliberate approach will help you prevent or manage a health concern in a way that is right for you.

PART ONE

YOUR HEALTHY PROSTATE

Life is not merely to be alive,
but to be well.

—Marcus Valerius Martial

CHAPTER ONE

PROSTATE 101: THE BASICS

For a considerable part of a man's life, the lowly prostate gland is taken for granted all too often. Unless it is acting up and forcing him to acknowledge it, the prostate flies under the radar, unnoticed and unappreciated. In my experience, it's the rare man who thinks about the health of his prostate, let alone knows where it is or what it actually does. Astoundingly, I even come across the occasional patient who doesn't even know he *has* a prostate!

MYTH BUSTER

Females do not have prostates! Only men and other male mammals do. However, women have Skene's glands around the urethra (the conduit for urine) that produce fluid similar to the prostate.

Yes, some men have heard of prostate-specific antigen or PSA—an enzyme produced by the prostate; elevated amounts detected in the blood can signal prostate cancer—but only because they may have had a PSA test by the age of fifty to check for the possible presence of prostate cancer and because, in recent years, this test has become the center of an international debate about its benefits and harms. An elevated PSA can often be a tipoff to prostate cancer, but other noncancerous conditions such as benign prostatic enlargement can also cause PSA elevations. Oftentimes a man will have the PSA test coupled with a doctor's digital rectal exam (DRE) to feel the prostate for any suspicious lumps, which can indicate cancer. With a normal PSA report and no sign of prostate cancer, any interest in the prostate often ends right there in the doctor's office—typically with no desire for more probing by the doctor.

All male mammals have some variant of the prostate; it's the way that we have all evolved over many millennia. Like the mysterious appendix, the prostate is a gland that you can live without, although minus its production of seminal fluid, reproduction through sexual intercourse isn't possible. Mammals differ widely in the amount of ejaculate volume they produce, from 1 milliliter (0.03 ounces) for a randy ram, to 250 milliliters (8 ounces) for a boar—the hairy animal, not the guy who always seems to buttonhole you in the corner at a cocktail party; that's a *bore*. That guy will produce about 3 milliliters, or 0.1 ounces, on a good day.

The prostate is diminutive compared with the kidneys, the liver, and other vital organs such as the heart and the lungs. Yet it's important that you know all about the gland: its primary functions, what can go wrong with it as you age, and how to lessen the chances of prostate disease—because the odds are very high that, with each passing day, you will get one step closer to either developing or being labeled as having a prostate disease.

My entire professional life, all thirty-plus years of it, has been spent investigating and treating all issues associated with this complex little powerhouse of a gland, and I still don't know what makes it so vulnerable. I think, however, that it really comes down to a combination of genetic propensity and the lifestyle choices that men make. The primary issues related to the prostate are problems caused by benign prostatic enlargement, which may result in lower urinary tract symptoms (a "going" problem), prostate inflammation, and prostate cancer. Each of these conditions, which are covered in great detail later in the book, is a disorder that can bring a man to his knees, to a hospital, or, in the case of advanced prostate cancer, to a medical oncologist who will help him decide which drug regimen he will follow to keep his cancer in check.

S-E-X: IT GETS MEN'S ATTENTION

When I was first speaking with publishers about writing this book, the one question that came up consistently was why I thought a healthy young man in his twenties or thirties would want to read this book and become proactive about his prostate health.

My answer was twofold: virtually every man, as he ages, will have to deal with issues involving urination, pelvic pain, or sexual dysfunction either caused by, related to, or blamed on the prostate. I went on to say that if proper steps were taken—mainly, steps having to do with awareness and lifestyle modification—these issues could be greatly reduced or, in some instances, prevented altogether.

The second part of my answer had to do with sex, plain and simple. I don't know any young man—or older man, for that matter—who is not interested in sex. Prostate issues vary in severity, but even the slightest problem with the prostate can have some impact on sexual function. The more serious conditions go hand in hand with significantly reduced sexual performance and, in some cases, the complete inability to have an erection ever again!

TAKING CARE OF YOUR PROSTATE

Let's start with proper pronunciation and spelling. The name of this gland is the pro*state*, not pro*strate*, as some men are wont to call it. But this gland, its name derived from the Greek word for "guardian," does anything but prostrate, or lie down, on the job. It's working all the time as a participant in urination and in helping to create a fulfilling sex life.

While the prostate is your guardian, you also have to be the guardian of your prostate. Changes in urinary habits or ejaculation, pelvic pain, and abnormal PSA results need attention before a treatable condition becomes more difficult—or impossible—to address effectively. Because the prostate is prone to microscopic malignant tumors, an inevitable part of aging for so many men, vigilance along with periodic testing after the age of forty is right for some men to ensure that they don't ever become a prostate cancer statistic.

All the while I've been describing the prostate, you've probably been wondering what it looks like. I want you to imagine a crabapple, stem side up. The prostate is typically about an inch and a half wide at the base, a little narrower in its vertical dimension, and weighs about 20 grams, or 0.7 ounces. Think of the protective skin of the apple as a stand-in for the outer portion of the prostate. The inner, fleshy fruit of the apple represents the prostate gland. The apple core, running from top to bottom, represents the urethra, the flexible tube that is buried within the prostate and transports urine and semen.

IMPORTANT MESSAGE FOR CONCERNED WOMEN

Since men of all ages typically don't know all the complex workings of their bodies and are often hesitant to respond to medical issues, you may find this prostate information invaluable as you try to help the various men in your life maintain optimal health and well-being. Helping your partner, father, brother, or son cope with prostate problems should include far more than just comforting. I've come to realize that a concerned woman acting as another guardian of a man's health—by offering daily encouragement or brushing up on prostate facts—can improve the quality of her man's life beyond measure.

HOW THE PROSTATE DEVELOPS

While tucked away in the womb, you and your grandmother, mother, sister, aunt, and wife were all indistinguishable from one another for the first two months of gestation: you all had the X (female) chromosome. But at the end of this time, you started to become male, thanks to the influence of your Y (male) chromosome. It's the presence of the Y chromosome that sets in motion the development of the testes, or testicles; without the Y chromosome, ovaries will develop. At about seven to eight weeks, the testes produce an inhibiting substance that prevents the development of female anatomy, and shortly thereafter, at around nine weeks, production of the male hormone testosterone (and its reduced counterpart, dihydrotestosterone, or DHT) leads to the development of the male anatomy, including the penis and the prostate.

In the developing female (with XX chromosomes), because of the absence of the inhibiting substance and male hormones from the testicles, tissues that would have become part of the male internal anatomy (prostate, seminal vesicles) wither away, and in their place, female structures (uterus, fallopian tubes, vagina) develop. Part of the vagina arises from tissues that would have formed the prostate had genetic shuffling not resulted in two X chromosomes.

By three months, the male anatomy is formed with ductwork intact, and in the last trimester, the testicles descend into the scrotum, and the penis starts to grow. Once you're born, the prostate lies relatively quiet for the next ten-plus years, until puberty, when a metamorphosis takes place. As testosterone levels begin to rise again, your voice deepens, hair begins to sprout in unfamiliar places, and the prostate begins to grow, eventually giving rise to the complex, mature prostate gland.

Prostatic hyperplasia, or benign prostatic hyperplasia (BPH), as pathologists like to call growth of the prostate gland that is not related to cancer, does not occur in men younger than age thirty. But after age forty, when most body functions are declining with concurrent drops in testosterone production, the prostate may start to grow in some men. The reasons for this growth are not clear but may be related to testosterone levels during fetal development in the womb, inherited genes, and lifestyle choices that lead to inflammation and alterations in growth factors, the protein molecules that regulate cell division and survival. Whatever the cause, prostates come in all sizes (much like breasts) and, after age forty, can enlarge from the size of that crabapple to a large orange or grapefruit over the decades.

As the prostate continues to enlarge in some men, it may begin to squeeze the urethra, pinching off urine flow. When severe cases of obstruction are ignored and left untreated, this problem can sometimes escalate to damage the bladder and kidneys or else cause other problems such as infections and stones within the bladder.

Although I have many patients who worry initially that this benign prostatic enlargement, or BPE, causes prostate cancer, they are greatly relieved to find that the two ailments are separate, apparently unrelated disorders that just happen to occur in the prostate. While prostate cancer is typically found in the gland's peripheral zone next to the rectum, prostatic enlargement that comes with aging begins in the inner transition zone of the prostate, compressing the urethra and causing bothersome urination issues.

ARE YOU A BOY OR ARE YOU A GIRL?

Shortly after a baby's birth, the doctor checks the status of the genitalia and reports the sex to the parents. In rare cases, a condition called ambiguous genitalia, in which the penis, scrotum, vagina, and clitoris are not distinct, makes it difficult to tell the sex of the baby.

What does this have to do with the prostate? The male hormone testosterone gets converted to a more potent hormone called dihydrotestosterone (DHT) in the tissues that before birth give rise to the prostate and male external genitalia. Without this conversion, the prostate and genitalia don't develop normally. In fact, the discovery that chromosomally normal males (XY) with an inability to convert testosterone to DHT had ambiguous genitalia and no development of a prostate eventually led to the formulation of the drugs you see advertised on TV for "shrinking" the prostate. These drugs inhibit the conversion of testosterone to DHT.

Of course, these medications wouldn't be very marketable if they also shrank the penis. That situation does not occur, thankfully, since the penis, unlike the prostate, is not sensitive to male hormones (androgens) such as testosterone later in life after it has developed fully.

WHAT THE PROSTATE DOES

The prostate is a mixture of dozens of microscopic, spongy, fluid-producing glands, ducts, and muscle all wrapped up in a neat, paper-thin wrapper of sturdy fibrous tissue, encased by a protective layer of fat. Its primary job description: produce fluid that makes up semen, allowing sperm to thrive. In fact, this fluid is initially thick, like hair gel (remember the comedy *There's Something About Mary* and how well that gel worked?), until acted upon by prostate-specific antigen (PSA), which liquefies the semen so that sperm, the male sex cell that contains genetic information, can swim all the way up the female reproductive system to fertilize a waiting egg and create new life.

The prostate may also have a role in preventing urinary tract infections. But this small organ can also produce big problems, since there is a lot of "high-priced real estate" nearby, including the bladder, the muscles that control urination to prevent urine leakage, the nerves that allow men to have erections, and the pelvic muscles involved in orgasm. Enlargement, inflammation, and cancer of the prostate can affect surrounding organs, leading to difficulty with urination, pelvic pain, and sexual dysfunction. That's a trifecta you don't want to win!

When it comes to sex, the prostate is also a crucial part of the male reproduction team, which is made up of the testes, where sperm are produced; the epididymis and vas deferens, which make up the conduit through which sperms passes from the testicles to the prostatic urethra; and the seminal vesicles, which produce part of the seminal fluid together with the prostate. It is not a sexual gland per se, but the prostate is vital in making sexual function possible by producing the fluid containing the hormones and proteins that protect sperm following ejaculation. This interesting mix contains numerous substances, including acid phosphatase, albumin, calcium, zinc, citric acid, and prostate-specific antigen (PSA).

Sperm are manufactured within the testicle in a system of small channels called seminiferous tubules. These tubules have the combined length of almost three football fields! After leaving the testicle, sperm undergo changes in the epididymis—like an athlete training for the triathlon—that will enable them to swim. Sperm are then stored in the epididymis and vas deferens and await their calling. (Check out Woody Allen in costume as a sperm waiting for the call to action in his 1972 comedy classic *Everything You Always Wanted to Know About Sex* But Were Afraid to Ask*.)

All of this activity from sperm production to "training" and then storage takes about two months—very inefficient when compared with other animals.

Following sexual arousal, and just before ejaculation, sperm are propelled upward from the epididymis via the vas deferens, a long tube that has the most muscle per tubular diameter of any organ in the body. From there, sperm are emitted into the urethra within the prostate, where they combine with the seminal fluid from the prostate itself and from the two-inch-long seminal vesicles, which are found behind the bladder and at the base of the prostate.

At the moment of climax, the contractions of the prostate and nearby muscles propel the semen through the urethra and out the penis.

Why out the end of the penis instead of backward into the bladder?

It's a one-way street because at the time of orgasm, the bladder neck closes tight, ensuring that the sperm head in the right direction: out. Nature has created various methods to guarantee that sperm meet egg. In male dogs, the erect penis has a bulb that "locks" the penis in the vagina and traps the ejaculate. In rodents, a seminal plug protects sperm. And in humans, seminal fluid is initially coagulated like blood or mucus and then liquefied through the action of PSA.

MYTH BUSTER

Sperm and semen are *not* the same. About three hundred million microscopic sperm cells, complete with heads and wiggling tails, are produced by the egg-shaped testes and make up part of normal seminal fluid. Semen, the milky white fluid manufactured mostly by the seminal vesicles, with contributions from the prostate and other glands, is the transport medium for sperm, carrying them through the urethra and out of the penis during powerful muscular contractions at the time of orgasm.

THE PROSTATE AND ERECTIONS

The erectogenic nerves responsible for signaling the penis to get hard run along the outside of the prostate with an overlay of a blanket-like covering of tissue, making the prostate an important bystander in erectile function. Diseases of the prostate that cause the gland to become inflamed or enlarged, as well as cancer, can adversely affect erections, so it pays to keep the gland healthy.

Dr. Patrick Walsh, chairman of the urology department at Hopkins when I arrived, was the first physician to discover that these fragile nerves did not run *inside* the prostate like most anatomists had thought, but rather *outside* the gland—a discovery that changed the history of prostate cancer treatment throughout the world. If prostate surgery is ever a necessity for you and you want to preserve your active sex life, in chapter 13 I'll explain just how important it is to find the right surgeon for the task.

MYTH BUSTER

You *can* have intercourse without a prostate. However, after radical prostatectomy, in which the prostate and seminal vesicles are removed, there will be no ejaculate produced during your "dry" orgasm.

SIZING UP THE PROSTATE

Prostates range in size over time. Babies have prostates the size of a pea, barely tipping the scales at the weight of a paperclip (1.5 grams, or 0.05 ounces) and continuing to grow very slowly. By the end of the teenage years and sexual maturation, the 1.5-inch-long prostate usually weighs in at around 18 grams (0.63 ounces) and generally has reached the size of a crabapple (or strawberry, walnut, plum, lime, or golf ball—the comparisons are many). With a third of the gland made up of muscular tissue, the prostate feels smooth, soft, and yet somewhat firm to the touch.

In the ensuing years of adulthood, the prostate gland grows slowly, from about 25 grams for men in their thirties, to 35 to 45 grams for men in their seventies. In some men, however, the prostate can grow to 100 grams or more. Or, getting back to the fruit analogy, those are good-sized crabapples, lemons, oranges, and even grapefruits.

An interesting aside to prostate growth is the fact that the gland actually continues to grow while another more prominent body part, the penis, will stop growing after puberty. I'm sure most men would rather have a larger penis and a smaller prostate, but apparently nature did not intend it to be that way.

The good news is that not all men's prostates will enlarge to be bothersome, and if they do, this benign prostatic enlargement has *nothing* to do with potentially lethal disease; it's just a big prostate. In fact, for unclear reasons, men with prostate cancer who have large prostates have *less* aggressive disease than those with smaller prostates. Does the large prostate produce a substance that provides protection from aggressive cancer? That's unknown at this time, but it's an interesting question that researchers at Johns Hopkins are pursuing.

When the prostate grows, it can do one of two things: it can enlarge and produce no symptoms at all, or it can enlarge and start to compress the urethra, the tube that runs from the bladder through the prostate and out through the penis. This compression causes lower urinary tract symptoms that can vary from mild and not warranting treatment to severe and requiring surgery. This is all covered in greater detail in chapter 5.

UMMM, WHERE IS IT EXACTLY?

The prostate is situated inside the pelvic area, just below the bladder and right in front of your rectum, about two inches up from the perineum, the region between your scrotum and anus. The base, which is the widest part of the prostate, is at the top, nearest to the urinary bladder, while the narrowest end of the prostate, where the urethra exits, is called the apex. This faces toward the perineum down below.

Since the prostate and bladder are so close to each other, you should not be surprised to find that many of the prostate disorders discussed in later chapters also have a major bladder—and urination—component to them.

Since the prostate is perched just in front of the rectum, urologists use the rectum as a window to evaluate the gland by way of a digital rectal exam (DRE) and by transrectal ultrasound (TRUS). DRE allows the physician to feel, or palpate, the part of the gland where cancers usually arise, while TRUS uses ultrasound waves to create two-dimensional images of the prostate. For this exam, a small ultrasound probe (about the size of two fingers) is inserted into the rectum. The DRE, along with the prostate-specific antigen (PSA) blood test, are the current mainstays for detection of prostate cancer.

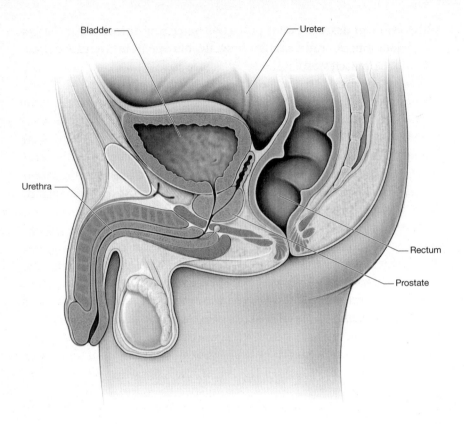

The adult pelvic area

YOUR PELVIC FLOOR: THE PROSTATE'S FOUNDATION

You know what a hammock is, of course. Well, you have your own internal hammock, made up of a collection of muscles that comfortably and securely hold your entire pelvic floor (the bottom of the pelvic cavity) together. These muscles attach to your pubic bone in front and your coccyx, or tailbone, in the back, and are linked from side to side by your "sit bone," or, as doctors like to call it, your ischial tuberosity. The pelvic floor muscles surround your anus and urethra, helping to support them, as well as the bladder, rectum, and prostate. What's more they help these organs maintain their proper function. One of the muscles also assists in propelling blood to the penis to create a more rigid erection.

In women, the pelvic floor becomes most important after childbirth, when the muscles weaken, allowing pelvic organs such as the bladder and rectum to descend, or prolapse, altering their functioning. Men's pelvic floor muscles can become irritated and spasm, causing pelvic pain, just as back muscles can spasm and trigger severe back pain. The cause of pelvic floor muscle irritation is usually not apparent, but it is believed to be caused by trauma from riding a bike, for example, or from organ inflammation brought about by an infection of the bladder or prostate.

Essentially, the pelvic floor muscles will shorten, tighten, and go into spasm. In turn, pain often centers in the perineum. Many a doctor still assumes that the man back to see him for the nth time with these pain complaints simply has prostatitis, an inflammation of his prostate gland. Unfortunately, that is true in less than 5 percent of cases, but for decades, that was the typical scenario. The painful condition, misdiagnosed as prostatitis, would be treated with antibiotics—which rarely worked, because you don't treat damaged muscles with antibiotics!—and, in some cases, surgery, which was not successful either.

Fortunately, today we have a better understanding of an ailment that we now call chronic pelvic pain syndrome (CPPS), which can be caused by muscle spasm and other conditions unrelated to the prostate. The ailment is now becoming less prostatecentric, and physicians are taking a multidisciplinary approach to treatment, incorporating physical therapy and a variety of medications to treat specific complaints.

PROSTATE ZONES

Two types of tissue comprise the prostate: glandular, or epithelial, cells that manufacture seminal fluid, including prostate-specific antigen (PSA); and stromal tissue, which makes up the majority of the prostate and provides support to its many internal glands. Made up of connective tissue and smooth muscle, stromal tissue contracts to release prostatic secretions during sexual activity.

Urologists like to divide the prostate into four specific anatomic zones:

ZONE 1
The transition zone. This part of the prostate encircles the urethra tube. Approximately 15 percent of prostate cancers lurk around here. While this area takes up only 15 percent to 30 percent of prostate volume, it enlarges with age. In some men, the transition zone grows so large that it forms masses called nodules that can squeeze off the urethra; imag-

ine stepping on a garden hose, significantly slowing the outflow of water. This can lead to bothersome lower urinary tract symptoms (LUTS) that frequently drive men to doctors in search of treatment.

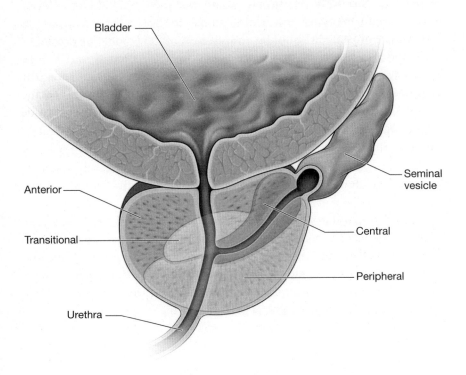

The prostate zones

ZONE 2

The central zone. About 20 percent of prostate real estate is located here, near the bladder and surrounding the region into which the ejaculatory ducts empty seminal fluid and sperm into the urethra; the central zone contains a significant number of glands that secrete prostatic fluid. Like the transition zone, this area can enlarge after men turn forty. It's unusual—but not unheard of—that prostate cancer is found here.

ZONE 3

The anterior zone. Think smooth muscle. The involuntary muscle fibers—those over which you have no control—are mostly found here at the front of the gland. It's rare for prostate cancer to lurk here, since there are no glands in this area.

ZONE 4

The peripheral zone. Think "danger zone." This is the back of the prostate, nearest to the rectum, encompassing about 75 percent of prostate tissue. This part of the prostate is the one examined during a DRE, when the physician manually examines the wall of the rectum and presses against the prostate. Most of the secretion-producing glands are located here, and it's where most prostate cancer typically develops; needle biopsies of the prostate most often sample this area to rule out cancer. The peripheral zone is the primary target for needle biopsies of the prostate, in which a hollow needle is used to withdraw samples of tissue, to be examined under the microscope for any evidence of cancer.

PROSTATE LOBES

The prostate gland is not divided anatomically into left and right hemispheres, but since it has a groove down its center called the median sulcus, it appears on examination to have right and left sides. We refer to these sides as lobes of the prostate gland. In describing prostate cancer findings on DRE, urologists will often refer to one or the other lobe (sometimes both) as being the troublesome area.

WHEN PROBLEMS DEVELOP IN THE PROSTATE

For its relatively tiny size, the prostate can cause monumental problems. Benign enlargement, infection, inflammation, trauma, irritation, and cancer growth within the prostate can quickly command a man's attention, with discomfort and pain registering from barely noticeable all the way to off the pain charts. Not only is the prostate pounding out "Help me!" messages, but so, too, are neighboring organs that are often affected when the prostate acts up. And when the prostate is eventually treated with drugs, heat therapies, surgery, or radiation, nearby organs can be affected as well, owing to their proximity to the prostate—unfortunately, not always for the better. Here's a thumbnail sketch of the three major problems involving the prostate that many men will have to confront:

1. LOWER URINARY TRACT SYMPTOMS (LUTS)

Frequent urination has men literally running in search of a toilet; stop-and-go urination leaves them stranded in front of the toilet, desperately trying to get all urine into the bowl without any dribbling when they're finished; and urination signals that awaken men throughout the night. All of these can be due to prostate problems but also to unrelated developments such as changes in the bladder, in urine production, or even in sleep. (See chapters 6 and 7 for more about how to deal effectively with the negative consequences of LUTS, benign prostatic enlargement, and overactive bladder.)

2. CHRONIC PROSTATITIS/CHRONIC PELVIC PAIN SYNDROME (CP/CPPS)

Formerly lumped together under the name *prostatitis*—only because no one knew any better and had no solutions for this vexing problem—CP/CPPS is a painful and often incapacitating ailment that still has many men wandering aimlessly from doctor to doctor (sometimes dozens of them) in search of relief. The recent name change, along with a group of dedicated researchers determined to find real solutions, has led to a multidisciplinary approach that encompasses urologists, physical therapists, psychiatrists, psychologists, and pain experts to provide the specialized lifestyle and medical care that men may need to find effective, long-lasting relief. Go to chapter 8 for information about prostatitis/chronic pelvic pain syndrome and read about innovative solutions.

3. PROSTATE CANCER

Death from prostate cancer, the most common cancer in men and the second leading cause of male cancer deaths, is an unfortunate reality, with more than thirty thousand men dying of it every year in the United States. That's more than three men every hour.

The good news is that the ability to detect prostate cancer early has prevented death in many men, and improved treatments have led to a reduction in treatment side effects.

The bad news is that in detecting prostate cancer, we are overtreating it, especially in older men. This book focuses on alternatives for detection and management that can reduce unnecessary treatments. The ongoing Johns Hopkins Active Surveillance Program, which I helped pioneer over sixteen years ago, is one step toward reducing the unnecessary treatment of prostate cancer. (See chapter 12.)

COMING RIGHT UP

Before we discuss the three specific prostate disorders in depth, however, I want to turn your attention to helpful ways that you can reduce urinary frequency problems and then introduce you to effective strategies utilizing changes in nutrition and exercise that will help you take control of your health. I have long been interested in the power of nutrition and physical activity, not only as effective ways to fuel and strengthen the body but also as helpful preventive strategies that may delay or prevent a decline in male health, including prostate disorders.

The important lifestyle changes that I recommend in the following chapters can dramatically improve your overall health and the health of your prostate.

Leading urologic researchers estimate that most prostate disorders, including cancer, are not related solely to genetics but also to personal lifestyle choices. This means that you have within your power the ability to minimize the effects and slow the course of the various prostate problems by implementing the lifestyle changes that I will detail for you.

THE TAKEAWAY

- The prostate is a gland of the male reproductive system that is tucked away in front of the rectum and just below the bladder, the organ that stores urine.

- The main purpose of the prostate is to produce the fluid that makes up semen, which helps transport and protect sperm during the male orgasm.

- The prostate consists of a base and a narrowed apex and is divided into different zones based on their function: the transition zone, the central zone, the anterior zone, and the peripheral zone.

- As a man ages, he may have to deal with some degree of prostate-related issues such as prostate inflammation, benign prostatic enlargement, and cancer.

- It is possible to reduce or prevent prostate problems that commonly occur with age by adopting a healthy lifestyle.

CHAPTER TWO

PROTECTING YOUR PROSTATE

Lack of activity destroys the good condition of every
human being, while movement and methodical
physical exercise save it and preserve it.

—Plato

The Washington, DC-to-Baltimore train was crowded, as it always seems to be whenever I'm on it. I was comfortably settled into my seat, reviewing my notes from presentations at the Prostate Cancer Foundation meeting that I had just attended in the capital. A few other passengers were boarding the car, and there was an empty seat next to me.

As the train slowly started to leave the station and everyone was apparently seated, I neatly folded my overcoat and placed my belongings on the empty seat beside me. The ride isn't too long, but a little extra room never hurts, and I take it when I can get it. No sooner had I done that when a heavyset middle-aged man who looked as if he were at the tail end of a hectic day came barreling down the aisle and made a beeline for the seat next to me.

I stood up and let him squeeze past me. As he eased his bulk down into the seat, he let out an audible "Aaaah!"

"I'm not the twenty-year-old buck I used to be," he said to no one in particular and quickly squirmed left and right to adjust his considerable backside into the small coach seat. Beads of perspiration dotted his brow and started to drip onto his pants, so I handed him the oversized paper napkin that was wrapped around my coffee cup.

"Thanks. I really had to hustle to get here," he explained, as he quickly mopped his brow.

After just a quick glance, it was clear that this man was a physical wreck. And the scary part was that he appeared to be only forty, at most. I could smell the stale cigarette smoke on him, and then my eyes instinctually moved to his yellowed middle and index fingers—a major tip-off to a longtime smoking habit. His flushed cheeks and rapidly rising and falling chest were dead giveaways to his lack of aerobic fitness. He was a big guy who carried a lot of weight; a warning for the overconsumption of calories that most likely came from consistently poor food choices.

"When you get to be my age, the body just isn't the same. It's not the well-oiled machine it once was. I used to be athletic, you know. All-sectional in baseball," he said matter-of-factly. "But once you reach forty, with a wife, kids, and job pressures, a few too many cocktails, you put on the pounds. There's not much you can do. You know what I mean."

REAL MEN MASTER THEIR OWN DESTINY

Actually, I didn't know what he meant, because I am from an entirely opposite school of thought. We live in a society that values and celebrates health, especially for those with spouses, kids, and jobs. Who wouldn't want to stay healthy indefinitely?

Once the train got up to speed, I put down my papers and looked out the window at the passing landscape. My seatmate was already dozing, his head resting on the windowpane, lulled to sleep by the rhythmic rattling of the steel wheels on the track.

I contemplated the various factors that have an impact on health and what makes us unhealthy. It then occurred to me that sleeping next to me could be the embodiment of a typical twenty-first-century American man. These are relatively young men who have become grossly overweight owing to bad eating habits and no exercise routine, leaving them in such poor health and so out of shape that "running" to catch a train leaves them sweating profusely and straining to catch their breath. Cigarette addiction and stress, coupled with a few too many cocktails, are just like pouring gasoline on a fire.

Contrary to what my fellow traveler had opined, age is not the main issue. Each one of us is master of his own body in terms of quality of life. When you believe in the power of physical activity and nutritious eating, you can make important changes in your life that will translate to huge gains in health. My patients are my proof.

ROGER THAT, OR GETTING INTO THE DRIVER'S SEAT

Whether you are concerned about optimal prostate health or concerned about your odds of developing prostate cancer, exercise and diet are tools that you have at your disposal to reduce your risks and enhance your quality of life. It's an important message of empowerment and one that places you squarely in the driver's seat. So often, people believe incorrectly that once the natural gifts of athleticism and physical fitness wash away with the years, their days of working out and exercising are over. Physical fitness might have come easier in one's younger days, but being physically fit is a lifelong pursuit, just like continuing education and learning, and it is one that the body is perfectly designed to handle.

I had a patient, Roger, on whom I performed a prostatectomy years ago. He recently came by to see me at my office to tell me that he was moving away, after a lifetime of living in Maryland. He wanted to say good-bye and thank me for the care that I had given him.

I asked Roger why he was leaving. "The company that I work for no longer has a position for me here, so I am being transferred out west," he said. "I'm not ready to stop working, so I'm moving."

Roger still looked like he was in his sixties. He was trim and robust and had a smile that lit up the room. He had recently celebrated his ninetieth birthday.

I asked Roger, "What's your secret to good health?" He didn't even pause: "I have not missed a day of exercise in my life."

Obviously, Roger had done a great job in choosing his parents—he had exceptional genes. But he had also remained vigorous with exercise and healthy life choices, which allowed him to remain in the workforce. I know of many other men like Roger, including a group of seventy-year-olds who enter sailing competitions in the middle of winter, racing along in the frigid air. They are filled with the spirit and enthusiasm of men half their age, and compared to the man sleeping next to me on the train, they are much healthier as well.

─────────────────────────MYTH BUSTER─────────────────────────

"My genes (parents) dictate my future health." The genetic cards that we are dealt are important, but healthy lifestyle choices can reduce the genetic predisposition to disease.

TURN OFF THE AGING SWITCH

The writer George Bernard Shaw once said, "We don't stop playing because we grow old; we grow old because we stop playing." If by "playing" he meant exercise, those were the most accurate words ever spoken. Our age in years has nothing to do with how "old" we are, how we feel, and what we can accomplish. However, not being in optimal physical condition can be a major drawback and a crucial aging factor. Not maintaining physical fitness and optimal health for the longest possible time increases the odds of developing chronic diseases, and those include an unhealthy prostate that can lead to inflammation, enlargement, and a higher risk of cancer.

Prostate enlargement and inflammation can also result in lower urinary tract symptoms, or LUTS. These symptoms can include urinary urgency and nocturia (nighttime urinary frequency) as well as generalized urinary frequency. I will go into much more detail on LUTS and BPE (benign prostatic enlargement) in chapters 5 and 6.

And then there is the negative impact that a poor diet and sedentary living have on the quality of your erections. If you cut back on exercise, increase caloric consumption, and put on excessive weight, faltering erections—the "canary in the coal mine"—may be the first visible sign you will get of underlying health problems, including heart disease. And for those younger men who are thinking of fathering children, it is crucial to note that a higher body mass index and unhealthful life choices have been associated with male infertility. (Body mass index is a measure of body fat, and a high BMI is an important indicator of an unhealthy lifestyle.) Furthermore, recent research shows that the combined effect of being overweight *and* sedentary increases your likelihood of developing aggressive prostate cancer.

MYTH BUSTER

Erectile dysfunction (ED) has traditionally been accepted as an older man's issue and that it is a natural part of growing older. However, ED can be a telltale sign of underlying cardiovascular disease that needs to be addressed.

COMMIT YOURSELF TO IMPROVEMENT

Contrary to what my seatmate might have believed—and anything else you might have heard to the contrary—you're never too old to exercise and improve your physical fitness. Regardless of how out of shape you are or how daunting the road to physical fitness might seem, it is never too late to get started. Once you decide to become more physically fit, you can make a significant impact on your quality of life as well as the health of your prostate. These changes in physical activity should go hand in hand with dietary changes regarding both food choices and quantities. I will discuss different food options and their impact on health in the upcoming chapter.

In the meantime, why not commit yourself to improvement by starting your quest for physical fitness today? What's stopping you? Feel free to come up with any excuse you can think of, but, believe me, I've heard them all before.

Let's be clear: you are certainly not going to become a triathlete overnight or even over the course of a year. Dispel all notions of incredible physical feats that you see in movies and on TV, where people seem to reach unachievable goals with little effort. The body doesn't work like that.

First, you will need to build a strong fitness base. You can't just jump right in, start exercising, and expect to see tremendous results. Building this all-important foundation is the key to sustainability. And, yes, brisk walking for a half hour a day counts. I will have a lot more to say about this later in the chapter when I outline a walking program, but consistent walking can build this solid base for you, reduce stress, whittle away fat, and rejuvenate the body, filling you with renewed vigor, greater confidence, and the glow of good health.

────────────────RED FLAG────────────────

Jumping right into the deep end and trying to do too much too fast when you have no exercise foundation is the perfect way to not only hurt yourself but also burn out.

EXERCISE CAUSES SOME DISCOMFORT, BUT SITTING ON THE COUCH CAN KILL YOU

Regular physical activity protects you from heart disease, the number one killer of men. Research has shown that exercise can lower blood pressure and cholesterol levels, reduce your risk of diabetes and some cancers, and protect your brain from Alzheimer's, the brain-robbing disease that is now becoming all too prevalent in our later years.

Want more? Regular exercise improves the odds of rock-hard erections in later years. I have never met a guy not interested in that!

Still not impressed? Need a little more convincing? Recent research also suggests that a healthy lifestyle may reduce your risk of death from prostate cancer, the most common cancer in men. And this protection also applies to patients who already have been diagnosed with prostate cancer.

These facts alone should be enough to motivate you to get off your duff and be physically active every day. An additional benefit is that walking, running, kayaking, swimming, tennis, squash, cycling, surfing, weight lifting, and in-line skating (feel free to fill in your favorites here) all promote good mental health, as they seem to reduce the risk of both the onset and the recurrence of depression.

LEADING CAUSES OF DEATH IN AMERICAN MEN

While many men fear prostate cancer, heart disease is the leading killer of American men. Prostate cancer kills more than 30,000 men annually in the United States and more than 250,000 worldwide. But heart disease kills roughly ten times as many American males, and, according to the World Health Organization (WHO, the agency of the United Nations responsible for providing leadership on global health matters), an estimated 17 million people die annually of cardiovascular diseases, particularly heart attacks, making it the leading cause of death in the world. The average age for a first heart attack for men is sixty-six and almost half of all male heart attack victims under the age of sixty-five die within eight years.

Table 2.1.

Leading Causes of Deaths, All Males, All Ages (2006)	Percentage
1. Heart disease	26.3
2. Cancer	24.1
3. Unintentional injuries	6.6
4. Chronic lower respiratory diseases	4.9
5. Stroke	4.5
6. Diabetes	3.0
7. Suicide	2.2
8. Influenza and pneumonia	2.1
9. Kidney disease	1.8
10. Alzheimer's disease	1.8

Source: US Centers for Disease Control and Prevention (CDC).

EXERCISE IMPROVES LOWER URINARY TRACT SYMPTOMS: WHAT THE RESEARCH TELLS US

We are finding out that, not surprisingly, exercise appears to play a key role in maintaining optimal prostate health. You probably never knew that there was a link between how much you exercise and your risk of developing moderate to severe lower urinary tract symptoms (LUTS) that can have you going to the bathroom all of the time. The most bothersome LUTS are urinary frequency that can occur day and night, and strong urges to urinate. The more physically active you are, however, the less time you may spend looking for bathrooms.

LUTS, a common complaint of men over forty, can be related to inefficient filling and storing of urine in the bladder. In some men, it's associated with an enlarged prostate. Over the years, many clinical studies, totaling tens of thousands of male subjects, have linked excessive weight and obesity with increased risks of LUTS and BPE. Many also highlight the importance of being physically active as a way to stave off lower urinary tract symptoms. For example, a 2006 study of thirty thousand Swedish men published in the *Journal of Urology* reported that the forty-five to seventy-nine-year-old male participants who were more physically active at work or at home were less likely to develop LUTS. As a matter of fact, not being physically active was associated with a twofold increased risk of LUTS compared with the risk in men who were physically active.

In 2006 several of my Hopkins colleagues published the results of their study of twin adult men with LUTS complaints. Drs. Alan Partin and Patrick Walsh and epidemiologist Dr. Elizabeth Platz had sent questionnaires that assessed LUTS symptoms, weight, height, alcohol consumption, cigarette smoking, and physical activity to 1,723 sets of twins who had LUTS complaints but no prostate cancer diagnosis.

Epidemiology is a branch of medical science that critically evaluates population studies, looking for trends. The Hopkins experts reported in the journal *Epidemiology* that while 72 percent of the variability in LUTS complaints was attributable to genetic factors in men with moderate to severe LUTS, modifiable lifestyle factors such as obesity and lack of physical activity explained 28 percent of the variability in LUTS. Physical activity was associated with a 40 percent lower risk of LUTS.

IMPORTANT NEWS FROM SAN DIEGO

A former Johns Hopkins colleague, Dr. J. Kellogg Parsons, who is now a researcher specializing in prostate disease at the UCSD Moores Cancer Center, in San Diego, published the most recent study examining the impact of exercise on urinary distress in 2008 in the journal *European Urology*.

Dr. Parsons began looking at exercise and prostate health because he noted in his work and in other research that modifiable lifestyle factors seemed to influence LUTS—both the risk of developing it and its severity. Specifically, he found that obesity and diabetes increase the risk—and that exercise and physical activity decrease the risk—of developing urinary complaints.

"This is all probably tied in with the Western lifestyle, which is high in fat-laden fast food and being sedentary," says Dr. Parsons. "That increases the risk of cardiovascular disease and other chronic diseases. This all seems to tie in with the prostate, which isn't that surprising, because obesity is basically a systemic disease. The excess fat cells in the body create an inflammatory state that definitely affects the heart. But what we are increasingly discovering is that it also affects the prostate and the bladder. What I had seen initially in a few studies is that there seems to be a decreased risk of prostate and bladder problems with exercise."

What Dr. Parsons did was to analyze previous major studies that examined the link between physical activity and LUTS. He then divided the exercise intensity levels that were reported by the men into three categories—light, moderate, and vigorous—and then ran the numbers.

His intriguing findings suggest that moderate to vigorous exercise can significantly reduce the risk of LUTS and prostate enlargement by as much as 25 percent when compared with physically inactive men. In addition, the more you exercise, the greater the benefit, and even light physical activity has a somewhat protective effect on the prostate.

According to this research, if you do nothing physically active in the course of your typical day, like the majority of American men, you will have a higher chance of eventually developing LUTS that can entail bothersome frequency of urination, day and night, and urgency to urinate.

"The overwhelming majority of men in the studies said that exercise was beneficial and that it decreased their urinary symptoms," says Dr. Parsons. "I have seen that in my medical practice as well. Most recently, Freddy, an extremely overweight patient of mine, asked what he could do that would not involve medication or surgery to relieve his prostate symptoms.

"I detailed some weight-loss suggestions and sketched out an exercise regimen for him to follow. Months later, he was exercising daily and had lost a good amount of weight. The next time he came to see me, his urinary symptoms had gone away completely."

What's surprising is that Dr. Parson's findings fly in the face of traditional thinking that LUTS is caused solely by aging and by changes in the size of the prostate. Granted, these can play a role in the development of urinary complaints, but regular exercise, as Dr. Parsons uncovered, appears to have a protective effect against the development of LUTS.

HOW EXERCISE PROMOTES A HEALTHY PROSTATE

How exercise enhances prostate health is still a matter of speculation, but it may be related to inflammatory changes that affect the vascular system in general, including the heart and the prostate. Animal studies have shown that high-fat diets—a major heart risk factor yet pretty much the picture of the Western diet—lead not only to cardiovascular disease but also contribute to bladder overactivity and increased prostate size, possibly through inflammation.

"I think that the prostate and the bladder are susceptible to microvascular disease due to overeating and lack of exercise, the same way that other body organs are," says Dr. Parsons. "But once you start exercising and losing weight, you are increasing blood flow to the pelvic region and diminishing the inflammatory state that you have in the prostate and the bladder. And if you have prostate cancer, I think you can also diminish the propensity for the prostate cancer to progress."

————————————————RED FLAG————————————————

The saturated animal fat found in the Western diet contributes to cardiovascular disease. A plant-based diet can reduce the risk of heart disease and, possibly, cancer.

INFLAMMATION: FANNING THE FLAMES OF
CHRONIC DISEASE AND PROSTATE DISORDERS

Human studies are reporting links between lifestyle choices and the development of LUTS and BPE, and it may have to do with metabolic syndrome, a medical condition that is associated with four medical issues: glucose intolerance, elevated cholesterol, hypertension, and obesity.

This syndrome is thought to set the stage for increased chronic inflammation within the body. This chronic inflammatory state is what occurs when inflammation has gone into overdrive in response to excessive calories, fatty foods, lack of exercise, and smoking. And unfortunately, chronic inflammation appears to increase the risk of all manner of prostate problems—including LUTS, BPE, and prostate cancer—as well as other cancers, atherosclerosis (so-called hardening of the arteries), diabetes, strokes, and possibly even Alzheimer's disease.

Inflammation has been thought of as an essential part of the body's healing system; its reaction to injury or infection. You experience inflammation as the reddening, warmth, and swelling around a cut or infection. However, it has become apparent that metabolic diseases can trigger inflammation, a process now referred to as metabolically triggered inflammation. The link between inflammation and high-fat diets, obesity, and a sedentary lifestyle appears to be promotion at the cellular level of the body's natural defense system for fighting infection. This system, characterized by a war zone of inflammatory cells that release signals calling for more inflammatory cells, creates an environment that is ripe for damage of "innocent bystanders" such as blood vessels, nerves, and the genetic material within glandular cells of the prostate, where prostate cancers arise. Chronic low-grade inflammation within the prostate over many years is thought to be one risk factor for the initiation of cancer, chronic pelvic pain syndrome, and prostatic enlargement that leads to LUTS.

And it's not only the prostate that's harmed by chronic inflammation. Over many years, ongoing inflammation causes serious damage on a cellular level that leads to many of the chronic diseases of aging, including cancer, vascular disease, and Alzheimer's. In essence, our modern Western lifestyle, characterized by the adoption of a high-caloric-density diet and a sedentary existence, has exchanged diseases associated with malnutrition with those associated with chronic diseases of age.

YOUR THREE BEST WEAPONS: USE THEM

Given the role that inflammation plays in diseases of the prostate, your goal is to prevent inflammation from beginning, or, if it is present, to reduce the inflammatory response caused by an unhealthy lifestyle. Your primary tools: regular exercise, weight control, and optimal nutrition.

All three are facets of your life over which you have complete control. By taking a much closer look at what you can do to make improvements on a daily basis, you will be giving yourself the best possible chance to protect your prostate and other organs of your body from the damage caused by long-term inflammation.

I will focus on the important, inflammation-dampening role of diet in the next chapter, but right now, let's turn to the benefits of exercise and how it can reduce the risk of both benign and potentially lethal prostate disorders.

ENHANCING PROSTATE HEALTH BY PREVENTING AND REVERSING METABOLIC SYNDROME

If you are walking around with a bulging belly, looking more like Bibendum, the Michelin Man, than Arnold Schwarzenegger in his heyday, you may already have metabolic syndrome, a potentially serious medical condition. *Metabolism* refers to chemical reactions that occur in the body, particularly those related to the conversion of food into energy. Metabolic syndrome, first described in 1988, is a grouping of metabolic risk factors that significantly increase the risk of developing cardiovascular disease, type 2 diabetes, or both. It appears now that other chronic maladies can be added to the list, including prostate disorders. It is estimated that possibly fifty-five million Americans or more have metabolic syndrome; if true, 20 percent to 25 percent of the population may be affected.

Without lifestyle changes and/or medical intervention, metabolic syndrome can lead to serious health problems, including heart attack, stroke, diabetes, and nonalcoholic fatty liver disease.

Experts at the National Cholesterol Education Program of the National Heart, Lung, and Blood Institute (NHLBI) say that you have metabolic syndrome if you exhibit at least three of the following five abnormalities:

1. **Abdominal obesity**, a waist circumference greater than forty inches, indicates central obesity and an "apple shape," which is a major risk factor for metabolic syndrome.

2. **A low HDL** ("good") cholesterol level (below 40 milligrams per deciliter of blood, or 40 mg/dl).

3. **A high fasting triglyceride level** (150 mg/dl or higher) indicates high blood levels of triglycerides (hypertriglyceridemia). Triglycerides, a type of fat found in your blood, is stored in fat cells and used later for energy.

4. **Higher-than-normal blood pressure** (130/85 mm Hg, or millimeters of mercury, or higher).

5. **Elevated fasting blood glucose level** (100 mg/dl or higher). This glucose, or blood sugar, level obtained following a fast is elevated but not high enough to constitute diabetes. Glucose levels above 126 mg/dl signify diabetes, the inability of the body to utilize glucose efficiently.

    Diabetes is a chronic disease in which high levels of glucose (sugar) build up in the bloodstream. The two most common types of diabetes are type 1 diabetes, which usually develops before age thirty and tends to come on suddenly, and type 2 diabetes, which accounts for 90 to 95 percent of diabetes cases and typically develops later in life, generally in people who are overweight. Type 2 diabetes, which is caused by an inability of the available insulin to work (referred to as "insulin resistance"), can often be controlled without insulin treatment through exercise, a proper diet, weight loss, and oral medications. That's why type 2 diabetes is also sometimes called noninsulin dependent diabetes.

CAUSES OF METABOLIC SYNDROME

Just as metabolic syndrome is not one specific disease, there is not one specific cause. However, abdominal obesity and insulin resistance are considered central metabolic defects leading to the syndrome, with physical inactivity playing a key role in its development. Some individuals are genetically predisposed to metabolic syndrome; nevertheless, adopting a healthy lifestyle can prevent it from developing. On the other hand, obesity and physical inactivity would promote its development. According to the American Heart Association, 70 percent of the American public is now considered sedentary; that's about 215 million people. Only 3 percent—a mere 9.2 million—follow healthy living advice to maintain a healthy weight, exercise regularly, eat five or more servings of fruits and vegetables each day, and avoid smoking.

It's not uncommon for men to develop a bit of a "spare tire" in middle age. The body doesn't metabolize food like it once did, but serving sizes generally don't go down as a way of counterbalancing that effect, nor does the average man's physical activity level increase. With further "inflation," the tire may become a pronounced paunch. In addition to that uncomfortable snugness around the belt line, your belly is sending you the message that it has become a threat to your health and requires attention. In fact, it has become a metabolic organ, one that produces inflammatory molecules that can lead to insulin resistance, cardiovascular disease, and higher rates of prostate disease.

Even though winning the battle of the bulge brings multiple benefits, many men choose to do nothing and instead seek refuge on the couch with the TV remote gripped firmly in hand. Against all odds and expectations, we must win this twenty-first-century battle of the bulge. The cost of losing this fight will lead to rising health problems and health care costs.

WHAT YOU CAN DO NOW

If you have three of the five risk factors associated with an increased risk of cardiovascular disease, you may have metabolic syndrome. But even if you have only *one* of the five risk factors, it's a wake-up call to do something now in order to reverse a dangerous trend.

Lifestyle modifications, including dietary changes that I will address in the next chapter, regular physical activity, quitting smoking, and avoiding excessive alcohol consumption will help eliminate the disorders that make up metabolic syndrome. Even when medication is required to lower your cholesterol or blood pressure to acceptable levels, lifestyle measures can help make medication *more* effective and may allow you to take a smaller dose or discontinue the drug altogether, which can reduce the risk of side effects such as erectile dysfunction.

———————————————MYTH BUSTER———————————————

If you don't make lifestyle changes that add up to a healthier life, drugs can certainly act as Band-Aids: they can help relieve the symptoms, but they are not going to "cure" the underlying problem.

———

Since physical inactivity and obesity are primary culprits in metabolic syndrome, the treatment plan that I recommend on page 39 is designed to get you moving every day and pare off excess weight. Stepping up your physical activity and losing even a modest amount of weight—in the range of 5 percent to 10 percent of body weight—can help raise HDL levels, lower blood pressure, decrease your triglyceride level, restore insulin sensitivity, and lower the chances that metabolic syndrome will evolve into a more serious chronic illness.

Although desirable, you don't have to reach your optimal weight to obtain benefits. Moderate weight loss, even if you're overweight, can help prevent the development and progression of metabolic syndrome.

In a 2007 study, researchers reported that the prevalence of metabolic syndrome was reduced by 30 percent in a population of overweight men and women who began an eight-month exercise program. Thirty minutes of moderate-intensity exercise (a brisk walk) a day was an effective strategy. Data from the National Health and Nutrition Examination Survey (NHANES) show that for every one thousand steps men take per day, there is a 6 percent to 11 percent reduction in their odds of having three of the risk factors for metabolic syndrome (large waist circumference, low levels of HDL cholesterol, and high levels of triglycerides).

When broken down by groups, those men who took ten thousand steps per day (active to highly active men) had a 69 percent lower chance of having metabolic syndrome than those who took fewer than five thousand steps per day (sedentary men). A mile is just over two thousand steps; take ten thousand steps a day, and you're covering about five miles.

EXERCISE: TOO MANY AMERICANS DON'T DO ENOUGH

How much do you exercise every day? Choose the broad category below that best describes yourself and your daily physical activities:

- Sixty minutes a day, seven days a week

- Sixty minutes a day, every other day

- Thirty minutes a day, seven days a week

- Thirty minutes a day, every other day

- Every now and then

- Never

If you checked "Never," then you need to seriously consider the future health effects and long-term consequences that are associated with doing no form of exercise.

According to the latest national figures, only one in four adults follow through with the recommendations from our national health officials to get at least thirty minutes of exercise most days of the week. Although most men say that they understand the value of exercise and claim to believe that it can help relieve stress and even prolong life, many nonexercisers say they don't have enough time for exercising. Yet Americans watch an average of 4 hours of TV every day of the week.

A 2011 study in the *Journal of the American Medical Association* (*JAMA*) reported that for every two hours of TV viewing per day, there was a 20 percent increase in the risk of diabetes, a 15 percent increase in the risk of developing cardiovascular disease, and a 13 percent increase risk of dying of any cause. TV viewing is just an indication of physical inactivity, and the less physically active, the greater the risk of chronic diseases, including prostate disease.

Do the math: Of the 168 hours in a week, most men spend an average of 50 or so hours sleeping and 40 to 50 hours working. That leaves about 68 "free" hours. If you set aside 3 of those 68 hours left in your week, or 180 minutes out of 4,080, that is less than 5 percent of your free time for exercise.

RED FLAG

Here is a little more math to consider: 4 hours of TV a day equals 1,460 hours a year. What do you have to show for it?

WEIGHT GAIN BEFORE PROSTATE CANCER SURGERY
INCREASES RISK OF RECURRENCE

Weight gain is never good, but when it comes before prostate cancer surgery, the surgical outcome is compromised when compared with no weight gain.

Johns Hopkins epidemiologists reported in 2011 in the journal *Cancer Prevention Research* that prostate cancer patients who gain five pounds or more near the time of their prostate surgery are *twice* as likely to have a recurrence of their cancer after surgery than patients whose weight is stable.

"We surveyed men whose cancer was localized, and surgery should have cured most of them, yet some cancers recurred. Obesity and weight gain may be factors that tip the scale to recurrence," says Dr. Corinne Joshu, a postdoctoral fellow at the Johns Hopkins Bloomberg School of Public Health.

Dr. Joshu and her colleagues sent questionnaires to 1,337 prostate cancer patients who had undergone surgery to remove their prostates at the Johns Hopkins Hospital. The men were asked to remember their dietary, lifestyle, and medical factors from five years before their operation through one year postsurgery.

It turned out that body weight did play a role in surgical outcomes. On average, the study participants who gained weight reported that they gained about ten pounds in the five years before surgery and one year following the operation. Those men whose weight increased more than about five pounds during that time had twice the rate of recurrence than men whose weight held steady.

Dr. Elizabeth Platz, one of the study coauthors, says that there are a variety of biochemical pathways—including metabolic, hormonal, and inflammatory—that could contribute to a recurrence of prostate cancer with weight gain. The impact of these pathways may vary depending on the stage and type of prostate cancer and the timing of the onset of weight gain and obesity.

Although this study could not determine whether weight loss would reverse the risk of cancer recurrence after surgery, men with prostate cancer should maintain their weight and do whatever it takes to avoid weight gain and obesity. Regular exercise certainly helps.

EXERCISE *IS* POWERFUL MEDICINE

Exercise is one of the best ways to improve health and reduce the risks of chronic age-related diseases that range from deterioration of the skeleton, damage to the circulatory system, and the development of cancer. But can exercise reduce the risk of prostate disease or, if it does develop, reduce its effects? Harvard researchers recently set out to get some answers about the relationship between exercise and prostate cancer.

In 2011 they reported that as few as twenty-five minutes of exercise a day could reduce overall mortality rates in men already diagnosed with prostate cancer. These findings were published in the *Journal of Clinical Oncology* (*JCO*).

Dr. Stacey A. Kenfield, an epidemiology research associate at the Harvard School of Public Health and the primary author of the study, and her colleagues reviewed the workout routines of more than 2,700 men diagnosed with prostate cancer since 1990; the authors then assessed the men's commitment and level of exercise intensity every two years for eighteen years. The men were asked if they participated in the following activities:

> Walking or hiking outdoors (including walking while playing golf)
>   at their usual pace
> Jogging (slower than ten minutes per mile)
> Running (ten minutes per mile or faster)
> Bicycling (including stationary biking)
> Lap swimming
> Tennis
> Squash or racquetball
> Calisthenics
> Rowing
> Climbing flights of stairs daily
> Doing heavy outdoor work
> Weight training

Exercise intensity was measured in METs, or metabolic equivalents of task. This is the energy expenditure during a specific exercise when compared with that at rest; 1 MET is the energy expenditure at rest,

2 METs indicates the energy expended is twice that at rest, 3 METs is triple that resting expenditure, and so on. Exercise physiologists use METs per hour as a measurement of exercise intensity.

In the Harvard study, each physical activity had a ranking, from fewer than 6 METs for less-than-vigorous activities and 6 METs and higher for the more intense workouts. Knowing this, the researchers were then able to determine how many METs patients expended during the week.

Over the course of the study, 548 patients died, with 20 percent of the deaths (112) linked directly to prostate cancer. Looking closely at MET results, the Harvard researchers discovered that the more physically active a prostate cancer patient was, the greater his chance of not dying of his cancer. Men with the lowest risk of prostate cancer death were those who exercised vigorously before and after their cancer diagnosis.

Dr. Kenfield says, "We saw health benefits at levels of physical exertion that most men could easily achieve if only they put their minds to it and made it a priority in their lives. And the more exercise the men did each week, the better the results for their prostate."

Exercise in the Harvard study didn't have to entail grueling spinning classes, either. Men who engaged in nine or more hours of workouts a week—which was equivalent to jogging, biking, swimming, or playing tennis for about ninety minutes per week—had a 33 percent lower risk of dying of any cause. More specifically, they had 35 percent lower risk of dying of their prostate cancer than men who exercised less.

Walking, the most basic of all physical activity, proved to offer benefits for those who walked seven or more hours a week when compared with those who walked less than twenty minutes a week. When compared with walking at an easy pace, walking at a normal pace or brisk pace was associated with a 37 percent to 48 percent lower risk of death from any cause. Walking at a brisk pace for seven hours or more per week was associated with a 56 percent lower risk of death from prostate cancer when compared with walking less than seven hours per week at a nonbrisk pace.

The researchers also found that the more strenuous exercise affected prostate cancer–specific mortality the most: when compared with men who engaged in some form of vigorous activity for less than one hour per week, those who exercised vigorously three or more hours a week had a drop in overall death rates of almost 50 percent. Deaths due to prostate cancer were 61 percent lower when these two groups were compared.

Critics will argue that men with advanced prostate cancer will naturally be less active, so that it is hard to determine whether exercise caused the reduction in prostate cancer death or, alternatively, that the men who exercised most vigorously had less extensive disease in the first place.

The researchers heard those complaints and went back and examined their spreadsheets even more closely. In particular, they looked at the effects of exercise on prostate cancer progression among 1,455 men after a diagnosis of localized prostate cancer, which is a cancer that has not spread out beyond the prostate. They recently reported their results in the journal *Cancer Research*. The study showed that brisk walking, independent of walking duration, provided the most benefit in terms of reducing prostate cancer progression. Brisk walking for three hours per week or more was associated with an almost 60 percent lower rate of prostate cancer progression when compared with walking at an easy pace for less than three hours a week. Still other studies have found a relationship between vigorous activities and a lower risk of developing advanced and fatal prostate cancer.

How does exercise exert this protective effect against prostate cancer progression?

The protective effect may be due to metabolic and hormonal changes that reduce the ability of cancer cells to grow and that increase the ability of the immune system to fight cancer. Exercise may also reduce inflammation that is promoted by excess fat deposits. Even if we can't pinpoint the exact mechanism, the evidence of exercise's protective effects is overwhelming.

The takeaway message from the Harvard study and others is this: a *moderate* amount of regular exercise may improve overall survival, while three or more hours per week of *vigorous* exercise—that's just twenty-six minutes a day—may decrease your chances of developing or dying from aggressive prostate cancer.

"I don't think that men exercise that much," observes Dr. Kenfield, "but if we can get them to reach these minimum exercise levels, it would be a move in the right direction. Hopefully, these study results will offer them both inspiration and encouragement."

INVEST $100 IN YOUR HEALTH

How much would you pay for a pill that would lower your risk of developing prostate cancer? And if you had prostate cancer, how much would you pay for a pill that would more than halve your risk of the disease's progressing? And how much for a pill that would reduce your overall risk of developing other chronic diseases? Let's see what some companies would like to charge you:

- A major multinational pharmaceutical company wanted to charge about $400 per year for a drug that they claimed could prevent prostate cancer; it supposedly reduced the likelihood of being diagnosed with prostate cancer by 25 percent—a claim that was subsequently rejected by the FDA.

- The maker of a particular brand of pomegranate juice might charge around 25 cents per ounce and claim a protective effect against prostate cancer—a claim that has prompted a recent lawsuit.

Millions of dollars' worth of selenium and vitamin E supplements have been sold over the years to millions of men who thought that taking them would reduce their risk of prostate cancer—a claim that was proven incorrect in a randomized trial sponsored by the National Cancer Institute. A randomized clinical trial is a study in which volunteers are chosen at random (by chance alone) to receive one of several treatments. The treatment group is then compared to a group not receiving treatment or a placebo ("sugar pill").

In the meantime, while everyone seems to be searching for the ultimate cancer preventive, human studies published in the most prestigious oncology journals in the world have demonstrated the importance of exercise in reducing cancer risk and disease progression. But this important news is such a hard sell to many men who look for pills and potions to protect against cancer—that is, until they get clobbered over the head with a diagnosis of a potentially lethal disease.

Your cost for reducing the risk of cancer and cancer progression is a mere $100 investment in a pair of comfortable exercise shoes. Make that purchase now and get moving to reap the maximum return on your investment.

MEN: CHOOSE YOUR EXERCISE

Exercise comes in a variety of forms, and the best advice that I can offer is to pick those that you enjoy, so that you will continue long term. Some people like to walk; others like to swim, row, or use a treadmill or elliptical machine; others like to garden, play tennis, or walk eighteen holes on the golf course.

The bottom line: whatever form of exercise you choose, you should do enough of it to help maintain a healthy weight. When it comes to prostate health, the more active you are, the better.

YOUR EXERCISE PLAN: PUTTING IT ALL TOGETHER

The task at hand is to figure out a way to incorporate exercise into your daily routine so that it becomes a lasting, fun, and meaningful part of your life. The key is to structure your work around your exercise program, not vice versa; exercise is the most important activity you will do every day. Why? I am convinced of the value of exercise in promoting health. And regular exercise is a habit that becomes addictive once you start.

There is no doubt that starting an exercise program is a challenge, especially if you've had unpleasant or unsuccessful experiences with exercise in the past. The following are tips that many of my patients have found helpful in successfully integrating a consistent exercise program into their lives:

Review the benefits of exercise. If you understand how you will personally benefit from exercise, you'll be more motivated to do it.

Write down all your personal reasons for exercising. Over the next few days, write down every reason you can think of to work toward overall fitness. Keep the list in a visible place—on your refrigerator or the bathroom mirror—so that you can review it regularly. You might include the following:

- Have more energy

- Be able to fit into my clothing

- Live a longer, healthier life with higher quality

- Feel more comfortable when I go out in public

- Be able to climb stairs without becoming breathless

- Prevent chronic diseases of aging, including cardiovascular and prostate disease

- Reduce or discontinue blood pressure, lipid-lowering, or glucose-lowering drugs

The list is important. If you should ever find that your enthusiasm for exercise is waning, review all the reasons for exercising that you wrote down.

Dedicate a time to exercise. Once you reserve part of your day for exercise, protect the time and make it a priority. Many people are most successful if they exercise first thing in the morning or dedicate their lunch hour to walking or working out. On the other hand, some feel better in the evenings after a later workout. An evening workout is a natural way to relax and unwind at the end of a stressful day. Decide what time of day works best for you. What's most important is consistency.

Be accountable. Find a buddy and exercise together. Research shows that people who exercise with a friend or group are more successful at sticking to a program consistently. Knowing you have to be in a certain place at a certain time to meet your workout partner is great motivation to show up. After all, someone else is relying on you.

Make exercise fun. Join a group of friends or go to a special place (such as a park or historical site) to exercise when you have time. Listen to your favorite music as you walk. Do whatever makes exercise most enjoyable. The more pleasant it is, the more likely you'll be to follow your program consistently.

MYTH BUSTER

While soreness can certainly be a part of the exercise experience, real pain never should be. A lot of us grew up hearing "No pain, no gain." Not true! Pain is a sign that you are doing something wrong that could cause harm.

Keep a log of your daily exercise routines. Progress is made when progress is measured. You can grade your efforts, from A—if you felt great and had an outstanding swim—to F—if you failed to meet your goal or didn't feel good while exercising.

If you're having a C day, cut back the intensity of your workout. Don't work so hard, or reduce the distance and time you walk. If you still feel it's a C day at your next session, cut the workout in half. If you have days you rank as Ds or Fs, skip the workout and get some rest.

RED FLAG

Take the rest when you really need it. Injuries occur when a person is fatigued and is trying to do too much, even with minor exercise.

PUMPING IRON

Resistance training prevents the loss of muscle mass and strength that occurs with aging. After a person reaches physical maturity, muscle mass and bone density begin to decline. The body of an average twenty-year-old man is about 18 percent fat, skyrocketing to 38 percent by age sixty. For a woman, the pattern is similar: A twenty-year-old woman's body is about 23 percent fat. Forty years later, it's gone up to 44 percent. But you don't just wake up one day and discover that you've lost muscle and gained fat; it's a gradual, lifelong process that you can alter significantly with weight training.

Loss of muscle mass—and the declining coordination, balance, and strength resulting in bone-shattering falls—is a major reason that older people end up in care facilities. Weight training three times a week can help prevent this.

Strength training is especially important for men with advanced prostate cancer being treated with androgen deprivation therapy (ADT). Medications used in ADT prevent the body from making or using androgens, hormones that support male sex characteristics and sexual organs. Testosterone, the principal male androgen, is the anabolic, or muscle-building, hormone. Withdrawal of testosterone can cause you to lose bone and muscle mass, but regular strength training can help to reduce the losses.

The bottom line: combine cardiovascular activities (walking, running, swimming) and resistance training to achieve the most benefit from an exercise program.

START WALKING

For people who don't exercise regularly, beginning a program of physical activity may seem daunting. It can conjure up images of expensive gym memberships, complex exercise equipment, and boring, physically strenuous workouts.

Walking, however, is none of these. It's free, simple, generally easy on your body, and proven to be effective at preventing chronic disease. It is a safe activity for almost everyone. It's something you can do on neighborhood streets and roads, in a park, on the local high school track, or even in a shopping mall. And walking doesn't require any elaborate, expensive equipment—just a sturdy, comfortable, well-fitting pair of shoes and a handy step counter (pedometer) that you can purchase at your local sporting goods store. This simple measuring device for calculating how far you walk costs about $25 and is the best investment you can make for achieving your long-term weight control and fitness goals.

Outlined below is a road map to follow for the next six weeks to get you started on the path to better fitness and improved health without fatigue. You will build a fitness base that can propel you to heights you may not have thought possible.

Studies suggest that walking ten thousand steps per day—about four to five miles—is an amount of exercise that will improve your health by reducing the risk of chronic diseases, including those of the prostate gland. To fulfill your daily walking goals, you can walk anywhere that you like, and it doesn't have to be nonstop; break it up if you wish. Twenty minutes in the morning, and you will cover a mile or two. Finish off the remaining steps after dinner.

RED FLAG

Use your pedometer all the time, not just when you work out. Put it on when you leave the house in the morning and take it off when you come home at night.

A twelve-year study published in the *New England Journal of Medicine* in 1998 showed that the death rate of older men who walked less than a mile a day was almost twice that of those who walked more than two miles a day, and the farther the men walked, the lower the rates of death.

Whether it is going to and from work, walking the dog in your neighborhood, or hiking a portion of the Appalachian Trail (or even its 2,181-mile entirety), walking is the perfect choice for a long-term physical activity. It is the best activity for getting into good cardiovascular condition and maintaining it for the rest of your life. Pleasurable, alone or with a partner, it is also easy on your joints, so that you won't be worrying about aches and pains when you are done for the day.

Sample Walking Program to Reduce Your Risk of Prostate Disease

Week 1 (initial goal). Establish your current walking baseline by finding out how many steps you take throughout the course of your everyday routines. Count your steps using your pedometer for the first four days, and then average it out. The result is your walking baseline.

For the remaining three days, add an additional two thousand steps per day. This is approximately a mile more of walking but something that you can accomplish with just two ten-minute walking sessions.

If you feel this is a bit too ambitious to start with, cut the recommended distance in half and gradually work up to the starting point of the program. Instead of going nonstop, break the sessions into shorter periods; you'll still be deriving a benefit.

Even multiple sessions of exercise in a day have a cumulative effect on building fitness. So if you can walk only for one or two minutes before you need to rest, do that. Later in the day, walk for another few minutes. Over time, you will be able to lengthen your exercise periods and intensify each session. Movement counts.

Week 2. Increase your daily walking by one thousand steps.

Week 3. Increase your daily walking by another one thousand steps, bringing the total to a minimum of seven thousand steps a day.

Week 4. Increase to eight thousand steps a day. As your strength and endurance are increasing as you enter your fourth week of walking, pick up your walking pace a bit.

Week 5. Increase to nine thousand steps a day.

Week 6. You finally reach your ten-thousand-step landmark this week. Congratulations!

Pushing beyond six weeks. At this point, your exercise routine should be part of your everyday life. In the ensuing weeks, vary your workouts, go to new places, walk in the opposite direction, and take in all the sites counterclockwise. You'll be amazed at what you missed when you were going the other way.

Why not try to increase your intensity and push yourself a little harder? You can maintain the same duration of exercise, or, if you're up to it, gradually increase the length of your walks. The health benefits will increase as you increase the intensity and duration of your workouts.

Most important, now that you have a solid fitness base, you can start to challenge yourself with other exercise or sports options. Join a gym and, if you can, get some help from a certified trainer to establish a lifelong program of cardiovascular, resistance, and flexibility training.

THE TAKEAWAY

- Being overweight or obese—especially amassing abdominal body fat—is a major health risk for men. Excess fat increases the odds of chronic aging diseases such as cardiovascular disease and diabetes as well as prostate disorders that include prostate cancer— the second leading cause of male cancer deaths.

- Chronic inflammation increases with excess body fat and can affect the prostate, leading to the cellular damage that promotes the development of prostate disorders, including cancer.

- Metabolic syndrome, a combination of disorders of weight, lipid and glucose metabolism, and blood pressure, increases the likelihood of cardiovascular disease (including heart attacks and strokes), diabetes, and prostate disease.

- Lifestyle modifications, including dietary changes and physical activity, can reverse metabolic syndrome and reduce the risk of chronic diseases of aging.

- A moderate amount of exercise, such as walking briskly thirty minutes a day, can reduce the risk of death from chronic diseases of aging and progression of prostate cancer in men with the disease.

- Make ten thousand steps a day your first exercise goal, and then take off from there.

CHAPTER THREE

NUTRITION AND MEN'S OPTIMAL HEALTH

My doctor told me to stop having intimate dinners
for four, unless there are three other people at
the table.

—Orson Welles

"Was it my diet that did me in?" asked Bob, a sixty-five-year-old patient with newly diagnosed low-grade prostate cancer and who now had some decisions to make. He had been initially referred to a urologist for evaluation of erectile dysfunction that had been worsening gradually over the years. His prostate cancer was found on a biopsy triggered by a PSA result of 3.5 nanograms per milliliter of blood (ng/ml), which was considered worrisome because it had gone up from 2.8 ng/ml a year earlier. Bob was overweight, with a body mass index of 29, putting him on the road to obesity. He was also prediabetic and hypertensive and, like most Americans and most patients who come to my office, had no established exercise program. He was living the sedentary life.

Countless other men whom I have counseled and treated over the years have wanted to know if there was something they could have done to prevent "this." The answer is yes: a healthy lifestyle can lower the risk of many diseases associated with a decline in male health—diabetes, hypertension, cardiovascular disease (CVD), and urologic issues that concern many aging males, including urinary symptoms and ED.

But the most concerning issue for Bob right now was prostate cancer.

He had been advised to have immediate surgery to get rid of the cancer. What Bob did not realize was that his prostate cancer was actually the *least* of his worries. For Bob, the risk of death from prostate cancer without any treatment could be as high as 5 percent over the next fifteen years, but his risk of death from chronic diseases associated with his other health issues—namely, heart disease, stroke, and diabetes—was higher than 40 percent.

My approach for Bob's consultation was the "sandwich" technique: good news, bad news, good news. Once I reassured him that his prostate cancer was not lethal (good news), I warned him about the risks of continuing with his current lifestyle (bad news), but emphasized that making the necessary changes would lower his risk of death from cardiovascular disease, reduce the likelihood that his prostate cancer would ever harm him, and improve his erectile function (all good news).

This we know: what we eat and how much we eat contribute to our risk of developing many of the chronic diseases that occur with age, including those that directly affect male health. Diet is linked directly to disorders of glucose and fat metabolism and to inflammation and disorders of the immune system—all of which lead to higher risks of chronic aging diseases such as cardiovascular disease, hypertension, diabetes—and, yes, sexual dysfunction and prostate diseases.

In the West, the death rate from prostate cancer is four to five times higher than in Asian societies. It is almost certain that lifestyle choices, including both food selections and the number of calories consumed, are linked to the disease. In societies where diets feature substantial amounts of whole grains, legumes (the class of vegetables that includes beans, lentils, and peas), a variety of colorful fruits and vegetables, and fish, there are much lower rates of common cancers such as breast and prostate cancers and lower rates of other chronic age-related ailments: heart disease and diabetes, for example.

When it comes to maintaining male health, the common American diet is not the smartest choice. Heavy on foods such as French fries, burgers, cookies, chips, soda, and other fast-food staples, our diet is calorie dense and provides excessive amounts of sugar, sodium, saturated fat, and refined (rather than whole) grains. Combine this with a sedentary lifestyle, and you have the perfect storm guaranteed to wreck male health.

YOU ARE WHAT YOU EAT

Diets high in calories, fat, dairy products, and grilled or processed meats are associated with metabolic disturbances that lead to an increased risk of fatal prostate cancer, prostatic enlargement and associated urination symptoms, sexual dysfunction, and prostatic inflammation. It may be that these foods promote the development of chronic disease through metabolic and hormonal changes that favor excess cell growth and reduced normal cell death. It's this uncontrolled cell growth that's a hall-mark of cancer. Alterations in nerve pathways, a reduced ability of the immune system to fight cancer, and increased inflammation also com-promises male health. In support of the inflammation theory of prostate disease, some studies—including our work with the Baltimore Longi-tudinal Study of Aging (BLSA)—have shown that anti-inflammatory drugs may protect against the development of prostate cancer.

In this chapter, I will detail the connection between what and how much you eat and its impact on male health. There is no doubt that poor dietary choices can lead to a cascade of metabolic disturbances (obesity, lipid and glucose disorders, hypertension) that can result in a decline in male health by leading to cardiovascular disease (CVD). But these same metabolic disorders are now recognized to also increase a man's risk of prostate disease, urination symptoms, and sexual dysfunction, among others.

We all recognize the overweight individual with the associated met-abolic abnormalities as one who is at higher risk for CVD, including heart disease. But there are other important aspects of male health that decline with the consumption of too many calories laden with sugar and fat, combined with a lack of physical activity.

Information gleaned from the Baltimore Longitudinal Study on Aging has provided much of this important information. Initiated in 1958, the BLSA is one of America's longest ongoing studies of aging. More than fourteen hundred men and women are study volunteers. Ranging in age from twenty to ninety, they are tested regularly every two years with a battery of medical exams and followed through into old age. Working with colleagues at the BLSA, we at Johns Hopkins have shown that an elevated BMI in men in their forties is associated with both prostate enlargement, which can lead to urinary symptoms, and erection problems two to three decades later in life. Early "sins"—the Western diet and a sedentary lifestyle—come back to visit men in the forms of erectile dysfunction and prostate disease, in addition to other chronic illness.

THE VANISHING ERECTION AND THE HEART ATTACK: ONE DISEASE OR TWO?

Tired from having too much sex? There is a solution. Supersize your meals with unhealthful foods while abstaining from physical activity, and do this with the same enthusiasm that you had when you first realized the "joys of sex."

The Western lifestyle, with high rates of hypertension, obesity, and metabolic disturbances, is associated with both sexual dysfunction and cardiovascular disease, and it will slowly bring your sex life to a halt. It might happen quicker if you have a heart attack.

In a study published in the *Journal of the American Medical Association*, researchers reported that compared with men without erectile dysfunction, those who had or developed ED over five years had a 45 percent greater risk of an event like a heart attack or stroke than those who did not have erection problems. Erectile dysfunction seems to carry the same risk of a future cardiovascular event as does smoking cigarettes or having a family history of a heart attack, because erectile dysfunction is an indicator of vascular disease throughout the body. And then there are the drug treatments for cardiovascular disease and metabolic disturbances that can cause erectile dysfunction. Why not prevent or correct these problems?

If you are already in the category of overweight or obese, and sedentary is an apt descriptor of the way you approach life, adopting a healthier lifestyle with exercise and dietary changes can certainly help reduce the risk of chronic disease later in life—and that includes both heart disease and erectile dysfunction.

TURN BACK THAT CLOCK

In a recent review, it was reported that even without weight loss, a well-balanced diet like the Mediterranean diet (see the discussion later in this chapter) reduced blood inflammatory and lipid markers that are associated with cardiovascular and other chronic diseases. Another review of published trials found that people who made lifestyle changes, including diet and physical activity, were less likely to develop cardiac disease or die than those who did not.

Dr. Carol Derby and her fellow scientists at the New England Research Institutes, a Watertown, Massachusetts, public health research group, evaluated whether changes in lifestyle, including obesity and a sedentary life, were associated with the risk of erectile dysfunction. Studying a random sample of almost six hundred men age forty to seventy who did not have erectile dysfunction, heart disease, or diabetes at the start of the study, the researchers found that baseline obesity predicted a higher risk of developing erectile dysfunction, even among those who *lost* weight. The highest erectile dysfunction rates were associated with remaining sedentary and the lowest, with remaining active or initiating an active lifestyle. The authors concluded that physical activity might reduce the risk of erectile dysfunction in midlife.

In another study, from Italy's Center for Obesity Management at Second University of Naples, Dr. Katherine Esposito studied 110 obese men between the ages of thirty-five and fifty-five with erectile dysfunction who did not have diabetes, hypertension, or hyperlipidemia (elevated cholesterol). Half of the men received detailed advice on how to lose 10 percent or more in total body weight by reducing caloric intake and increasing physical activity; they belonged to what was called the intervention group. The other half, known as controls, were given only general information about healthy food choices and exercise. After two years, when compared with the control group, the intervention group exhibited a greater reduction in body mass index and inflammatory markers in the blood and a greater increase in physical activity.

The gain? Erectile function scores improved more in the intervention group than in the control group, and when considering all factors, changes in BMI, physical activity, and blood markers of inflammation were associated with improvement in erectile function. About one in three men in the study showed improved sexual function by altering their lifestyles. But consider this: the intervention group had an average decrease in BMI of only 15 percent and, on average, was still overweight. I would speculate that a greater reduction in BMI would be associated with even more health benefits. And a bigger improvement in sexual function, too.

Lifestyle factors that contribute to obesity and diabetes have also been linked to a greater risk of prostatic enlargement and lower urinary tract symptoms, while increased physical activity and a healthy diet have been associated with a lower risk of these problems.

The bottom line: the Western lifestyle of high-calorie foods, excess calories, and being sedentary is associated with declines in male health—a decline that can be prevented or diminished by adopting a healthy lifestyle.

LIVING THE ANTICANCER LIFESTYLE

While there are those who, after a diagnosis of cancer, continue to indulge in disease-causing behaviors such as smoking and overeating, many change their outlook on life. They come to view their cancer diagnosis as a call to arms and seek, if possible, to make their bodies inhospitable to these microscopic cells threatening to put a premature end to their existence. In addition to regular exercise, many men switch from calorie-dense foods that are high in animal and dairy fats to meals rich with plant-derived foods. These include red, orange, green, and yellow vegetables; plenty of fruit; whole grains; and beans, lentils, and soy, which are mainstays of the legume family.

SAY YES TO VEGETABLES

Many men are awakened to the health value of colorful and nutrient-rich fruits and vegetables after their diagnosis of prostate cancer or a heart attack, when the damage of poor food choices is evident.

To be clear, food choices alone don't cause cancer; it is more likely a combination of genetic predisposition and lifestyle choices—including diet—that increases the odds that your health will suffer. The problem is that you don't know for certain whether or not you are vulnerable to any particular health problem, including cancer, and which particular micronutrients might benefit you. The smart play is to diversify your diet as you would your investment portfolio and eat a wide variety of micronutrients, especially those found in plants.

My short answer for those who continue to overeat and choose poorly, like my patient Bob—and the hundreds of others like him I see every year in my office—is that, yes, the diets we choose can cause big problems. In animal studies performed years ago by Dr. William Nelson, a molecular biologist and director of the Sidney Kimmel Comprehensive Cancer Center at Johns Hopkins (one of forty centers awarded this designation by the National Cancer Institute), it was found that overcooked red meat produces substances called heterocyclic amines (HCAs). These are similar to the carcinogens found in cigarette smoke, and they promote the development of prostate and colon cancer. According to the US Department of Health and Human Services, HCAs are "reasonably anticipated to be human carcinogens."

One of these HCAs produced by cooking meats at high temperatures is PhIP (2-amino-1-methyl-6-phenylimidazo<4,5-b>pyridine), a substance that accumulates in the prostate, damaging DNA, inducing inflammation, and eventually leading to a higher risk of cancer. It has been estimated that the average American diet leads to consumption of a similar amount of carcinogens from charred meats as would be inhaled from one and a half packs of cigarettes per day! African Americans, with higher rates of prostate cancer incidence and death, are thought to consume almost double the amount of PhIP that white males consume.

Dr. Nelson believes that since the liver can't metabolize the carcinogens from the overcooked meat, they get sent off to the prostate, which puts some men at much higher risk for developing prostate cancer.

Switching to alternate protein sources that won't form carcinogens when cooked—soy and beans, for example—is an easy and tasty way to minimize inflammation and other damage to the prostate caused by eating charbroiled meat. Asians, whose diet is based predominantly on soy and other plants, not only have far less prostate cancer than Americans, but also have less prostate inflammation than American men do.

MYTH BUSTER

Many men die *with* prostate cancer, not *from* it. The lifetime chance of being diagnosed with prostate cancer is 16 percent to 17 percent, but the chance of dying of the disease is about 3 percent. Most men with the disease will die of something else—cardiovascular disease, most likely. The risk of death from prostate cancer depends, in large part, on the age at which it is diagnosed and its aggressiveness.

According to Dr. Elizabeth Platz, who is nationally recognized for her work in cancer prevention, "What you eat can definitely affect whether or not you develop prostate cancer. Based on epidemiological studies, in which researchers use food diaries, diet recalls, or questionnaires to examine closely what people eat, it's now believed that diet is one of the most important lifestyle factors that can influence cancer rates of many organs. The problem is that we haven't been able to specifically identify which components of the diet have the most effect."

Cancer experts now speculate that diet plays a role in cancers of the prostate, colon, breast, and pancreas and that even lung cancer may have a dietary link. While we may not know what specific foods help protect against prostate cancer, we do know that people who consume plenty of vegetables, fruits, and grains and exercise regularly are less likely to develop various cancers—like cancer of the prostate—than those who don't.

A wide-ranging diet and regular exercise help reduce chronic inflammation. Recall from the previous chapter that it's inflammation that plays a significant role in many of the diseases that compromise male health, including cardiovascular and prostate disorders as well as sexual health. A healthy diet plus exercise can lower the risk of changes in glucose and lipid metabolism that promote chronic disease. Wise food choices such as fruits, veggies, whole grains, and legumes help reduce the risk of chronic diseases that threaten male health.

EAT THE RAINBOW

When it comes to fruits and vegetables, keep it simple and think color. Include orange, red, green, blue, purple, and yellow. The powerful anti-inflammatory nutrients found in these colorful foods can help protect against prostate disease and other disorders. If you follow a 2,000-calorie-a-day diet, the US Department of Agriculture (USDA) recommends that you eat nine servings of fruit and vegetables daily—at approximately 1 cup per serving, or, for you metric-minded men, 100 grams.

THE SIX MAJOR RISK FACTORS FOR PROSTATE CANCER

Risk factors are conditions or even lifestyle choices that make a person more susceptible to a particular condition. In addition to promoting disease development, risk factors can increase the chances that any existing disease, including cancer, will worsen or progress. While many men with one or even more risk factors *never* develop prostate cancer, there also are some men who develop the disease despite having *no* known risk factors. Scientists are still trying to explain this phenomenon. The major risk factors for prostate cancer include the following:

Risk Factor 1: Advanced Age: Prostate cancer is not commonly diagnosed in men under age fifty, but the rates of diagnosis increase dramatically as men age, with 85 percent of cases diagnosed after age sixty-five. Other than having a Y chromosome (male sex), age is the strongest risk factor for a prostate cancer diagnosis.

Table 3.1. Rates of Prostate Cancer Diagnosis per 100,000 Men

Age (years)	Rate per 100,000 males
40–44	9
45–49	41
50–54	140
55–59	333
60–64	585
65–69	885
70–74 (peak ages for prostate cancer)	984
75–79	951
80–84	790
85+	681

From the National Cancer Institute's Surveillance, Epidemiology, and End Results (SEER) program.

Risk Factor 2: Family History and Genetics: Prostate cancer often clusters in families. If you have a father or brother with prostate cancer, your risk doubles, whereas your risk quadruples if your father and brother were diagnosed. Your risk is especially high if the disease was discovered at a younger age among your relatives. There is a growing list of genes that are associated with a man's risk of prostate cancer by making him more susceptible to infection, DNA damage, inflammation, or cell proliferation.

─────────────────────RED FLAG─────────────────────

If you have a family history of prostate cancer, speak with your doctor about scheduling prostate-specific antigen (PSA) and digital rectal examination (DRE) testing.

Risk Factor 3: Race: The incidence of prostate cancer in African Americans is among the highest in the world and is 1.6 times higher than for Caucasian Americans. They are also twice as likely to die of their disease. These differences are likely attributable to multiple factors that are still being researched, including genetic links, diet, and other lifestyle choices. Greater access to health care services for white males compared with African Americans probably plays a role in this disparity as well. By contrast, prostate cancer occurs less often in Asian Americans and Hispanic/Latino men than in non-Hispanic whites.

Risk Factor 4: Nationality: Prostate cancer is common in North America, the Caribbean, northwestern Europe, and Australia, and less common in Asia, Central America, and South America. Incidence rates (new cases per one hundred thousand men) around the world vary as much as a hundredfold; mortality rates (deaths per one hundred thousand men), over fivefold, with the highest rates in North America and Scandinavia, and the lowest in Asian countries. (See table 3.2.) Lifestyle (physical activity and diet) differences and more intensive PSA screening may partly explain this difference. But most experts agree that lifestyle choices play a large role in explaining differences, because first-generation immigrants from a low-risk area (Asia) to a high-risk area (United States) are at substantially increased risk for prostate cancer development.

Risk Factor 5: Diet: Although the exact role of diet in prostate cancer has not been confirmed, there is growing evidence for a link between the development of prostate cancer and dietary excess and calorie-dense diets. Supporting this link is the finding that the rates of death from prostate cancer in countries around the world correlate with both fat consumption and excess calories: the higher the per capita fat and sugar consumption, the higher the prostate cancer death rates. The relationship between diet and prostate cancer is reviewed throughout the rest of this chapter.

Table 3.2. Relationship Between Dietary Intake and Prostate Cancer Mortality

Country	Prostate cancer mortality (rate per 100,000 men)	Fat intake	Sugar intake
(Per capita consumption in calories per day) +			
Sweden	27	240	414
Norway	27	235	398
Switzerland	27	237	415
Denmark	23	203	397
United Kingdom	19	163	399
United States	18	158	306
Israel	14	125	403
Italy	12	106	282
Japan	5	48	227
Turkey	4	36	296
India	3	24	127
Cambodia	2	20	21
Vietnam	1	12	50
China	1	9	73

Adapted from Janet L. Colli, et al., "International Comparisons of Prostate Cancer Mortality Rates with Dietary Practices and Sunlight Levels," *Urologic Oncology* 24, no. 3 (May–June 2006): 184–94.

Risk Factor 6: Obesity: Some studies have reported that having a body mass index of over 30 increases the risk of more aggressive prostate cancer, while other studies point out that obesity increases the risk of more advanced prostate cancer and of dying of the disease. The prostate cancer grade, which is quantified by the Gleason scoring system utilized by a pathologist studying a prostate biopsy, is a measure of how abnormal the prostate cancer cells appear. The more abnormal the cells, the higher the Gleason score (Gleason 8 to 10, for example), and, the more aggressive the cancer. Prostate cancer is advanced if it has spread beyond the prostate gland and the area around the prostate.

POMEGRANATES AND CANCER PROTECTION

Preliminary results from a scientifically-rigorous eighteen-month study led by my colleague Dr. Michael A. Carducci, professor of oncology and urology at the Sidney Kimmel Comprehensive Cancer Center at Johns Hopkins, showed that treatment of men with rising PSA levels after primary cancer treatment with either one or three POMx capsules (a commercially available pomegranate extract) daily was associated with a more slowly rising PSA, a possible indication of a more slowly progressing cancer. But the results are very preliminary, and since there was no comparison, or placebo, group—for example, a group with people taking apple, grape, or cherry pills—it is difficult to know if pomegranates are beneficial in reducing cancer growth.

NATURE, NURTURE, AND PROSTATE CANCER

For years, researchers have stated that about one-third of cancers are related to diet, one-third are related to tobacco use, and the other one-third are due to a variety of factors (genetic inheritance, viruses and other infections, occupational carcinogens, among others) or unknown causes. This means that two thirds—or 66 percent—of cancers may be preventable.

An age-old question is whether nature (genetics) or nurture (lifestyle) is more influential in the development of prostate cancer. The question was recently addressed in a comparison of the prostate cancer rates among identical twins and nonidentical twins. Identical twins share all the same genetic information, whereas nonidentical twins share 50 percent of the same genes, on average. In a Scandinavian study published in the *New England Journal of Medicine*, the researchers postulated that lifestyle factors might account for as much as 60 percent of prostate cancers. This study backs up my own belief that a healthful diet and regular exercise can reduce hormonal changes and inflammation that promote disease and enhance the body's protective mechanisms for fighting disease—including prostate cancer.

THE INTERHEART STUDY AND WHAT IT MEANS FOR YOU

Lifestyle modifications can help overcome genetics when it comes to heart disease, and that is almost certainly the case for prostate cancer and other age-related diseases that are linked to metabolic disturbances. Results from the Interheart Study, which was conducted by the World Health Association in fifty-two countries, were first published in 2004 in the medical journal *Lancet*.

In this study, the researchers reported that a series of factors—regardless of what country a person lived in—explained 90 percent of his or her risk of a heart attack, no matter his ethnic group, gender, or age. Men and women without any of the risk factors had an 80 percent to 90 percent lower risk of heart disease. The major risk factors for a heart attack were abnormal lipid levels, smoking, hypertension, diabetes, abdominal obesity, and psychosocial factors such as depression and stress. According to the investigators, eating fruits and vegetables, exercising, and avoiding smoking can lower the risk of a heart attack by an estimated 80 percent.

What this tells me is that it's never too late to make changes in your lifestyle. Over time, depending on the age that you start to implement change, you can reduce both cardiac risk and, likely, the risk of other age-related diseases—including prostate cancer.

FREE RADICALS AND INTERNAL DAMAGE

Human beings are made up of cells that are organized into tissues and organs, and each cell contains a master control center: the genetic material, or DNA, that provides the information for normal cell function. At the molecular level, chemical reactions requiring energy and oxygen are constantly going on within living cells. The more we learn about these chemical processes, the more clearly we see that along with normal cell chemistry, there is a continual process of damage and repair—a business that continues over the life span of the cell.

Living cells require large amounts of energy to function, with oxygen being an essential part of the reactions involved in cellular energy production. We call this energy production metabolism, or cellular respiration. Without oxygen, our cells die within minutes. During metabolism, the oxygen atom is broken apart, forming molecules called free radicals that can be toxic and dangerous to our cells. How living cells deactivate free radicals is an important evolutionary adaptation that allows the cells to function normally.

In the cells, oxygen is constantly involved in chemical reactions in which electrons (atomic particles) are shifted around. To generate energy, cells remove electrons from sugars, fatty acids, and amino acids (an amalgam of oxygen, hydrogen, nitrogen, and carbon that are the building blocks of protein) and *oxidize* these substances—by adding the electrons to oxygen. This forms highly reactive compounds, unstable and electrically charged in such a way as to combine readily with other elements. That's because electrons prefer to exist in pairs, not as single units.

When oxygen finally combines with hydrogen, a stable compound, water is formed. But some of its intermediate pairings are not so benign. A molecule with an unpaired electron must either acquire an additional electron from some other molecule or rid itself of the odd one. As oxygen combines and recombines and electrons are exchanged, other unstable molecules are generated, containing unpaired electrons. These reactive molecules are known as free radicals, and as they acquire reactive oxygen from other compounds, they will often set off a chain reaction that creates even more free radicals. The process never stops and is influenced from both inside and outside of the cells.

The normal process of cell metabolism that allows us to exist inevitably produces free radicals, which cause molecular damage to protein, DNA, and other compounds. The number of such damaging "insults" produced daily in each cell may run into the tens of thousands. Damage to genetic material may, if unrepaired, promote the initiation or growth of a cancer.

FREE RADICALS AND INTERNAL DAMAGE

Many external factors also can promote free radical formation in the human body: cigarette smoke, alcohol, and air pollutants such as nitrogen dioxide and ozone. Tobacco smoke is a well-known source of free radical damage that can overwhelm the body's defenses and cause cancer. Smoking is one of the worst lifestyle choices you can make. In a study of patients with prostate cancer who were or were not cigarette smokers, the risk of death from prostate cancer among smokers was small when compared with nonsmokers. But that's because those who smoke often die of other causes and *not* prostate cancer.

RED FLAG

If you smoke, quit immediately. If you are thinking about starting, don't!

There's no way to avoid producing free radicals: the cells themselves, without any aggravating environmental factors, produce them. White blood cells manufacture them as weapons against infectious organisms such as bacteria and viruses. If DNA damaged by free radicals isn't repaired, the damaged genetic material is replicated in new cells. This genetic damage contributes in part to cancer development and proliferation. DNA damage that is passed along to future generations of cells increases the risk of cancer. Why not decrease the likelihood of DNA damage by consuming a diet rich in antioxidants?

ANTIOXIDANTS TO THE RESCUE

Just as our body has methods of fighting infections, it also is equipped to systematically battle free radicals and repair the molecular damage. These chemical warriors are called antioxidants. The cells themselves manufacture some antioxidants, and others found in the nutrients of certain foods ramp up the protective mechanisms within cells to help avoid DNA damage.

Well-known antioxidants are vitamins C and E, the carotenoids beta-carotene, alpha-carotene, and lycopene (substances that give vegetables and fruits their red, yellow, and orange colors), and chemicals in plant-based foods called phytochemicals. Most experts believe that the greatest value of antioxidants is obtained from consuming natural sources—fruits and vegetables—and not supplements.

We have only scratched the surface of what is known about the valuable nutrients in healthful foods that may prevent disease, but I agree that supplements will shortchange you. This is one time that your parents and grandparents were correct when they admonished you to eat your fruits and vegetables.

VITAMIN SUPPLEMENTS AND PROSTATE HEALTH: YOU MEAN THERE'S NO PILL TO FIX THIS?

Some experts believe that about 40 percent of deaths in the United States could be prevented by modifying unhealthy behaviors, such as consuming a poor diet and being physically inactive. Men often believe that there are supplements that can prevent diseases caused by these unhealthy behaviors; no doubt, taking a supplement is much easier than changing your bad habits.

Patients often ask me what vitamins they can take to protect them-selves from prostate cancer and to ensure optimum prostate health. My answer is brief and direct: they don't exist. But what we do know is that some supplements can cause harm.

The SELECT (Selenium and Vitamin E Cancer Prevention Trial) study, the largest-ever prostate cancer prevention trial, confirmed the potential danger of taking supplements that have no proven benefits. Previous studies had suggested that selenium and vitamin E, alone or in combination, might reduce the risk of developing prostate cancer. (Selenium is obtained mostly from plant sources, tuna, and some meat; vitamin E, in whole grains and nuts.) This intrigued researchers, so the National Cancer Institute sponsored SELECT to evaluate both nutrients

However, the study was halted after five years, when it became appar-ent that vitamin E and selenium, alone or in combination, did not prevent prostate cancer. More disturbing, investigators noted a slight increase in the number of prostate cancers in subjects who were taking only selenium or vitamin E.

The news about selenium doesn't get better: A recent study in the *Journal of Clinical Oncology* by Dr. June Chan, of the University of Cali-fornia, San Francisco, reported that higher selenium levels in the blood may actually worsen prostate cancer in some men. Dr. Chan found that men who carried a special gene variant called SOD2 and had high levels of selenium in their blood, were twice as likely to develop an aggressive type of prostate cancer as compared to men with low selenium levels.

BUT IF YOU WANT TO TAKE A MULTIVITAMIN . . .

Millions of Americans take multivitamins because of a belief in their potential health benefits. A recent study of multivitamins and prostate cancer in the *Journal of the National Cancer Institute* (*JNCI*) reported that while regular multivitamin use is not linked with early or localized prostate cancer, taking too many multivitamins may be associated with an increased risk of advanced or fatal prostate cancers.

Dr. Karla Lawson of the National Cancer Institute and her colleagues followed 295,344 men enrolled in the National Institutes of Health–AARP Diet and Health Study to determine the association between multivitamin use and prostate cancer risk. After five years of follow-up, 10,241 men were diagnosed with prostate cancer, including 8,765 with localized cancers and 1,476 with advanced cancers.

The researchers found no association between multivitamin use and the risk of localized prostate cancer. But they did find an increased risk of advanced and fatal prostate cancer among men who used multivitamins more than seven times a week, compared with men who did not use multivitamins. Men who took too many multivitamins saw their risk of aggressive cancer jump by one-third, with the risk of fatal prostate cancer doubling. The association was strongest in men with a family history of prostate cancer and men who also took selenium, beta-carotene, or zinc supplements.

This study suggests that while a daily multivitamin may be healthful for some, more than the recommended daily dose is definitely not better for men looking to enhance prostate cancer protection. Researchers speculate that excessive intake of vitamins may actually speed the growth of existing tumors in some men.

The US Preventive Services Task Force (USPSTF) is an independent panel of experts that develops recommendations—based on scientific evidence—for preventive health services. The USPSTF evaluated the use of supplements for prevention of cardiovascular disease and cancer in general and concluded that the "evidence was not sufficient to recommend for or against the use of supplements of vitamins A, C, or E; multivitamins with folic acid; or antioxidant combinations for the prevention of cancer or cardiovascular disease." In addition, the USPSTF recommends "against the use of beta-carotene supplements, either alone or in combination, for the prevention of cancer or cardiovascular disease."

I believe that, instead of supplements, a more effective source of protection against age-related diseases such as cancer and cardiovascular disease is wise food choices. By obtaining nutrients from natural food sources, you will diversify your levels of protection while taking advantage of a sophisticated defensive system that has evolved over millions of years. But, having said that, there are some people who don't eat well because they either don't have access to healthful foods or have chosen not to. In such cases, supplements might be beneficial.

THE SKINNY ON FATS

You may be wondering how anything fatty could possibly be good for your heart. So let's start with the difference between the "good" fats and the "bad" ones. There are four major categories of fat found in food and one that is produced artificially (trans fat):

Cholesterol. Substance found in fats circulating in the bloodstream and present in all cells of the body.

HDL (high-density lipoprotein) is "good" cholesterol; helps rid the body of cholesterol consumed in fats

LDL (low-density lipoprotein) is "bad" cholesterol; builds up in arterial walls

Saturated fatty acids. Substances that are solid at room temperature, such as butter and cheese; raise blood cholesterol levels, increasing risk of cardiovascular disease.

Monounsaturated fatty acids. Substances that are liquid at room temperature and turn solid when chilled, such as olive oil; healthful in moderation by lowering LDL cholesterol and providing antioxidants.

Polyunsaturated fatty acids. Substances that are liquid at room temperature and when chilled, such as oils from vegetables, nuts, and oily fish; healthful in moderation by lowering cholesterol levels and providing essential fats that the body cannot produce.

Trans fats. Liquid vegetable oils that have been modified to be solid at room temperature and referred to as partially hydrogenated; raise bad LDL cholesterol and lower good HDL cholesterol, increasing the risk of cardiovascular disease.

The first group, cholesterol, can itself be divided into "good" cholesterol (or high-density lipoproteins) and "bad" cholesterol (low-density lipoproteins). Too much bad cholesterol promotes a buildup of plaque in the arteries, which in turn can lead to a heart attack or a stroke. Of the categories of fat, saturated and trans fats are guilty of raising bad (LDL) cholesterol levels.

Saturated fats are found primarily in meat and dairy products, which have become staples of the American diet. These fats are associated with high cholesterol levels, an increased risk of cardiovascular disease, and, in some studies, an increased risk of prostate cancer.

TRANS FATS: AN INDUSTRIALIZED
WEAPON DESIGNED TO KILL

A dramatic and upsetting shift has taken place over the past one hundred years or so in how people in this country get their food. The replacement of seafood, wild greens, and free-range animal meat with processed and fast foods as the mainstays of the average American's diet has led to a marked decrease in healthy polyunsaturated and monounsaturated fats in our diets, with a soaring increase in saturated and—worst of all— trans fats, the artificial killers.

Well, maybe *killers* is a bit too strong a description of trans fats. They were not originally designed to kill, but rather were intended to extend the shelf life of liquid vegetable oils and improve their texture. They also taste good: think French fries, doughnuts, cookies, piecrust, and more. But trans fats raise bad cholesterol levels and lower good cholesterol levels. In a recent review in the *Journal of the American Dietetic Association*, researchers noted that a 2 percent increase in energy from trans fat is associated with a whopping 23 percent increase in the risk of cardiovascular disease.

Thankfully, the word has gotten out, and consumers are paying more attention to trans fats. Better yet, food manufacturers have cut back on their use. In 2006, trans fat labeling became mandatory in the United States. On food labels, you will see the words *trans fat* or *partially hydrogenated oils* and the number of grams per serving. Unfortunately, the FDA rules allow a label to state 0 grams of trans fat if there is less than 0.5 grams. It is easy to consume more than the trace amount per day recommended by the American Heart Association while believing that you are eating none. Look at the food label and add up the saturated, monounsaturated, and polyunsaturated fat, and if the total fat number is greater than the number for total fat on the label, the difference is probably the trans fat that you want to avoid.

————————————————RED FLAG————————————————

A diet rich in processed foods is the enemy to a healthy life. Eat fresh foods that are close to the source.

FAT: REDUCE YOUR LEVELS OF SATURATED FAT

Epidemiologists, such as my colleague Dr. Elizabeth Platz, suspect that diets high in fat, especially fats from animal sources, may promote prostate cancer as well as cancer of the colon, among others. They have found that the risk of prostate cancer is high in countries such as the United States and Finland, where high-fat diets predominate, and is extremely low in countries such as China and Japan, where fat is not a major dietary component.

Animals are often used in scientific experiments to test the efficacy and safety of new drugs but also to learn more about certain diseases. Results in animals don't always apply to people, but many studies in animals have supported the cancer-dietary fat link. In general, human studies demonstrate that animal fat, especially red meat, is associated with an elevated risk of developing prostate cancer. And animal and dairy fats, high in saturated fat, have been associated with a greater risk of advanced prostate cancer in some studies.

Prostate cancer risk may increase because fats enhance tumor growth by promoting cell proliferation and by suppressing apoptosis, the usual process by which damaged cells die off. Fats may also influence hormone levels that promote cancer growth and increase inflammation, resulting in DNA damage that brings about cancer progression.

A caveat: research on nutrition and cancer is a complex field, and progress and results come with difficulty. Food studies—what men eat and how much—are challenging to conduct and extremely complex to analyze. For example, if men eat a predominantly meat-based diet and develop prostate cancer:

- Was it the type of meat that was the problem?

- Was it the meat or the way it was cooked (broiled, grilled, roasted, fried)?

- What were the fat percentages of the particular cuts of meat?

- Was it something else in the diet that was commonly omitted among the meat consumers—for example, a lack of accompanying fruits, grains, and vegetables?

- Was it that high-fat diets provide excess calories?

HOW TO REDUCE FAT IN YOUR DIET

While cancer researchers continue their work, trying to pin down exactly how excess fat intake might cause harm, here are three important things that you can do right now that will enhance your heart health, help keep your weight in check, and possibly reduce your risk of prostate cancer.

Before beginning, here is a quick two-step way to determine your daily fat intake of 20 percent: Assume that you eat 2,200 calories per day. Since at least 20 percent of these calories should come from fat, here are the numbers:

1. 2,200 calories per day multiplied by 0.2 equals 440 calories. This is the maximum number of calories from fat you should eat daily.

2. Fat is more calorie laden than carbohydrates or protein. Each gram of fat contains 9 calories (as compared to 4 calories for 1 gram of protein or carbs). Thus 440 calories divided by 9 calories per gram equals 49 grams of fat.

1. DON'T EXCEED 10 PERCENT

Keep saturated fat intake to less than 10 percent of daily calories. These fats are found in products that are solid at room temperature. Think butter, margarine, high-fat cheese, fatty meat, and products containing palm oil, palm kernel oil, or coconut oil. Make all your dairy choices low fat; skip whole-fat dairy products. For cooking oil, rely on olive oil or go for canola oil if the taste of olive oil is too strong for you. And when it comes to meat, choose lean varieties; remove skin from chicken and say no to fried foods and fatty meats such as beef unless it's a lean cut.

2. DON'T EXCEED 30 PERCENT

Essential fatty acids play a vital role in energy production, stabilizing blood sugar, balancing hormones, and controlling hunger. To maintain good health, your diet must contain adequate amounts of fat sources that supply essential fatty acids.

Fats commonly contribute as much as 45 percent of the calories in the typical American diet, and this leads to excess calories. Lower your fat consumption to 20 percent to 30 percent of total calories, with 10 percent or less of that total coming from saturated fat.

Good fat sources are those that are unprocessed and occur naturally in foods. High-quality fat sources include olive oil, fish and fish oils, vegetable oils, and all types of raw nuts and seeds.

3. INCREASE YOUR OMEGA-3 FAT CONSUMPTION

Doctors have been searching for years for heart protection breakthroughs. Now it appears that they may have finally found one called EPA and DHA (eicosapentaenoic acid and docosahexaenoic acid). We know them better as omega-3 fatty acids, a specific type of polyunsaturated ("good") fat that is found in abundance in oily fish such as salmon, tuna, and sardines, as well as walnuts and flaxseeds.

Research supporting a role for omega-3s in reducing heart disease has been accumulating since the 1970s, when population studies showed that Eskimos and Japanese fishing families tended to have low rates of atherosclerosis and heart attacks.

Researchers suspected that the omega-3 fatty acids in the fish helped reduce plaque inside artery walls, decreased blood clotting, lowered triglyceride (blood fat) levels, and decreased both blood pressure and blood vessel inflammation.

The sinking levels of omega-3s in the American diet may be related partly to the rise in heart disease. Scientists reporting in leading medical journals have noted that the higher the intake of omega-3s, the lower the likelihood of coronary artery disease and sudden death due to cardiac ailments. These findings form the basis for the recommendation from the American Heart Association to consume fish, especially oily fish, at least twice a week.

——————————————RED FLAG——————————————
Avoid packaged and fast foods to limit trans fats.

GETTING YOUR OMEGA-3S: FROM THE SEA, HEALTH FOOD STORE, AND PHARMACY

A number of trials have proven the benefits of dietary and supplemental omega-3 fatty acid consumption in reducing cardiovascular disease. There is also evidence—albeit less convincing, because it comes from nonrandomized studies, where subjects are not randomly chosen to receive one or other of the alternative treatments under study—that fatty fish is associated with a reduction in the development of and death from prostate cancer.

In one study of 6,272 Scandinavian men followed over thirty years, those who ate no fish had a two to three times higher risk of a prostate cancer diagnosis than those who consumed moderate or high amounts. And in the large Health Professionals Follow-up Study, which tracked 47,882 men for twelve years, eating fish more than three times per week was associated with about a 40 percent reduction in the risk of metastatic prostate cancer compared with eating fish less than twice per month.

If you believe that you are at higher risk for cardiovascular disease and may need more omega-3s because of a personal or family history, elevated cholesterol levels, diabetes, or obesity, speak to your physician about fish oil supplements. Lovaza, a prescription fish oil product, is a more concentrated (and guaranteed) source of DHA and EPA than any other omega-3 product.

MYTH BUSTER

What's on the label and in the bottle may not be the same. Since supplements aren't closely regulated, unlike pharmaceuticals, it's possible for potency to vary from batch to batch. If going the supplement route, be sure to stick with well-known manufacturers.

LEGUME CONSUMPTION, SOY, AND PROSTATE CANCER

Plant proteins are a beneficial way of getting dietary protein while avoiding the saturated fats often found in meat. Legumes such as soybeans, lentils, chickpeas, string beans, split peas, mung beans, red kidney beans, and cannellini beans are also good sources of fiber. While we most often think of peanuts as nuts, they too are actually legumes.

Try to incorporate beans into your diet on a daily basis. Make soups—lentil, black bean, navy, and cannellini—for starters. This is a great way to create protein-rich meals with multiple vegetable servings as well, depending on the varied and interesting recipes you use. Use beans in salads with onions and parsley, or create dips by grinding beans in your blender with a little canola or olive oil and fresh garlic and herbs. Be creative!

When you get the hang of this, you can even try a bean-based mock meat loaf, with brown rice and nuts to create texture. Look for bean offerings in vegetarian cookbooks.

These inexpensive, delicious, vitamin-rich "poor man's meats" might reduce cardiovascular disease and lower the risk of prostate cancer, although the evidence for this is not so strong as for other foods. Researchers became interested in soy—consumed regularly in Asia—when it was discovered that Asians had not only lower rates of heart disease but also less cancer when compared with people raised on the meat-rich Western diet. The focus has been on isoflavones present in soybeans, which are plant-based estrogen compounds thought to be responsible for its benefits. Research over twenty years is only suggestive at best that soy protein reduces cardiovascular disease and prostate cancer.

HUMBLE HUMMUS

An easy-to-prepare dip for raw veggies or use as a delicious mayo substitute sandwich spread. Keep some on hand in your fridge. It's a surefire way to introduce legumes to your diet.

- 1 15-oz can chickpeas

- ¼ cup water

- ¼ cup lemon juice

- 2 Tbsp extra-virgin olive oil

- Pinch of salt

- 2 cloves minced garlic

- 1 tsp black pepper

Drain and rinse chickpeas. Add all ingredients to a blender. Puree for 3 minutes.

Nutrition Information
21 grams protein, 70 grams carbohydrate, 10 grams fat

SOY PROTEIN SMOOTHIE

If you're looking for a tasty, nutrient-dense drink with plenty of vitamins and protein, a breakfast smoothie is an excellent on-the-go morning meal that gives you 25 to 50 grams of high-quality soy protein. It's also a great postworkout snack that will help refuel your tired muscles.

- 2 Tbsp instant chocolate milk

- 1 cup soy or 1 percent milk

- ½ oz soy protein powder

- 3 to 5 ice cubes

In a blender, combine the ice cubes, instant chocolate milk, milk, and soy protein powder. Process until the ice is all crushed and the drink is smooth. If the chocolate or protein powder is stuck to the inside of the blender, use a spatula to scrape it off and blend for another 10 seconds. There are all kinds of combinations of smoothies. Add fruit, flaxseeds, or nuts; the choice is yours.

Nutrition Information
30 grams protein (with 1 oz of powder and milk; 50 grams with
2 oz of powder), 30 grams (approximately) carbohydrates

FLAXSEEDS: TASTY—AND THEY MIGHT PROTECT YOUR PROSTATE, TOO

Flax is a particularly interesting plant that is being studied for its effects on prostate and breast cancers.

The flax plant yields the fiber from which linen is woven, as well as seeds and oil. Like olive, canola, and most other plant-derived oils, flaxseed oil is highly unsaturated and is thus a healthful choice to replace saturated fats such as butter and lard. Flaxseeds, from which the oil is extracted, can be eaten whole, sprinkled over cereals, or ground into a flour and spooned into fruit smoothies or used in baking.

Flaxseeds have a mild, nutty flavor, and are the richest source of all plant-based omega-3 fatty acids that have caught the attention of cancer researchers. Nutrition scientist Dr. Wendy Demark-Wahnefried, who is now the associate director of the University of Alabama at Birmingham Comprehensive Cancer Center, got together with researchers from the University of Michigan, the University of North Carolina, and Duke University Medical Center to study the impact of daily flaxseed consumption on men at least one month before they were scheduled to undergo a radical prostatectomy to surgically remove their cancerous prostates.

The men were stratified into four groups of about forty each, with one group taking three tablespoons of ground flaxseeds daily and mixing it with their food, and another group eating flaxseeds in conjunction with a low-fat diet. Flax suggestions and various recipes were provided to the men in the multisite study, but most simply mixed the ground seeds into a glass of water or juice and drank it down in one sitting. The volunteers in the third group followed a low-fat eating regimen, while those in the fourth group kept to their normal eating habits.

Once the men's prostates were removed, the researchers examined the tumor cells under a microscope and were able to determine how quickly the cancer cells had multiplied over the one-month span. The results, published in the journal *Cancer Epidemiology, Biomarkers & Prevention*, showed that those men who took just flaxseeds as well as those who combined daily flaxseeds with low-fat eating had the slowest rates of tumor growth, which indicated that flaxseeds were safe and might be associated with a therapeutic effect on prostate cancer.

What is it that boosts flaxseeds into the power food category? Dr. Demark-Wahnefried believes that flaxseeds play a part in halting the cellular activity that leads to cancer growth and spread. "The omega-3 fatty acids in the tiny flat seeds help alter how cancer cells lump together, which can help put the brakes on their proliferation," she says. "In addition, the lignans in the seeds may have definite antiangiogenic properties, which means that the seeds can possibly help choke off the abnormal blood supply to the tumors and keep them from growing." Lignans are a unique group of plant chemicals known as phytoestrogens that are beneficial to human health through their antioxidant activity.

Dr. Demark-Wahnefried is continuing her flaxseed research and is planning upcoming clinical trials for men who have experienced a recurrence of prostate cancer following prostate surgery, and for men undergoing radiation therapy for prostate cancer.

"The studies on flaxseed and cancer are limited," she acknowledges, "but of all the studies we have done in mice and men with prostate cancer, we have seen consistent results that are very supportive of flaxseeds."

A SPOONFUL OF HEALTH

"Keep an open mind about flaxseeds," says Dr. Wendy Demark-Wahnefried. "They are tasty, nutritious, readily available, inexpensive, and prostate friendly. Since flaxseeds are sometimes difficult to digest in their whole form, they can be easily ground up with a coffee grinder or blender and used in a variety of dishes."

Men in Dr. Demark-Wahnefried's 2008 prostate study consumed 30 grams (three tablespoons) daily in order to have a major impact in the short time before their scheduled surgery, but she now recommends reducing that to one tablespoon a day for men with or without prostate cancer hoping to improve their prostate health. Here are her recommendations for incorporating flaxseeds into your daily diet:

- Stir ground flaxseeds into juice, water, sports drinks, or fruit smoothies.
- Add ground flaxseeds to cookies, muffins, and cornbread recipes.
- Add ground flaxseeds to yogurt or cottage cheese.
- Stir flaxseeds into applesauce, jellies, and jams.
- Mix flaxseeds into your salad dressing or sprinkle them over your salad.
- Sprinkle flaxseeds over cold cereal or oatmeal.
- Mix flaxseeds into pancake or waffle batter.
- Sprinkle flaxseeds over your favorite soup.

DON'T GO SWEET ON ME

Not only has sugar been linked to the rise in obesity and diabetes in this country—especially all the sugar that has been dumped into processed foods—but now there is also evidence from animal studies confirming that sugar is a primary fuel used by prostate and other cancers to grow (See table 3.2 on page 55 showing the relationship between sugar intake and prostate cancer death rates around the world.)

What's good for the heart is good for men's health and the prostate: the American Heart Association now recommends that men consume no more than 37.5 grams of sugar daily—that's 9 teaspoons and 150 calories. Your typical American male, however, will take in 90 grams of sugar per day (360 calories), which is a heaping 22 teaspoons of the sweet stuff. The sugar doesn't come straight from the sugar bowl but principally from soda. Sugar is also consumed in breakfast cereals, candies, and commercially prepared desserts.

Nutrition labels on these products list sugar in a variety of ways, so read carefully if you are serious about reducing your sugar intake. In addition to raw or brown sugar, other forms of sugar include malt syrup, corn and high-fructose corn syrup, fruit juice concentrate, evaporated cane juice, molasses, honey, and agave nectar.

DIABETES AND PROSTATE CANCER LINK

Diabetes has reached epidemic proportions in the United States, primarily because of overeating and lack of physical activity. This disease, which now afflicts around twenty-six million Americans, can be considered a metabolic disorder, caused by either an inadequate amount of insulin production or the cells' inability to respond to insulin (insulin resistance). Insulin is a hormone produced by the pancreas that regulates the uptake of glucose—an important energy source—from the bloodstream into cells. The signal for insulin release is blood glucose levels, usually highest after a meal.

There are two types of diabetes. In type 1 diabetes the immune system attacks and destroys cells so that the pancreas can no longer produce sufficient amounts of insulin. Often called juvenile-onset diabetes because it typically begins in childhood, people with type 1 diabetes must take insulin injections several times a day to prevent dangerous rises in blood glucose and to avoid any long-term complications, which can include heart disease, kidney disease, blindness, and nerve damage.

The most common form of diabetes, type 2, results from a combination of genetic factors, excess body weight, and lack of physical activity. Fat reduces the ability of cells to respond to insulin, and when the hormone is not effective in moving glucose into cells, blood glucose levels rise—a major cause of the damage from diabetes. Type 2 diabetes can often be managed successfully without insulin treatment with dietary changes, weight loss, regular physical activity, and a variety of oral medications.

Elevated glucose levels and insulin resistance are one part of metabolic syndrome, mentioned in a previous chapter, which also includes elevated blood pressure, elevated blood lipids, and excess weight. There appears to be an association between disorders of metabolism (lipid and glucose) and prostate cancer. Researchers exploring the effects of weight on cancer now suspect that there may be a link between diabetes and obesity and aggressive prostate cancer.

Dr. Stephen Freedland's recent research, published in *Cancer Epidemiology, Biomarkers & Prevention,* has shown that white men who had both diabetes and obesity had more aggressive prostate cancer than men who had diabetes but were not obese. In addition, among men with diabetes and prostate cancer who had the best glycemic control as measured by hemoglobin A1C levels, those with poorer glycemic control were more likely to harbor aggressive prostate cancers at surgery. A1C is an important test that measures what percentage of your hemoglobin is coated with sugar. Hemoglobin is the protein molecule in red blood cells that carries oxygen. The higher the A1C level, the poorer the blood sugar control.

"We really don't know what mechanisms might be in place that can account for this aggressive cancer in obese men with diabetes," says Dr. Freedland, an associate professor of urology at the Duke Prostate Center at the Duke Cancer Institute, but he has some ideas that need to be explored further. "Diabetes is associated with low levels of insulin and testosterone, which makes for an inhospitable environment for tumor growth. However, if a tumor is powerful enough to survive in such a hostile environment, then it's probably a very aggressive one."

Being overweight or obese is the major contributing factor to type 2 diabetes, but this is a disease that responds to lifestyle modifications. With aggressive prostate cancer now a possible consequence, it's yet another reason men have to change their diets, drop the extra weight, and begin exercising on a daily basis.

CALORIC CONSUMPTION: DON'T EAT SO MUCH

Many leading researchers believe that the number of calories you consume daily can affect the growth of prostate cancer cells. In experimental studies, restricting the calories consumed by rodents has been shown to decrease tumor burden and to prolong life. Also known as tumor load, tumor burden refers to the number of cancer cells, the size of a tumor, or the amount of cancer in the body.

A recent study showed that prostate tumors implanted in rodents grew less when the animals were fed a diet consisting of 20 percent to 40 percent fewer calories. In studies of men, Dr. Elizabeth Platz of Johns Hopkins has reported that the subjects who usually had the higher caloric intake were more likely to develop prostate cancer than those men who took in fewer calories. Furthermore, many researchers now believe that high caloric intake appears to be associated with the most aggressive cases of prostate cancer.

The caloric story is certainly complex. The number of calories a person needs daily depends on body size and activity level. It may turn out that the balance of energy in and energy out is what is important rather than just total number of calories consumed. It's all relative, so that means if you are an Olympic-caliber swimmer like Michael Phelps, and you consume about 8,000 calories a day but are burning through more than that in your daily swimming workouts, that alarmingly high number of calories is necessary.

The typical U.S. male who exercises daily should be consuming approximately 2,200 calories a day. Unfortunately, Americans are taking in many more calories than ever before in recorded history and are less active, making us some of the fattest people in the world. While we as a nation have many incredible achievements to boast about—from technological innovations to advances in medicine—being among the fattest is one of our least notable accomplishments.

Fast-food outlets, the huge increase in food and beverage portion sizes at restaurants, and the many hours spent watching TV or using computers are all contributing to this epidemic of obesity not only here in the United States but also in developing countries such as India and China.

Put in simplest terms, we all need to be aware of energy balance. Eating too many calories for our needs leads to obesity, which is associated with many chronic diseases, such as heart disease, and that leads to less than optimal male health. The US Centers for Disease Control and Prevention (CDC) is the federal agency that works to protect public health and safety by creating and providing the expertise, information, and tools that people and communities need to protect their health. According to a survey by the CDC, 61 percent of Americans weigh too much, and about 26 percent of them are obese. This means they are at least thirty pounds or more over a healthy weight for their height.

EATING, OVEREATING, AND OBESITY: THE ROLE OF EXCESS WEIGHT IN PROSTATE CANCER

Maintaining a healthy weight might be one of the most important things you can do to reduce the risk of developing prostate cancer and to slow progression of the disease if diagnosed. The rates of prostate cancer diagnoses and deaths around the world mirror the rates of caloric intake and obesity. Those countries where energy intake and obesity are highest have the highest rates of prostate cancer. And recent studies suggest that those who maintain a healthy weight have lower rates of disease progression after a diagnosis of prostate cancer.

Obesity is associated with metabolic disturbances that change the hormonal environment of the body and increase inflammation, and these may promote more aggressive tumors in some men. Alterations in the production of insulin, sex hormones such as testosterone and estrogen, and growth factors that occur in obese men may also be involved in the development of more aggressive tumors.

Needless to say, more research is needed. In the meantime, the choice to live better, healthier, and longer is yours. Don't wait for scientific validation as a reason to make healthful changes in your life. Commit now to eating right and injecting regular doses of vitality into each day with physical activity. If this is a choice you are ready to make, but you are simply overwhelmed by the prospect of beginning, then consult chapter 2, which contains exercise suggestions; I address many of these concerns.

HARA HACHI BU

"Eat until you're 80 percent full," the translation of *hara hachi bu*, is a Confucian-inspired philosophy of eating followed by most people in Okinawa, an island chain to the south of mainland Japan. The Okinawans, who are famed for their longevity (average life expectancy for women is eighty-six; for men, seventy-eight) and have one of the world's highest numbers of centenarians—people who live beyond one hundred years—eat about 200 grams (7 ounces) of fish and 100 grams (3.5 ounces) of meat daily, with antioxidant-rich vegetables comprising the greatest part of their diet.

What separates Okinawans from other world cultures, however, is the gentle prayer that many say before eating in which they say they will stop eating when they are 80 percent full. Since it takes sensory receptors in the stomach at least twenty minutes to get the message to the brain that it's actually full, the Okinawan self-imposed limits of *hara hachi bu* serve as a good strategy that we Americans could use to avoid overeating.

In Okinawa, cholesterol levels are less than 180 milligrams per deciliter (mg/dl), on average, and cancer rates, including prostate cancer, are 50 percent to 80 percent lower than in the United States. Diet and limited consumption play major roles in these incredible results, but the Western lifestyle has come to Okinawa, and the next generation may not fare so well.

The most inexpensive way to keep your weight in check safely is to reduce your daily caloric intake. It's a win-win situation all around: eat less and improve your health, while spending less money on food. Although it may not be easy at first to push away from the table with food still on your plate, do as the Okinawans do: *hara hachi bu!* Your overall health will benefit.

MYTH BUSTER

It's okay to leave food on your plate. The concept of "clean your plate" began during a time when megaportions of food and drink did not exist.

WHY PEOPLE IN ASIA HAVE LOW RATES OF PROSTATE CANCER: IT STARTS WITH THEIR DIET

Scientific evidence strongly suggests that differences in diet and lifestyle may account in large part for the variability in prostate cancer rates around the world. Researchers are now hard at work examining the foods that we eat to see exactly what they contain and what effect they have on the prostate.

We do know, for example, that the mortality rates from prostate cancer are four to five times lower in Asian countries—where vegetables are treated as meals in their own right—than in the United States, where large portions of fast food and heavily processed foods high in saturated fats and sugars are mainstays.

Japanese men typically consume a diet high in soy-based foods such as tofu, tempeh, and soy milk, and they eat plenty of fruits and vegetables. According to the World Health Organization, between 1990 and 1993, only four in one hundred thousand Japanese and Chinese men died of prostate cancer; that's less than one-fourth the US mortality rate from this disease.

Table 3.3. Top Foods Contributing to Energy Intake in the United States Versus China

United States	China
Soft drinks	Rice
Cakes, rolls, pastries	Wheat flour
Hamburgers, meat loaf	Coarse grains
Pizza	Pork
Potato chips, corn chips	Eggs
Rice	Edible oils

Data from the National Health and Nutrition Examination Survey (NHANES) and China Health and Nutrition Study.

Are Asians genetically more resistant to prostate cancer than Americans? Not likely, because when men migrate from Japan to the United States, their rates of prostate cancer and the rates for subsequent generations rise noticeably—something that is almost certainly linked to their adopting an American diet and a lifestyle that's often devoid of regular physical activity. In fact, within two generations, the incidence of prostate cancer among Asian immigrants to the United States equals that of native-born Americans.

THE ASIAN WAY OF COOKING

For thousands of years, soybeans have been an important part of the crop cycle in Asia. Only about two thousand years ago, with the discovery of fermentation, did soy become a staple of the human diet, mostly in pastes and sauces. Sometime after 200 BC, the Chinese developed a way to mold soy products in blocks, and what we now know as tofu became the primary source of protein in Asia.

In recent years, nutritionists and research scientists have been able to confirm what Asian families have known for hundreds of generations: the soybean—tofu, tempeh, natto, yuba, soy milk, soy flour, and bean sprouts—is the vegetable that most closely provides the complete diet necessary for good health.

"Soybeans are rich in vitamins, minerals, and the unsaturated fats that help the body break down cholesterol," says Grace Young, a noted Chinese cooking expert and cookbook author. "Soybeans are high in B vitamins, folic acid, lysine, iron, zinc, and calcium. Soy protein also contains an isoflavone called genistein that might interfere with the reproduction of prostate cancer cells."

CHINESE COOKING: LESSONS FROM THE MASTER

Traditional Chinese meals are high in fruits and vegetables, fiber, minerals, vitamins, and antioxidants, and low in saturated fat and total fat. Foods are typically stir-fried or steamed and while a traditional Chinese diet is primarily cooked vegetables, rice, and noodles and small portions of meat, you'd never know that from going to many Chinese restaurants in the United States. Catering to American diners, the chefs at many restaurants have changed their menus to give Americans what they want: twice-fried pork, beef and broccoli, orange chicken, and other deep-fried and fat-laden delicacies.

Grace Young, a great cook in her own right and the author of three award-winning books on Chinese cooking, is confident that most men who know their way around the kitchen can learn to cook healthful Chinese meals at home. Her most recent book, *Stir-Frying to the Sky's Edge* (Simon & Schuster, 2010), won the prestigious James Beard Foundation Best International Cookbook Award in 2011. "Cooking requires patience, thought, time, and knowledge," Grace says. "But preparing tasty food that is healthful takes no more time or effort than cooking food that's not healthful for you—provided you have the right ingredients and use an easy technique, such as stir-frying."

The cook and author grew up in San Francisco surrounded, on the one hand, by the immigrant Chinese traditions of her family and, on the other, by innovative American culture. Her Chinese roots reinforced the importance of the freshest ingredients, while her discovery of Julia Child on television exposed her to cooking a variety of dishes.

Grace doesn't believe in foods that take hours to prepare. Try the two delicious recipes that she has provided here for you. They are designed to help you enjoy the pleasure of food while helping you to prevent prostate cancer.

STIR-FRIED GINGER CHICKEN AND TOFU

Firm tofu is generally sold in 3-inch squares or in one rectangular block. Rinse the tofu before cutting. It should have a clean, nonsour smell. When cooking the chicken, spread the pieces in a wok and allow them to sear thirty seconds before stir-frying, to create a nice caramelized crust. If the chicken is stir-fried without this step, it will not brown.

- 3 squares firm tofu (about 12 oz), rinsed

- 1 Tbsp plus 2 tsp peanut or vegetable oil

- 8 oz skinless, boneless chicken breast cut into ¼-inch-thick, bite-sized slices

- 1 Tbsp ginger, minced

- 1 tsp reduced-sodium soy sauce

- 1 tsp Shao Hsing rice wine or dry sherry

- 2 tsp cornstarch

- ½ tsp salt

- ⅛ tsp sugar

- ⅓ cup reduced-sodium chicken broth

- 2 Tbsp oyster sauce

- 2 scallions, cut into 2-inch pieces

Pat dry the tofu squares with paper towels. Cut each square of tofu into 1-inch cubes. Heat a 14-inch flat-bottomed wok over high heat until a bead of water vaporizes within 1 to 2 seconds of contact. Swirl in 1 tablespoon of the oil, and add the tofu and panfry until light golden, about 3 minutes, turning midway through cooking. Transfer to a plate.

Put the chicken in a shallow bowl and add the ginger, soy sauce, rice wine, salt, sugar, and 1 teaspoon of the cornstarch. Set aside for no more than 10 minutes. In a small bowl, combine the broth, oyster sauce, and the remaining teaspoon of cornstarch.

Heat the unwashed wok over high heat until hot and a faint wisp of smoke rises from the pan. Swirl in the remaining 2 teaspoons of oil and carefully add the chicken, spreading it in the wok. Cook, undisturbed, 30 seconds, letting chicken begin to brown. Add the scallions, then, using a metal spatula, stir-fry 1 minute until the chicken is lightly browned but not cooked through. Add the tofu and stir-fry 30 seconds. Stir the cornstarch mixture and swirl into the wok and bring to a boil, stirring constantly or until the chicken is just cooked and the sauce has thickened, about 1 to 2 minutes.

Serves 3 as a main course with rice or 4 as part of a multicourse meal.

Nutritional Information (Per Serving)
Calories, 332; fat calories, 138; total fat, 15 grams;
carbohydrate, 12 grams; protein, 37 grams.

SPICY VEGETARIAN FRIED RICE

The secret to great fried rice is to use cooked rice that's been chilled. Hot, freshly cooked rice results in gummy, sticky fried rice. If you want to increase the protein content, you can add 1 cup of diced firm tofu, cooked chicken, or ham to the rice.

- 2 Tbsp peanut or vegetable oil

- 1 Tbsp garlic, minced

- 1 Tbsp jalapeño chili, with seeds, minced

- 1 cup ¼-inch red bell pepper, diced

- 3 cups cold cooked brown or long grain rice

- 1 cup cherry tomatoes, halved

- 1 Tbsp reduced-sodium soy sauce

- ½ tsp salt

- ¼ tsp freshly ground black pepper

- ½ cup pine nuts, toasted

- 2 tsp sesame oil, toasted

Heat a 14-inch flat-bottomed wok over high heat until a bead of water vaporizes within 1 to 2 seconds of contact.

Swirl in the oil and add the garlic and chilies, and stir-fry 10 seconds or until fragrant. Add the bell peppers, and stir-fry 30 seconds or until just combined.

Add the rice, tomatoes, soy sauce, salt, and pepper, and stir-fry 2 to 3 minutes, separating the rice with a metal spatula until the rice is heated through.

Remove from heat. Stir in the pine nuts and drizzle on the sesame oil.

Serves 4 as a main dish.

Nutritional information (per serving)
Calories, 292; fat calories 126; total fat, 14 grams;
carbohydrate, 36 grams; protein, 5 grams.

SIX ESSENTIAL STIR-FRY TIPS FROM GRACE YOUNG

1. Invest in a flat-bottomed carbon-steel wok and season it to create a slick surface. Season the wok by rubbing it with a thin coat of vegetable oil to fill in the microscopic pores in the metal and then remove any excess oil with a paper towel. Heat the wok in a 450-degree oven for thirty minutes. Once it is seasoned, the wok's natural nonstick surface allows meat, poultry, shellfish, tofu, vegetables, rice, and noodles to stir-fry with minimal oil.

2. Preheat the wok before adding the oil. This prevents chicken, beef, pork, lamb, shrimp, scallops, tofu, rice, and noodles from sticking to the wok. If the pan has been preheated correctly, the oil will shimmer upon being added, without smoking.

3. Use an oil with a high-smoking point such as peanut, canola, or grapeseed. Avoid low-smoking-point oils such as extra-virgin olive or sesame oils, which are unstable at high temperatures.

4. Be sure tofu and vegetables are completely dry. Wet ingredients cause spattering and bring down the temperature of the wok, turning a stir-fry into a soggy braise.

5. Don't crowd the wok with too much meat, or the ingredients won't sear and seal in the juices; never put more than 1 pound of chicken, pork, shrimp, or scallops into the wok. More than 12 ounces of beef at one time will turn gray and release foam from the meat.

6. Swirl liquid ingredients in a thin stream down the sides of the wok. Pouring liquids into the center brings down the pan's temperature.

PROSTATE HEALTH AND THE
MEDITERRANEAN WAY OF EATING

We all know that there's certainly no scarcity of dietary advice in the United States. From best-selling books and popular magazines to the nightly news reports and the Food Channel and its twenty-four hours of cooking shows, we are inundated with nutrition information on a daily basis. It's not surprising that you might feel confused about what you really should be eating to increase the likelihood that you will live a long and healthy life.

But if the statistics about the lower rates of heart disease and heart-related deaths in nations that border the Mediterranean Sea are any indication, you may also want to focus your attention on the Mediterranean diet, with its emphasis on fruits, vegetables, fish, and little meat.

Of course, natives of the sun-soaked Mediterranean region have eaten this way for thousands of years, but their diet became popular in the United States only in the 1980s, when some results from the Seven Countries Study were published. This epidemiological study of men, the first to look at the link among lifestyle, diet, and heart disease, reported that people living in Greece and southern Italy—who typically eat plenty of fruits, vegetables, and whole grains, and who get most of their fat from foods high in monounsaturates (olive oil, almonds) and omega-3 fatty acids (fish, walnuts)—had a lower risk of heart disease than residents of countries such as the United States and Finland. In those two countries in particular, fruit and vegetable consumption is lower, and most of the fat in the diet is saturated, from sources such as dairy products and red meat.

More than a quarter century later, studies are still reporting the heart benefits for those who follow a Mediterranean-pattern diet—whether or not they live in southern Europe.

If you're interested in optimal heart and prostate health, consider replacing those supersized American meals high in saturated fat, cholesterol, and sugar with a heart-healthy diet that includes antioxidant-rich fruits and vegetables along with fish, avocados, canola oil, olive oil, nuts, and other foods rich in monounsaturated and omega-3 fats. It may take some discipline, but your meals can be varied, satisfying, and delicious, and there is no downside to following a healthier diet.

Here are seven tips to help you get started with this health-enhancing Mediterranean way of eating:

1. Instead of meat, base your meals around fruits, vegetables, whole grains, and legumes. The meat aisle may start calling your name when you get to the supermarket, but fight it!

2. Use monounsaturated fats such as olive and canola oil instead of solid fats such as butter, margarine, and vegetable shortening. Sauté or broil in these oils but don't deep-fry. Drizzle the oils

over vegetables and use in salads with lemon or your favorite vinegar as well.

3. Eat fish at least twice a week, and choose these protein sources much more often than red meat and poultry.

4. Incorporate fresh, vibrant herbs and also items from the allium group in your recipes, including onions, garlic, shallots, chives, leeks, and scallions, for flavor and antioxidant power.

5. For snacks, try mixing cereals with less than 5 grams of sugar per serving and more than 5 grams of fiber per serving together with nuts and dried fruits without added sugar. Wean yourself off traditional snack foods like potato chips.

6. Choose fruit, raw or poached, for dessert rather than cakes, cookies, or ice cream. There is still plenty of sweetness after dinner with no fat.

7. If you drink alcohol, enjoy it in moderation: a glass of red or white wine with dinner.

EATING FOR YOUR HEALTH: NIBBLING VERSUS GORGING

Instead of three meals a day, with the main focus on dinner, try five minimeals instead. In addition to breakfast, lunch, and dinner, you should have healthful midmorning and midafternoon snacks.

In a study published in the *New England Journal of Medicine* in 1989, investigators compared two identical diets that were consumed either by nibbling or by gorging. In one group (nibblers), the subjects ate seventeen snacks per day, while the gorgers group had three meals per day. The nibblers had lower levels of total cholesterol, bad LDL cholesterol, and apolipoprotein B (a component of LDL that increases cardiovascular risk), as well as lower insulin levels. The authors concluded that the frequency of meals—not just the amount and type of food—may be important in determining lipid levels in the blood.

—MYTH BUSTER—

Eating as little as possible in an effort to lose weight is an age-old *mistake*. Starving yourself is unhealthy. Evidence shows that eating five minimeals will be more effective at controlling weight and hunger.

EAT THIS, SKIP THAT

Eating healthy means making better choices about food purchases, preparation, and cooking. When deciding on what to eat—and what not to eat—consider these recommendations from the American Heart Association:

- Balance calorie intake and physical activity to achieve or maintain a healthy body weight.

- Consume a diet rich in vegetables and fruits.

- Choose whole-grain, high-fiber foods.

- Consume fish, especially oily fish, at least twice a week.

- Limit your intake of saturated fat to 7 percent of calories, trans fat to 1 percent, and cholesterol to 300 milligrams per day by choosing lean meats and vegetable alternatives, selecting fat-free (skim), 1 percent-fat, and low-fat dairy products, and minimizing your intake of partially hydrogenated fats (trans fats).

- Minimize your intake of beverages and foods with added sugars.

Here are some dietary changes you may want to incorporate into your new lifestyle to help you achieve the goals set by the AHA.

BREAKFAST SUGGESTIONS

Don't skip breakfast. We all tend to race out of the house in the morning, and oftentimes breakfast gets sacrificed or compromised, but studies report that people who eat breakfast every day take in fewer calories throughout the day.

A common item on most Americans' breakfast menus is that breakfast cereal with low nutritional value. Packed with sugars that contribute to obesity and its associated metabolic disturbances, those cereals make it difficult to stick to the AHA recommendation to keep sugar consumption below 37.5 grams a day. Say no to most boxed cereals from your grocery store that are targeted at children. If cereal is on your menu, find one that has less than 5 grams of sugar and more than 5 grams of fiber per serving.

As an alternative to cereal, here are some healthful and tasty breakfast alternatives:

- Try an omelet, but not a whole-egg omelet. Instead use two egg whites or an egg substitute.

- Go for tomatoes and skip the potatoes with your omelet or scrambled eggs.

- Opt for whole-wheat toast or a whole-wheat muffin. Skip the white bread.

- With your dry toast, use jam and pass up the butter.

- Select either turkey bacon or turkey sausage, not pork bacon.

- Look for whole-grain cereals, pancakes, and waffles. Use raisins, fresh fruit, and maple syrup. Avoid products with white sugar and high-fructose and regular corn syrups.

- Embellish your breakfast with an array of fresh fruit. Eliminate sugar-laden pastries such as doughnuts, which are deep fried, packed with calories, and high in trans fats.

LUNCH SUGGESTIONS

Your midday meal, whether at home or at the office, can include a wide range of healthful and interesting fresh-food choices that are readily available.

- It's just a fact of life that sandwiches make great lunches. Use whole-grain breads and try hot sauces and mustards for condiments. Try the Humble Hummus recipe on page 68. Nix the butter and mayo.

- Consider veggies and tofu with brown rice. Skip the cheese and processed meats.

- For extra flavor for your low-fat meats and vegetables, sauté in a little olive or canola oil rather than frying.

- Use salsa on eggs and fish in place of the butter. Salsa adds flavor.

- Sardines, which are high in omega-3s, are tasty with fresh lemon and whole-grain flatbread. Say no to the mayo-laced chicken salad.

- Soup is tasty and filling; just make sure to skip the buttery cream varieties.

- Go for white-meat chicken instead of processed meats.

- Use tuna packed in water, not oil. Add to salads instead of something more fattening.

- For salads, use fat-free or light dressing. Skip the commercial ranch or bleu cheese varieties. Better yet, make your own dressing with some Dijon mustard, extra-virgin olive oil, and lemon juice or balsamic vinegar.

- Pizza is a delicious lunchtime comfort food. If you must indulge, make sure that it has low-fat cheese and is topped with lots of vegetables. Leave off the sausage and pepperoni toppings.

- Make a wrap and be sure to pack it with plenty of vegetables; skip hot dogs and hamburgers.

SNACK SUGGESTIONS

When food is around, you'll have a tendency to want to eat. A good rule of thumb is to keep food out of sight except at meal times, so that what you can't see can't hurt you. Snacks are an exception, however. Most meals satisfy your hunger for about two to three hours before hunger returns. As your blood sugar levels begin to dip, you may notice a slight decrease in your energy levels. Your goal is to never feel hungry throughout the day. Healthful snacking at the first signs of hunger pangs will help you achieve this aim. Snacking on nutrient-rich foods such as fruits, vegetables, yogurt, and nuts allows you to bridge the gaps between breakfast, lunch, and dinner easily.

Think of your snacks as simple, easy-to-prepare minimeals that help rejuvenate. Unlike eating fast food or junk food, nutritious snacking takes some thought, so when you're making your weekly shopping list, be sure to include some of the items listed below. Keep these tasty items handy, whether in your cupboard, refrigerator, briefcase, glove compartment, or office refrigerator.

- Have an apple or banana as your go-to snack; ditch the chocolate candy bar.

- Have some whole-grain crackers with low-fat cheese rather than greasy potato chips.

- Cut whole-grain pita bread into small triangles and sprinkle with olive oil, then bake until crisp; they're so much better than packaged bagel chips.

- Cottage cheese (2 percent fat or lower) with salsa is tasty; skip the ultrahigh-calorie commercially prepared dips.

- Raw vegetables with fat-free salad dressing or a simple hummus hit the spot; steer clear of the nachos with melted cheese.

- Low-calorie fudge bars are great snacks, and they sure beat cookies and pastries.

- Berries added to yogurt will take the edge off your appetite; skip the ice cream bars.

- Unsweetened fruit juices can easily quench your thirst; keep away from soda, diet or otherwise.

- Add a tablespoon of ground flaxseeds to your unsweetened fruit juice instead of ordering a calorie-dense protein bar.

- Fruit smoothies are easy to make and tasty. Use fresh or frozen fruit and mix with low-fat milk or water rather than with whole milk. Add protein powder for extra punch.

─────────────────────────RED FLAG─────────────────────────

As reported in the medical journal *Circulation*, just one sugar-sweetened (high-fructose corn syrup) carbonated soda a day can contribute to the development of metabolic syndrome.

───

DINNER SUGGESTIONS

In the United States, as in most Western cultures, the majority of calories come at the end-of-the-day meal. For too many men, this is a time of overeating. Here's a way to reduce portion size and calories without sacrificing taste.

- Fish, chicken, and turkey are the leanest animal protein sources available. Leaner cuts of beef have less saturated fat. Skip the hamburger with lots of fat.

- On the weekend, make a pot of lentil soup with carrots, onions, celery, and tomatoes and use it during the week. Each time that you warm up a portion, throw in a handful (or two) of a different green (spinach, Swiss chard, kale, collards). Drizzle with extra virgin olive oil and fresh pepper. Don't go for the fried chicken and dumpling takeout.

- Fish is high in usable protein and has vitamins A, B, and D; skip the all-you-can-eat Buffalo wings at your local sports bar.

- For fish or chicken, add zest and flavor with lemon instead of butter.

- Create a medley of sweet potatoes, parsnips, and turnips. Julienne and microwave in a bit of water, toss with a dash of olive oil, freshly ground garlic powder, and turmeric. Who needs the potatoes au gratin?

- Fill your plate with salad and vegetables in a varied assortment of shapes, sizes, and colors. Limit the meat portion to what can fit in the palm of your curled hand. Pass up the prime rib.

- Eat whole-grain pasta with garlic sautéed in a tablespoon of olive oil, topped with fresh tomato and basil. Shun Alfredo and carbonara pasta sauces.

- Stir-fry fresh vegetables and tofu in low-sodium soy sauce and serve with brown rice. Say no to the cheese risotto.

- Choose a glass of red wine or sparkling water with a lemon, lime, or orange wedge to accompany lunch or dinner. Explore flavored seltzers in place of soda.

- Whip low-fat ricotta with cinnamon, lemon zest, and a touch of maple syrup. Skip the puddings and ice cream.

- Blueberries, raspberries, and strawberries make a fine dessert. Avoid the high-fat cakes and pies. And that includes the non-fat cakes and cookies that are made with corn syrup, sugar, and other unhealthy ingredients.

- Enjoy herbal teas with a half teaspoon of honey for dessert. Skip the after-dinner cordial.

I hope that the recommendations above help point you in the direction of some simple and tasty food choices that, once put into place, will begin to reduce your caloric intake naturally and lead to gradual but permanent weight reduction and maintenance of a healthy weight—something that dieting rarely does.

Incorporate thirty minutes of physical activity into your day, every day, and you will see even more reduction in body weight. Do not attempt drastic measures to lose weight. You are destined to fail. Granted, the weight will come off, but it will come back—plus some.

CREATING A SHOPPING LIST TO MAINTAIN OPTIMAL MALE HEALTH

In writer Michael Pollan's fascinating book *Food Rules: An Eater's Manual,* he has done a masterful job of distilling the complex and confusing food messages that we are bombarded with on a regular basis. He says: Eat food. Not too much. Mostly plants. That made a lot of sense to me when I read it, and it's a message that I have been conveying to patients for a long time.

Start shopping now for real food on a regular basis and veer away from prepared, frozen, canned, and packaged foodstuffs. Empty your fridge and pantry of sugary, salty, preserved, and processed foods. The more natural the product is, the better it is for you. Buy fresh food more frequently. Try to find out where your food comes from. Use organic, local products whenever available.

To improve your overall health, you'll need to create a healthful shopping list. Phytochemicals in plants protect them against bacteria and fungi. Eating brightly colored fruits and vegetables, whole grains, and beans will ensure that you are getting the phytochemicals and other nutrients associated with a reduction in many age-related diseases, including cancer. Here are some of the basic healthful foods that you can incorporate into your diet:

Apples	Carrots	Onions
Apricots	Celery	Pears
Arugula	Chili peppers	Raspberries
Asparagus	Cranberries	Red wine
Avocado	Fennel	Soy nuts
Banana	Flaxseeds	Spinach
Beets	Garlic	Tomatoes
Bell peppers	Ginger	Turmeric
Blueberries	Grapes	Turnips
Broccoli	Green tea	Watermelon
Brussels sprouts	Kale	Whole grains
Cabbage	Legumes	
Cantaloupe	Olives	

WHERE TO GET ADDITIONAL NUTRITION HELP

You might need help learning more about healthy portion sizes and food choices. Most physicians have had little, if any, training in nutrition. Nutritionists are registered dietitians (RDs), who have expertise in nutrition and can make dietary suggestions that will help you improve your health.

To make sure you receive advice from a qualified nutrition expert, consult a registered dietitian who is a member of the Academy of Nutrition and Dietetics (formerly the American Dietetic Association). For free referrals to registered dietitians in your area, go to its online Find a Registered Dietitian service: www.eatright.org/programs/rdfinder.

THE TAKEAWAY

- An unhealthful diet that is high in saturated fats and fast foods and low in fruits and vegetables, whole grains, and fish (the "Western diet") is associated with high rates of overweight and obesity.

- Being overweight or obese increases the risk of hypertension, diabetes, and lipid disorders that are associated with diseases of aging that adversely affect male health, such as cardiovascular disease and cancer.

- The Western lifestyle of high-calorie foods and a sedentary existence increases the risk of metabolic disorders that have been associated with a decline in male health due to sexual dysfunction, urinary symptoms, and prostate disease—a decline that can be prevented or diminished by adopting a healthy lifestyle.

- A healthy diet features portion-controlled meals that are low in animal and dairy fat and high in fruits, vegetables, whole grains, and fish.

- The smart play is to diversify your diet and get a wide variety of micronutrients, especially those found in plant-based foods.

PART TWO

WATERWORKS

Water is the driving force of all nature.

—Leonardo da Vinci

For the longest time, the prostate was blamed for just about every urination issue, including frequency, hesitancy, interrupted stream, urgency, retention, pain, nocturia, leaking, and dribbling. Each of these conditions might have occurred separately or overlapped with one another. Even so, the urologist invariably told patients that they had BPH, which is shorthand for benign prostatic hyperplasia, a term that soon came to stand for an enlarged prostate and the host of urination problems for which it was blamed.

Not only is that not the case, but the terminology is incorrect as well. BPH is a histological term stemming from the microscopic study of tissue. It denotes that the cells of the prostate, while nonmalignant (benign) and not enlarged, are proliferating at an abnormally fast rate (hyperplasia).

Times have changed, and so have our definitions. We have refined and clarified the cluster of bothersome symptoms that we now refer to as lower urinary tract symptoms. LUTS has replaced BPH as the umbrella term that best describes a man's urinary complaints, and does so without indicating the cause. These complaints may or may not be related to the prostate, but they definitely involve symptoms related to the storage of urine or urination. For the most part, they are common among aging men—and also women.

This constellation of symptoms—LUTS—increases with age and can negatively impact a man's quality of life. Due to increased longevity, most men will most likely develop some changes in urination with age but most are manageable. Managing lower urinary tract symptoms demands painstaking work on the part of the doctor and the patient in order to determine the exact cause of the underlying problem.

A man with LUTS may have one or more of the following conditions:

- **Frequency.** The need to urinate more often than normal, the most common symptom of LUTS, is caused many times by how much a person eats or drinks. When you have frequency symptoms, in most cases the bladder is not storing urine properly, and/or there is increased urine being made. In some cases, however, frequency could be a sign of a urinary tract infection or an early sign of type 2 diabetes, which is why a proper urologic evaluation is needed. Much more on frequency problems in healthy men is found in chapter 4, including a simple presentation on how urine is produced and stored.

- **Benign prostatic enlargement (BPE)**—Also called BPH, this disorder is a condition that results from prostate enlargement and often leads to LUTS, typified by a slowing of the urinary stream due to blockage of urine flow through the urethra. BPE does not cause cancer, although men with BPE can develop prostate cancer. When blockage occurs and becomes chronic, it is referred to as bladder outlet obstruction (BOO), described below. Benign prostatic enlargement and its treatments are covered in depth in chapter 5.

- **Bladder outlet obstruction (BOO)**—This refers to any condition that blocks urine flow from the bladder into the urethra. When left untreated, urine can back up into the pair of ureter tubes that carry urine from the two kidneys to the bladder, as well as the kidneys themselves. This can lead to infection, and the potential for permanent damage to the bladder and kidneys. Possible causes of BOO include BPE, certain medications, narrowing or scarring of the urethra due to infections, surgery, or injury, bladder stones, or prostate cancer. I will focus on the effects of BPE on the bladder and how problems can be resolved.

- **Overactive Bladder (OAB)**—This is a syndrome of urinary urgency (the strong sensation that you have to urinate) and occasional urge incontinence (a sudden urge to urinate immediately, sometimes leaking urine before getting to a toilet) as a result of the inability to delay urination. It is typically accompanied by daytime and nighttime frequency. For all that you need to know about OAB, including an eight-week program designed to retrain your brain and bladder and eliminate urgency, go to chapter 7.

I have found that many men have no idea how or why they urinate and what can be done to help them when they have urination problems. Therefore, part 2 of the book is for men who urinate too much at night, who map out their daily activities around bathroom locations, who don't urinate enough and retain urine, and whose urination difficulties are due to a prostate or bladder problem.

I am going to address men's common urinary complaints, describe the symptoms, explain how a doctor will diagnose them, and offer a variety of possible management options, including simple lifestyle changes, medications, minimally invasive surgical therapies, and surgery. Using this information, my hope is that men will then be able to make better decisions about putting an end to their own vexing symptoms.

CHAPTER FOUR

FREQUENCY PROBLEMS

No disease that can be treated by diet should be
treated with any other means.
—Maimonides, physician and philosopher (1135–1204)

Gotta go all the time?

Some of this might sound vaguely familiar. You are awakened once, sometimes several times, by the need to go to the bathroom in the middle of the night. Your sleep and your partner's sleep is interrupted constantly, and your sex life becomes a memory. You have to urinate more than usual at work and squirm your way through important business meetings, just praying for them to end so that you can make a break for the nearest bathroom. You make sure that you always sit on the aisle in planes, at the movies, and at the theater, because you know you will need frequent bathroom breaks. You're constantly annoyed within the first mile of your daily jog because you feel the strong urge to go—even though you emptied your bladder before you left home. You debate about whether or not to have that second drink at dinner. You decide that you will, and four hours later, you're roused from a deep sleep and find yourself hurrying to the bathroom yet again.

I'm sure you have your own story. Everyone does. But let me be the first to tell you that you can change all that, become empowered, and play a central role in combating your frequent urination problem.

Before we go on, I understand that anything having to do with your voiding (peeing) habits is neither the easiest nor the most glamorous topic to discuss, but believe me, urinary frequency is a very common problem for healthy men. Not a day goes by that I don't talk about urination on some level or see patients with urinary complaints. For those with more serious voiding problems related to overactive bladder or lower urinary tract symptoms linked to benign changes in the prostate, there will be more in-depth information detailing symptoms and the latest advances in therapies, including medications, laser therapies, and surgical intervention, beginning in chapter 5.

In this chapter, we're going to take a close look at the urinary system. I'll examine the structures that comprise it, explain how urine is made, and what role—if any—the prostate plays in urinary disorders.

WHERE IT ALL GOES

Fluid that ends up in your bladder originates with the breakdown or metabolism of all the proteins, fats, and carbohydrates you've consumed during the day. Metabolism of food produces water, among other things, and some foods are made up mostly of water. All the water, coffee, soda, sports drinks, beer, wine, and liquor that you have taken in also contribute to the total amount of urine produced.

Urine, the end product of kidney filtration, is composed mostly of water, salts, and urea—a by-product of food metabolism—and is produced and then eliminated from the body about six times a day, with about 250 milliliters (almost 8.5 ounces) going down the toilet with each flush. For many people, however, urination is more like a seven-times-a-day (or more) activity, with many additional times at night. That's what life is like when you have frequency problems.

———————————————RED FLAG———————————————

If you are urinating more than seven times a day and are bothered by urinary frequency, speak to your doctor.

HOW THE URINARY SYSTEM WORKS

A review of how the urinary system works will provide a good background for the more in-depth information that follows. The seemingly

simple act of urinating is actually the end result of a complex and deli-
cately balanced biological process. Urine is produced by the two kidneys
that lie underneath the rib cage on either side of the back. The bean-
shaped organs filter the blood and send the unwanted liquid waste (fluid
not reabsorbed by the kidney) to the balloon-like bladder by way of a
pair of tubes called ureters. The bladder then stores the urine until it is
eventually eliminated.

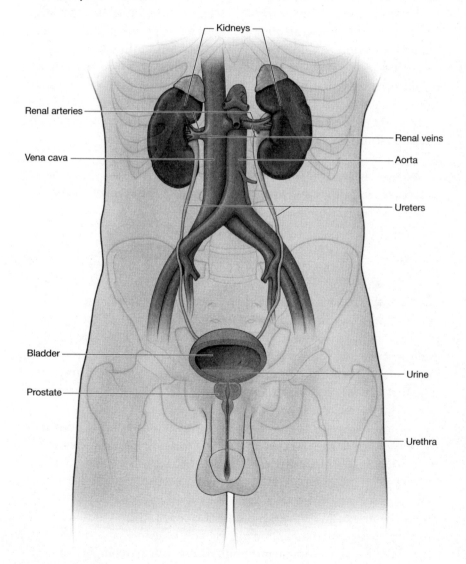

The male urinary system

Each ureter, a thin, hollow, eight- to ten-inch length of muscular tube, contracts its walls to propel the urine downward, with small amounts of urine dripping into the bladder about every fifteen seconds. When completely filled and expanded, the bladder has a capacity of about 300 to 500 milliliters, or one-third to one-half a quart. However, once it contains a little less urine than that, you start to sense the urge to relieve yourself because the bladder's stretching sends a signal to the brain.

If urine cannot leave the kidneys, or if it backs up from the bladder into the kidneys, due to an obstruction or nerve problems, kidney damage and infection can develop. As much as constantly having to go to the bathroom is a problem for you, *not* going is even worse and can land you in the hospital. The urinary tract functions normally when urine moves freely from kidneys to bladder and out of the body, whereas any obstruction of this process can give rise to infection, kidney stones, and possible kidney damage.

RED FLAG

If you are not urinating, or you notice a substantial decrease in the amount of urine you produce each day, see a doctor promptly.

EMPTYING YOUR BLADDER

The bladder is located within the pelvis behind the pubic bone and above your prostate. Sphincter muscles, both at the neck of the bladder (where the bladder and prostate connect) and below the prostate, closer to the penis, keep urine from leaking out of the bladder by creating resistance. The bladder is connected to the tip of the penis by the urethra, a thin tube that runs from the bladder, passes through the prostate and penis, and allows urine to pass outside the body.

Urination directly involves the detrusor muscle—the smooth muscle in the wall of the bladder—as well as the sphincter muscles. When the bladder is filling, the detrusor muscle relaxes while the urethral and bladder neck sphincters remain closed—a mechanism that keeps urine from proceeding through the urethra. During urination, the detrusor muscle contracts and squeezes out the urine while the sphincters relax, opening up the outlet and allowing the flow of urine.

Although urine storage and emptying require a complex interplay among the urinary outlet muscles, the bladder, and the brain and spinal cord, Dr. Alan Wein, the codirector of the Voiding Function and Dysfunction Program and the Chief of the Division of Urology at the Hospital of the University of Pennsylvania, has simplified the way we think about voiding symptoms. He emphasizes that whatever their cause, all urinary symptoms—day or nighttime frequency, urinary urgency, incontinence, and obstruction—can be thought of as problems with either urinary storage or emptying, or a combination of the two. An exception would be urinary frequency due to increased urine production.

FREQUENT URINATION: IT'S *NOT* ALWAYS A PROSTATE PROBLEM

While this is a prostatecentric book, it is important to dispel common misconceptions held by physicians and nonphysicians alike that the prostate is to blame for all male frequency problems. Urinary frequency can develop for a variety of reasons, but it is often *not* a sign of disease, nor is it always a prostate problem. As we age, the bladder becomes less efficient as a storage organ, and urinary frequency increases as the signal to urinate occurs more often when the bladder is only partially full. For example, at age forty, a man's bladder typically holds 13 to 15 ounces of urine, with urination occurring five to seven times a day. But in older men, the ability to store urine when the bladder is only partially full begins to diminish, and the need to urinate more often begins to increase.

This is a direct result of the aging bladder and occurs in both men and women. It can be due to changes in the bladder wall, changes in nerve signals that instruct the bladder to relax, or both. Just as you may find that your joints and muscles are not as flexible as they once were, the aging bladder changes as well, losing some of its elastic properties that allowed the bladder to fill up under low pressure. With less elasticity, pressure within the bladder rises at lower volumes, and the brain receives the signal more frequently that the bladder is full, triggering a trip to the bathroom. Changes in relaxation signals to the bladder may lead to bladder contractions at lower volumes and result in increased frequency and urgency.

In addition, the biological clock in the brain that is responsible for daily rhythms is tightly wired to the area that produces the hormone signals for water retention. With age, these signals that once peaked at night—telling the body to reabsorb water so that we can sleep undisturbed—

become altered. Interestingly, this is especially true for people who live in settings where there is a loss of diurnal signals (for example, those representing daylight and darkness), such as nursing homes. The result is more nighttime trips to the bathroom for both men *and* women. The prostate, especially an enlarged prostate, often takes the blame for these frequency problems, but women don't have prostates, so the blame is often misplaced—and, more importantly, prostate-directed treatment is often ineffective.

Rather, the culprit in urinary frequency is often the excessive consumption of liquids and thus increased urine production, which rapidly fills a bladder that has lost some of its ability to store efficiently with age.

FREQUENCY: TIMING MATTERS

A key issue for the person with urinary frequency is the timing of the problem. In general, men who have frequency only during the daytime don't have a prostate problem.

- If frequency is a morning-only or daytime-only issue, you should be thinking about fluid intake as the culprit. Perhaps it's the amount of coffee, juices, water, or other beverages that is being consumed during the day that is causing the problem.

- If frequency is a nighttime-only problem, the excess fluids in the body that are mobilized when lying down in bed could be the instigator.

- Another cause could be that more urine than usual is being made at night, owing in part to a loss of nighttime antidiuretic hormone (ADH) secretion. ADH acts on the kidneys and causes them to conserve water. ADH levels modulate the amount of water reabsorption in the kidneys, maintaining the body's osmolality (the concentration of dissolved substances in water). ADH action plays a key role in how much urine is produced each day.

- If frequency is a daytime and nighttime bother, the underlying cause could be either an overactive bladder or an enlarged prostate that is literally putting the squeeze on the urethra. Issues involving an enlarged prostate and the treatment options that are available for it are covered in great detail in chapter 5's section on benign prostatic enlargement.

• The good news is that we have effective solutions to most frequency problems, no matter when they occur.

THE FREQUENCY CONTROL NERVES: KID STUFF

After the kidneys produce urine, it is first stored in the bladder and then emptied by bladder contraction that propels the liquid out through the urethra. As infants, when this intricate nerve pathway that controls urination was not yet fully developed and in operation, we emptied our bladders by reflex. When the bladder filled and stretched beyond a certain point, it sent signals via the sacral nerves of the pelvis to the spinal cord, which triggered the urinary sphincter to relax and the bladder to contract. It was time for a diaper change.

As young children, we gradually developed control over the voiding reflex. Bladder stretching registered consciously, and our brains learned to suppress the reflex to urinate until we found an appropriate place to relieve ourselves. For some, control of the voiding reflex takes longer to develop than for others, but it eventually happens, even though, as any parent will remind you, there are plenty of slipups along the way.

As a healthy adult, you have control over your own bladder. It fills painlessly and unconsciously, and normally we urinate every three to five hours, five to seven times during any twenty-four-hour day. The signal to urinate usually occurs when the bladder has filled with approximately eight ounces of urine, or about a quarter of a quart. After we empty our bladder, the whole process starts all over again: storage and emptying.

WHY WE URINATE MORE AT NIGHT AS WE AGE— AND WHAT WE CAN DO ABOUT IT

Antidiuretic hormone (ADH) is secreted in the body rhythmically over a twenty-four-hour period through a process known as diurnal variation, with a peak at night. This nighttime peak results in a smaller proportion of urine produced at night for most people. We were designed to sleep through the night, but as with the graying of hair and the loss of muscle mass that come with age, so, too, is the diurnal variation in ADH secretion reduced with age in some men and women. The end result is less ADH in the evening and more urine production at night. This change, together with the aging bladder that stores less efficiently, can result in bothersome nighttime urination, or nocturia, for some men.

Nocturia is not only inconvenient for you and any bed partner, waking you up countless times to march from bedroom to bathroom, but if not treated effectively, it can also have considerable health-related consequences. These may include significant sleep disturbances leading to increased daytime sleepiness and fatigue along with impaired perception and balance, which can, among other things, lead to falls. One study reported that two or more nocturnal bathroom visits led to a twofold increase in falls compared with people with fewer than two nighttime voids.

In a recent study reported in the *Journal of Urology*, Dr. Patricia Goode, the Gwen McWhorter Endowed Professor of Geriatric Medicine at the University of Alabama at Birmingham, and her colleagues analyzed data for 5,297 men aged twenty and older who had to get up at night at least two or more times to urinate. Here's the latest snapshot of male nocturia that was captured by the researchers:

- 21 percent of the men had nocturia.

- Nocturia increases with age, from 8 percent for all men twenty to thirty-four years old to 56 percent for men seventy-five and older.

- More non-Hispanic black men had nocturia (30 percent) than other racial/ethnic groups.

- The significant factors that boosted nocturia included:

  - a ten-year increase in age,

  - non-Hispanic black race/ethnicity,

  - fair/poor self-rated health,

  - major depression,

  - hypertension, and

  - arthritis.

- Among men forty and older, benign prostatic enlargement (BPE) and prostate cancer were associated with nocturia.

MANAGING NOCTURIA

Nocturia comes in varying levels of severity as we age. For most men, the first thing that needs to be done to reduce nocturia complaints is to incorporate one or more of the following changes:

Stop drinking at night. Eliminate or significantly reduce all beverage consumption in the evening, especially drinks containing caffeine or alcohol.

Wear compression stockings. If you have fluid retention in your lower legs and feet, wearing compression stockings before going to bed could help reduce the fluid retention and increased urination at night. The specialized stockings made of strong elastic material apply pressure in a gradient fashion, with the most pressure around the foot and ankle and less pressure as they go up to the knee or thigh. It's this gradual pressure that helps move pooled fluids back up the leg toward the heart. Compression stockings come in various strengths and over-the-counter stockings can be purchased in most pharmacies and medical supply stores. Prescription-strength stockings also are available.

Change your diuretic schedule. The use of diuretic (water pills) medication for treating high blood pressure or other heart-related illnesses can cause a significant increase in nocturia. If you regularly use diuretic medications, speak to your doctor about the timing of the medication.

Use a CPAP device every night. If you have obstructive sleep apnea, be sure to use your continuous positive-flow airway pressure (CPAP) device as directed. Sleep apnea causes reduced levels of oxygen in the blood. The right side of the heart then undergoes increased stretching in response to these reduced oxygen levels, which, in turn, increases the release of a diuretic called atrial natriuretic peptide (ANP). This results in increased diuresis, or urine production, at night.

Ask your physician about drug therapy. After excluding causes of nocturia like heart or kidney disease, drug therapy may be an option. While there are no FDA-approved medications for nocturia, ask your doctor about desmopressin (brand names include Minirin and DDAVP), which is a vasopressin, or antidiuretic hormone, administered by a nasal spray. In addition, for those with an overactive bladder that causes day and nighttime frequency, antimuscarinic drugs can be useful. (See page 205.)

NOCTURIA

Most people are able to sleep through the night without having to wake up and urinate. Getting up more than twice to urinate after going to sleep for the night—nocturia—is considered abnormal.

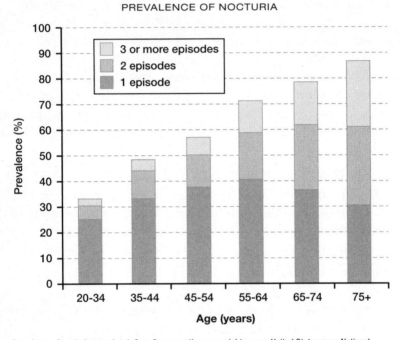

PREVALENCE OF NOCTURIA

Prevalence of nocturia occuring 1, 2, or 3 or more times per night among United States men, National Health and Nutrition Examination Survey, 2005–2006 and 2007–2008.
Adapted from Markland, A. D., et al., *J. Urol.* 2011; 185:998–1002.

THE SKINNY ON H₂O: HOW MUCH IS ESSENTIAL? HOW MUCH IS TOO MUCH?

Drinking too much water is the cause of many daily frequency problems, but it's not the only cause. An average-sized adult with healthy kidneys, living in a temperate climate, needs no more than one quart (about one liter) of fluid per day. That's about four eight-ounce glasses—half the current recommendations that you'll most often find in nutrition articles. It's also the amount that most Americans get in just the solid food they eat every day! In short, many of us could cover our bare-minimum daily water needs *without* drinking anything at all, although I don't recommend it.

Each day, Americans drink an average of 6.1 cups of water, 3.7 servings of soda or sports drinks, 3.2 cups of coffee and tea, 1.9 cups of juice, and 1.7 cups of milk. Add to that an alcoholic drink—or a couple, in some cases. Even without the alcohol, that's 15 cups of hydrating fluids.

What do we do with all this excess water? We eventually run to the bathroom—and sometimes frequently. Blaming this on the prostate and directing treatment at the prostate (like you see on TV ads) are not likely to decrease urinary frequency, despite advertisers' claims.

ONE LAST POINT ABOUT WATER

Many men ask me how much water they should be drinking every day. This seemingly simple question has no simple response because your hydration needs depend on a variety of factors, including your physical activity level, where you live, and what foods you consume.

Eight glasses a day?

There's no question that we now live in a water-obsessed society, with everyone from schoolkids to busy execs lugging around water bottles wherever they go. More than 8.5 billion gallons of bottled water are sold annually in this country at a cost per gallon that is significantly higher than the gas you pump into your car. During your next trip to the supermarket, take a close look at how many different brands of water are on the shelves. That's mainly because of the "8 x 8" rule," an old wives' tale that urges everyone to drink eight 8-ounce glasses of water a day.

You don't have to drink eight glasses daily—nothing close to it, actually. Like so many old wives' tales, this water consumption "fact" has no scientific basis. What is a fact, however, is that most Americans are drinking *too much* water, which is a major reason behind the frequency complaints that patients bring up with their physicians.

MYTH BUSTER

Do we need to drink bottled water? In the United States, we are blessed with fine drinking water in just about every municipality. Drink tap water and put the savings into supporting clean drinking water efforts worldwide.

How much to drink? When it comes to water consumption, drink whenever you are thirsty. If you exercise and begin to sweat, you will need to drink more to make up for the fluid lost through perspiration.

Your thirst mechanism is exquisitely tuned to maintain fluid balance, and when you need to drink, your body will let you know through thirst.

While carefully adjusting what you eat and drink works effectively to treat some frequency issues, its degree of success may vary among men. Should the various behavioral and dietary strategies I have outlined bring only limited relief, it's time to contact your physician for more detailed testing to rule out other medical conditions.

For men who have urinary frequency that by history may be related to neurological disease or chronic bladder dysfunction due to prostate enlargement and obstruction, urodynamic tests may be performed by a urologist to evaluate the storage of urine in the bladder as well as the flow of urine from the bladder through the urethra. In the upcoming chapters, I will cover these issues in greater detail: LUTS begins in chapter 5; overactive bladder, in chapter 7. Although prostate cancer rarely presents any more with urinary symptoms because the cancers are being detected much earlier when they are still microscopic, it can cause urinary symptoms when it is advanced. Prostate cancer is covered in chapter 9.

THE TAKEAWAY

- The urinary system consists of the kidneys, the ureters, the bladder, and the urethra.

- Urination or voiding is under the control of the nervous system and the frequency of urination is associated with fluid intake, regulation of urine production by the kidneys, and the ability of the bladder to store urine.

- Urinary frequency, the most common cause of lower urinary tract symptoms, can easily affect quality of life.

- Urinary frequency can be caused by excess urine production, reduced ability to store urine in the bladder, or a combination of both. The prostate is most often not the culprit.

- Urinary frequency that occurs only during the day or only during the night is usually not caused by prostate disease.

- Most of us barely need four 8-ounce glasses of water a day—and certainly not eight.

- If you're bothered by frequency problems, a daily voiding diary (see page 208 for instructions) will help pinpoint how much fluid is being consumed and voided every day.

CHAPTER FIVE

LOWER URINARY TRACT SYMPTOMS

Going Too Often Day or Night, Dribbling and Dripping, Straining, Hesitating, and Leaking

> Water, taken in moderation, cannot hurt anybody.
> —Mark Twain

Reggie was fifty-three when his urination problems began. This posed a lot of problems for him, since he was a long-haul trucker. Time was money, and stopping for anything but fuel and food cut into his paycheck. He used to tell me all the time, "If I'm not rolling down the street with a load on the back, I'm not making any money, Dr. C."

Reggie had obstruction problems, and it took him a while to urinate. Since he couldn't use the tried-and-true trucker trick of urinating in a bottle while driving, many times he found himself standing in front of a truck-stop toilet waiting, and waiting, working his way through the Baltimore Orioles lineup, staring intently at the porcelain bowl, and then waiting some more. While he had the sense that his bladder was full and his brain was telling him he needed to go, nothing much happened. When Reggie finally did urinate, sometimes he had a weak stream. *Dribbling* was the operative word, however, not *urination*.

Nighttime wasn't much better. That's when the powerful wake-up calls from his bladder began, and he found himself careening toward the bathroom two, sometimes three times a night. But, again, he would just stand there and wait some more for something to happen.

"I just thought it would get better. That's my usual response, and it has always worked pretty well for me," he told me with a strained grin, "and kept me out of the doctor's office most of my life. But after a few months, I knew this pissin' problem wouldn't go away, and it actually got worse. Now I am completely helpless, and for the first time in my life, I can't control this darn thing at all."

————————————————RED FLAG————————————————

Urinary issues will not go away on their own, so don't be afraid to talk to your doctor about them and get help.

PROSTATISM . . . BPH . . . LUTS . . . BPE

It seems like yesterday, but back in the early 1980s when I first started my urology training, *prostatism* was the term used to describe Reggie's symptoms—not to mention pretty much the symptoms of every man over the age of fifty who complained of a weakening urinary stream, problems with urinary frequency and urgency, a feeling of incomplete bladder emptying, and getting up to urinate two or more times a night. Men with these symptoms were all said to be suffering from prostatism, a voiding problem originating in the prostate.

I was pretty precise about language back then—and still am—and the term *prostatism* never really made much sense to me because it could describe almost anything.

"You have to go a lot? It's prostatism for sure."

"Can't go when you want to? Well, it certainly must be prostatism."

"Having issues with the strength of your stream? You guessed it: it's prostatism."

More than anything, the word *prostatism* bothered me because it also inferred that whatever urination symptoms were present, they originated in the prostate. But I knew that many urinary complaints had nothing to do with prostatism, or for that matter, with the prostate itself.

Over the years, the word *prostatism* fell out of favor, only to be replaced with yet another all-encompassing term, *benign prostatic hyperplasia.* Again, the imprecision of the term was quite evident since BPH describes what prostate cells look like under a microscope.

When it comes to voiding issues, the public perception is that it's a problem that only affects men, when in reality, men and women have similar voiding issues with frequency and urgency, especially as they pass the half-century mark. Since men have prostates and women do not, we need a more accurate description of these conditions than BPH.

The better term to describe these urinary complaints is *lower urinary tract symptoms,* or simply *LUTS.*

LUTS certainly does not get as much attention as BPH, but there are several important reasons why both physicians and patients should understand this new nomenclature. And it's not simply a matter of semantics. *LUTS* best describes a man's urinary complaints without indicating the cause. Many conditions both inside and outside of the prostate, for example, may cause LUTS; it's a nonspecific descriptive term.

On the other hand, *BPH,* which has become the umbrella term for men's voiding symptoms, is actually a specific term describing the increased growth of prostatic tissue seen under the microscope. Furthermore, benign prostatic enlargement (BPE) is a medical diagnosis that can be made based only on the results of a digital rectal exam or an imaging study that measures the size of the prostate. Men with BPE may have bothersome lower urinary tract symptoms due to an enlarged prostate.

I know you've seen the popular TV commercials with the embarrassed man having to race off the golf course to go to the bathroom, or the one with the flustered man out in the middle of a lake with his guy pals who has to paddle back to shore quickly to relieve himself. The soothing voice-over reassures us that an enlarged prostate caused by BPH is behind these problems.

But in reality, BPH may cause BPE that may result in urinary symptoms due to obstruction of the urethra. Confused yet? Then read on.

Maybe the prostate was the cause for the problems depicted in the TV commercials, but the forty-five-second sound bites are an overly simplistic representation of the many causes of LUTS. Generally speaking, until a detailed history is taken by a urologist and some office exams performed, these men are suffering from LUTS—lower urinary tract symptoms. While the TV commercials want you to believe that all men's urination symptoms can be solved by simply taking any one of the popular prescription medications for BPE, that's just not true. This would not be good medical practice, and moreover, it is simply unrealistic to think these drugs will be effective for every man.

LUTS: THE NEW PARADIGM

Granted, prostate enlargement could be the cause of a man's voiding complaints, just like those TV commercials suggest, but these lower urinary tract symptoms could also be related to an overactive bladder that does not relax with filling and is unrelated to the prostate. (See page 185.) Other conditions that cause LUTS include:

- prostate cancer,

- urinary tract infection,

- bladder cancer,

- prostatitis,

- age-related changes in the bladder, and

- neurogenic bladder, a condition caused by an abnormality in the nerves of the bladder.

I want you to think of LUTS as you would a headache. There are several different types of headaches (tension, migraine, cluster), each with different causes and specific treatments that come after a doctor has made a careful assessment based on complaints and a medical history. Yet, more often than not, when someone is talking about it, she will simply say, "I have a headache."

Like a headache, LUTS is a symptom that could indicate an underlying condition, and it's up to your doctor to figure out exactly what's causing the symptom and then offer the appropriate management solution.

Although urologic researchers still have a long way to go in developing "perfect" remedies for all LUTS, they are developing therapies that will hopefully reduce your bathroom adventures. And that's the good news I am about to share.

LUTS COMPLAINTS

By the time a man reaches forty, it's not uncommon that he will develop LUTS. Symptoms typically start very gradually, and stealthily, too, so that a man may not really take notice of anything unusual going on until he is in his fifties. The symptoms fall into these broad categories of storage and emptying:

STORAGE SYMPTOMS

The following *irritative* symptoms can occur as the bladder is filling and storing urine:

Frequency. While you used to be able to hold your water like a camel, bathroom breaks at work become more frequent, and you find yourself going every ninety minutes or so, hoping that no one notices.

Urgency. Not only do you have to go to the bathroom, you *really, really* have to go. As in right now, so get out of my way, please.

Urgency incontinence. Oops! Try as you might, there are times when you've just got to go but can't hold it in as you race toward the bathroom. Before you can even get your zipper halfway down, it's too late. Urine has already leaked out.

Nocturia. In the middle of a great sleep and an even better dream, your body suddenly alerts you that it's time to get out of bed and go to the bathroom. The unlucky ones receive this urination alert several times or more per night.

EMPTYING SYMPTOMS

The following *obstructive* symptoms can occur at the time of urination:

Hesitancy. Between innings, you are standing at the urinal in the crowded men's room at the ballpark, all ready to urinate. You definitely want to go, but nothing happens for quite a while, and men waiting in line behind you start grumbling. And then, finally, the magic happens, and the urine starts to flow. What's happening is that it now takes longer for the bladder muscle to generate enough force to push urine past the obstruction that's usually caused by the prostate.

Poor flow. Your once powerful urine flow has been significantly reduced, and you need to move even closer to the urinal or risk wetting your shoes.

Intermittency. You're standing there in the process of going, like you have countless times before, and the urine flow suddenly stops—and then starts up again unexpectedly. The cause can be that the bladder muscle is not producing a coordinated contraction to empty the bladder smoothly, and multiple inefficient contractions are now needed to get the job done.

Straining. The only way to get the flow going is by concentrating and then squeezing the abdominal muscles or contracting the pelvic floor muscles.

Unfortunately, a man with LUTS can have one or more of these symptoms. The only way to sort them out is to have a proper evaluation by a urologist, a doctor who specializes in lower urinary tract disorders. Prostate growth is *one* contributing factor to LUTS in the aging male. But because of the long-held belief that the prostate causes all LUTS, some doctors often ignore the possibility that something else is to blame, such as the aging bladder and nervous system, as well as lifestyle habits (too much fluid consumption and the resulting urinary frequency). Instead of investigating further, they write a prescription for a drug that will shrink or relax the prostate to ease urine flow.

WHEN IT'S MORE THAN LUTS

Pete started having irritative symptoms in 2008 and soon consulted a urologist a few weeks after he noticed blood in his urine. He was treated for his LUTS from 2008 until 2012 with a drug commonly advertised on TV for "going" symptoms. Even with the daily medication, however, Pete always carried a receptacle with him because his urinary frequency was so extreme he was afraid he wouldn't always make it to a restroom in time.

Pete finally came to see me when his LUTS worsened and his quality of life was at new lows. When he admitted that he had been a cigarette smoker most of his life, a red flag immediately went up. Tobacco smoking is a significant risk factor for bladder cancer, with current smokers at four times greater risk than people who have never smoked.

When I examined his urine under the microscope, blood was in evidence. Moving into my examination room, I then used a cystoscope and looked into his bladder. It was there, just inside the neck of the bladder located near the prostate, that I discovered the bladder cancer that had been causing his symptoms.

The lesson here is that men should never assume that their LUTS are nothing to be concerned about. Rather, be proactive in questioning the doctor about the cause, and get other opinions if there is no clear explanation given. Above all, don't ever ignore worsening LUTS.

Table 5.1. Causes of LUTS

Symptoms	Causes
Urinary frequency, daytime or nighttime (nocturia)	Undiagnosed or poorly controlled diabetes Excessive urine production Overactive bladder Medications
Weak or interrupted stream and/or hesitancy	Urethral obstruction and/or impaired bladder muscle (detrusor) function
Urgency and/or urge incontinence	Overactive bladder and/or bladder inflammation (urinary tract infection)

THE PROSTATE AND LUTS

It may not be easy for a man to accept the fact that he is aging, but the signs of aging are certainly easy to spot: Joint pain and sore muscles after running out some grounders at the company softball game? Check. Graying hair? Check. Less hair? Check. More body fat at the belt line? Check. Smile lines at the eyes and mouth? Check.

Here's another telltale sign for you: problems urinating that are possibly caused by changes in the bladder or prostate.

Men, the joke goes, spend the first part of their lives making money and the second part making water. Or trying to make water. Or else constantly thinking about trying to make water.

As a man ages, it's almost guaranteed that he will notice a change in urination (LUTS), and in some cases the prostate may be the primary cause. In many cases, my job is to figure out what the problem is and try to help resolve it.

Benign prostatic enlargement, together with age itself as a contributor, is a common cause of LUTS in older men. As some men age, if the prostate grows in size in the transition zone (see illustration on page 14), pressure is placed on the urethra, the tube transporting urine from the bladder through the prostate. This can lead to LUTS or a host of complaints that not only can make urination difficult but also can send you to the bathroom more times than you ever thought possible.

Good news: BPE will not kill you. And it doesn't lead to prostate cancer.

Bad news: Left untreated, BPE *can* diminish your quality of life, and for some, it can lead to serious health problems.

My longtime patient William, sixty-three, assured me that getting up six to eight times a night to go to the bathroom was never a problem. "It's just who I am. I was never a really heavy sleeper anyway," he'd told me confidently, although he did mention that his wife had moved to the spare bedroom after being awakened one too many times.

But then William went into painful retention when he was in the hospital following knee replacement surgery. The combination of anesthesia and increased IV fluids were too much for his bladder, and he had to be catheterized immediately to drain the urine from his swollen bladder that would not empty. That's when William finally realized that he had to deal with his urination problem before it got a whole lot worse.

PROSTATE ENLARGEMENT: IT'S A GROWING PROBLEM

The prostate, snuggled at the base of your bladder, just in front of the rectum and behind the pubic bone, is about the size of a pea at birth. At puberty, the prostate begins to grow with an increase in testosterone levels. It reaches normal adult size—likened to that of a crabapple weighing almost an ounce—in young adulthood. After age forty to forty-five, different patterns emerge, with some men experiencing continued prostate growth, while in others the prostate remains the same size or even decreases in size.

These patterns are related to the balance of cell death and proliferation, with continued growth of the prostate in some men attributable to the loss of the normal "brake" on cell growth. The fact that the prostate continues to grow in some men but not in others appears to be due in part to genetics and in part to lifestyle choices.

Prostate tissue keeps responding to androgens because with age androgen receptors continue to remain active within the prostate.

WHAT HAPPENS WHEN PROSTATE ENLARGEMENT OCCURS

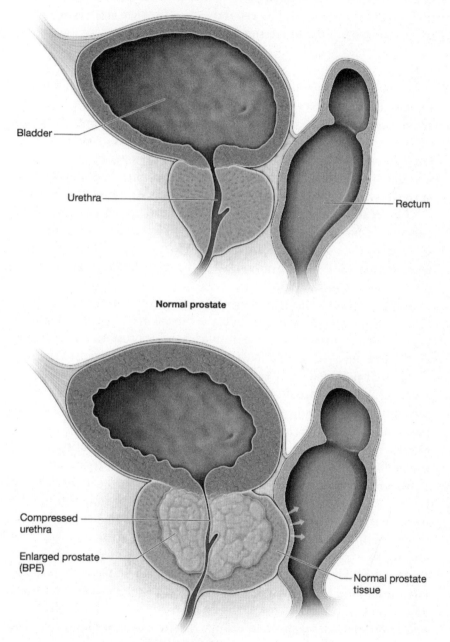

Bladder

Urethra

Rectum

Normal prostate

Compressed urethra

Enlarged prostate (BPE)

Normal prostate tissue

Prostate with BPE

And although androgens are necessary for prostate growth, they are not sufficient in and of themselves. Other growth factors, and possibly inflammation from foods you eat and lack of physical activity, also play important roles in the process of prostate growth.

WHAT CAUSES BPE

Why some men develop prostate enlargement and others do not is still somewhat of a mystery. As with so many things that make us who we are, genetics appears to play a role in prostatic enlargement. We know this because surgery for BPE is more common in first-degree relatives (a family member who shares about 50 percent of their genes with a particular individual in a family; this includes parents, offspring, and siblings) of those with prostate enlargement than in men with no family history of BPE. In addition, the likelihood that the brother of an affected individual with prostate enlargement will have BPE is higher if the brothers share all of their genetic information (monozygotic, or identical twins) when compared to sharing only a part of their genetic information (dizygotic, or nonidentical, twins).

While there is no strong evidence that any one dietary factor is responsible for enlargement of the prostate, the typical meat-heavy and fat-rich Western diet appears to increase the likelihood of prostatic enlargement, LUTS, and the need for prostate surgery for obstruction caused by BPE.

In a well-designed study, researchers investigated Asians who adopted a Western diet for an average of seven years after moving to a Western culture. Seven years of eating and living like Westerners caused the migrants to have larger waistlines and bigger prostates when compared to Asians who remained in Asia. The prostates of migrating Asians resembled Westerners who had always lived in a Western culture.

These data suggest that dietary factors culminating in an elevated body mass index can influence prostate growth, probably through an increase in growth factors within the prostate and perhaps also through increased inflammation due to weight gain and diet, together with androgens.

As you will recall from the prostate illustration on page 14, the prostate is composed of four specific zones: peripheral, central, transition, and anterior fibromuscular (stroma). After the age of forty, this once relatively small gland starts to change for the worse in many men. For those affected, the prostate may continue to grow at a rate of 2 percent per year—even higher for those with larger prostates—and can reach the size of a very large apple. In some men with BPE, bladder outlet obstruction (BOO) caused by prostate enlargement can cause urinary symptoms. That's because nodules of enlarging tissue in the transition zone begin to squeeze the urethra and cause obstruction as the gland increases in size. This can lead to storage (urinary frequency and nocturia) and emptying (poor flow and straining) symptoms.

At least 33 percent of middle-aged men will lodge complaints with their doctors about a host of voiding problems that in many turn out to be caused by their prostates. It's been estimated that about 8 percent of men thirty-one to forty years of age start to complain, 40 percent to 50 percent of men in their sixties are actively complaining, and over 80 percent of men in their eighties suffer distress from LUTS.

THE SMOOTH MUSCLE EFFECT ON BPE

Another cause of the urinary symptoms related to benign prostatic growth is abnormally increased smooth muscle tone in the prostate. There is a lot of smooth muscle within prostate tissue and at the bladder neck—muscle over which we have absolutely no control. The more well-known smooth muscles are those that control the iris of the eye, allowing it to contract and expand involuntarily as light levels change, and the smooth muscles throughout the gastrointestinal system that allow the undulating action known as peristalsis to push food through the system.

Smooth muscles in the bladder and prostate contract when the nervous system sends unconscious signals. For example, at the time of orgasm, smooth muscle at the bladder neck contracts so that seminal fluid does not go backward into the bladder but gets propelled into the urethra from the prostate and seminal vesicles and forward out of the penis. Smooth muscle tone within the prostate can increase abnormally in some individuals—even those without an enlarged prostate. This creates a resistance to urine flow or bladder outlet obstruction that restricts urine flow. End result: LUTS.

THE HIGH COST OF PROSTATE ENLARGEMENT PROBLEMS

Although prostate enlargement is not a synonym for prostate cancer—nor does it increase your odds of developing prostate cancer—it's still an ailment that comes with both a human and economic price tag. It's estimated that as many as 14 million American men have symptoms from BPE. So bothersome is benign enlargement of the prostate that treating this chronic and progressive condition is responsible for more than 4 million annual doctor office visits, 117,000 emergency room visits, and more than 100,000 hospitalizations. The prostate problem in this country also rings up an annual medical tab, directly and indirectly, of close to $4 billion.

THE PROSTATE: BIGGER IS NOT ALWAYS BAD

Though it makes perfect sense to assume that having a prostate the size of a Granny Smith apple would cause some issues with bladder outlet obstruction, that is actually not the case. The size of the prostate does not always correlate with the degree of obstruction and LUTS. That's because we have now come to realize that the degree of smooth muscle tone and the prostate capsule itself can contribute to the degree of symptoms. (The capsule is the outer covering of the gland.) Men with smaller prostates can have more smooth muscle tone that creates obstructive symptoms than those with larger prostates and less smooth muscle tone.

As the prostatic tissue begins to grow due to aging and other factors, it begins to press against the outer capsule. This pressure is then retransmitted to the transition zone, the small area of the inner prostate that surrounds the urethra. It's thought that this constriction of the urethra is what leads to LUTS and bladder problems in some men and eventually the need for treatment.

We know this about BPE because the dog, the only other species that develops an enlarged prostate, does not have a capsule encircling its prostate gland. Even though a dog's prostate will grow in size as it ages, it's extremely rare for a dog to develop LUTS or bladder outlet obstruction. In the aging man, a whole host of symptoms surfaces with urination complaints and the growth of the prostatic nodules that squeeze the urethra like a boa constrictor.

BLADDER OUTLET OBSTRUCTION

The bladder is certainly not immune to what's going on downstairs with the prostate and urethra, because this muscular storage receptacle now has to work extra hard to force the urine through the much smaller urethral opening past an obstruction. When I first started in medicine and was training, urologists believed that this caused an increase in the detrusor muscle size, much like the bulging biceps you get from curling a twenty-pound dumbbell through three sets of fifteen repetitions.

Now we know differently. The increased workload that the bladder takes on actually leads to a stiffening of the bladder due to collagen deposition in the bladder wall. Collagen is the scaffolding system of tissues that holds things together. The urologist sees this when he or she examines the bladder with a cystoscope and sees trabeculations, or ridges of excess collagen, within the wall of the bladder. This in itself might not pose a problem, if not for the fact that the stiffening of the bladder wall decreases urine-storing capacity. Add these changes to an already aging bladder that is undergoing some of the same changes independent of bladder outlet obstruction (BOO), and the ultimate outcome is:

- **You're shortchanged.** The amount of urine the bladder can hold without a strong signal to urinate is reduced, sometimes significantly, and as it loses its ability to empty completely, it leaves urine in the bladder, which can lead to urinary retention.

- **Signals are crossed.** The bladder begins to signal you that it is full and that you need to void long before it's actually full.

- **Urinary frequency increases.** Not only are your daytime bathroom trips increased, but also nocturia sets in, and you can count on being awakened numerous times throughout the night.

Like my patient William, who wasn't too bothered initially by his increased frequency or nocturia until he eventually went into urinary retention, many men are loath to contact their doctor about their new urination problems. Unfortunately, this neglect may come with a price, as it did for William. Over time, some men's bladders fill but don't empty, causing urinary retention requiring emergency catheterization to allow the bladder to empty. Retained urine can also lead to the development of calculi (bladder stones), but the urine can also become infected, leaving you feverish and with chills.

URINARY RETENTION

Urinary retention, the inability to pass urine, typically strikes without warning. The pain can be excruciating when you can't urinate, and, not surprisingly, this is a medical emergency that calls for prompt treatment. It is not just a bladder issue but a serious medical condition that can also cause anxiety and high blood pressure. Other complications of untreated urinary retention include damage to the bladder and chronic kidney failure. The quicker you are treated, the lower your risk of complications.

While I have heard many men with acute urinary retention let out very audible "Aaaahs!" from the almost instantaneous abdominal pain relief that catheterization can bring, I have also seen others go on to become—understandably—extremely frustrated and angry that catheterization, something they now have to do several times a day, is the only way they can drain their bladders fully.

Acute urinary retention, or the complete inability to urinate, can be spontaneous or precipitated. When men with an enlarged prostate go into retention spontaneously, about three in four of them will eventually require an operation to remove prostate tissue. This is described in chapter 6.

Urinary retention in men with an enlarged prostate can also be caused by medications. The most common offenders are over-the-counter cold and allergy medications.

Rapid hydration, especially with alcoholic or caffeinated beverages can also trigger retention. Delaying urination during a long airline flight, for example, is another common way to get into big trouble. I once had a patient returning from a business trip to Brussels who was sitting in a window seat. He had two beers en route, as well as a coffee, and had also taken a cold medication that morning for a cough. When he finally felt the urge to urinate, he decided to wait until the plane had landed instead of bothering his two sleeping seatmates.

By the time he finally made it to the bathroom in the airport terminal, not a drop of urine came out. In a panic, he zipped up and went through customs, and headed to the first bathroom he could find. Again, nothing happened. He was in retention. His bladder had become overstretched from rapid filling from the beverages he had consumed, while the cold medication caused an increase in smooth muscle tone in the prostate that increased resistance to urine flow. This combination resulted in no flow whatsoever. Instead of heading home, he went straight to the hospital emergency department and had his bladder catheterized.

Delaying urination and rapid hydration overstretch the bladder, which then decreases the ability of the detrusor muscle to contract. This is why men with prostatic enlargement often complain about hesitancy and slow flow more in the early morning, when the bladder is full.

In order to avoid urinary retention, here are my three rules for all men with LUTS and prostatic enlargement:

1. Avoid over-the-counter cold and allergy medications containing antihistamines or decongestants, such as pseudoephedrine or phenylephrine. See a complete list below of other anticholinergic medications to avoid. These drugs will slow or stop urination and can cause you to go into retention.

2. Do not drink copious amounts of liquids over a short period. This will stretch the bladder and can cause you to go into retention.

3. Do not delay urination. When you feel that you have to go, go! Wait too long, the bladder becomes overstretched, and you may go into retention.

Table 5.2. Drugs That Slow or Stop Urination

Antihistamines	chlorpheniramine (Chlor-Trimeton, Alermine)
	cyproheptadine (Periactin)
	diphenhydramine (Benadryl)
	hydroxyzine (Atarax, Vistaril)
Antidepressants	amoxapine (Asendin)
	amitriptyline (Elavil)
	clomipramine (Anafranil)
	desipramine (Norpramin)
	doxepin (Sinequan)
	imipramine (Tofranil)
	nortriptyline (Pamelor, Aventyl)
	paroxetine (Paxil)
Anti-nausea/vomiting	prochlorperazine (Compazine)
	promethazine (Phenergan)
Antipsychotics	chlorpromazine (Thorazine)
	clozapine (Clozaril)
	olanzapine (Zyprexa)
	thioridazine (Mellaril)
Antivertigo	meclizine (Antivert)
	scopolamine (Scopace)

Cardiovascular	furosemide (Lasix, Uremide)
	disopyramide (Norpace)
Decongestant	pseudoephedrine (Sudafed)
	pseudoephedrine and dexbrompheniramine (Drixoral, Dimetapp)
Gastrointestinal	diphenoxylate and atropine (Lomotil)
	clidinium (Quarzan)
	chlordiazepoxide (Librium, Mitran)
	hyoscyamine (Levsin, Levsinex)
	propantheline (Pro-Banthine)
Muscle relaxants	cyclobenzaprine (Flexeril)
	dantrolene (Dantrium)
	orphenadrine (Norflex)
Overactive bladder medications	oxybutynin (Ditropan)
	propantheline (Pro-Banthine)
	solifenacin (Vesicare)
	tolterodine (Detrol LA)
	trospium (Sanctura)
Antiparkinsonian medications	amantadine (Symadine, Symmetrel)
	benztropine (Cogentin)
	biperiden (Akineton)
	trihexyphenidyl (Artane, Trihexane, Tritane)

TAKING CHARGE: IT'S TIME TO MAN UP

Too many men are doctorphobic when it comes to lower urinary tract symptoms, and, unfortunately, this can lead to health problems not only for LUTS patients but also for those who care about them. Men's reluctance to take care of their health and realistically confront their health problems exacts a toll on relationships as well.

I find that too many men take a hands-off approach about their health, and this includes LUTS. They will often ignore the signs of frequency and nocturia. In the process, their "prostate problem" and all the potentially scary thoughts that it conjures up, worries their significant others. In some cases, it even compromises their partner's health, due to the anxiety and stress that come with it.

In general, women appear to be much more realistic and matter-of-fact about health issues. They undergo routine gynecological check-ups and yearly pap tests, deal with urinary tract infections, and then many go on to experience pregnancy. All of this helps to create a deeply ingrained awareness about their bodies.

Unfortunately, for the most part, men do not have this awareness—that is, until a medical emergency develops. Men will often take a laissez-faire approach to their own health. They think that going to a physician is a nuisance or inconvenience, no matter how sick they are, and take the "It'll go away, like it always does" attitude toward healing. They are not accustomed to thinking about early disease detection, especially when it concerns their prostate. If men don't have any symptoms, they tend to think they are fine.

Bottom line: listen to the messages that your body is sending you. Acknowledge that there could be an issue, face it directly, get checked out early, deal with it, and move on!

LUTS AFFECTS YOUR PARTNER TOO!

Unfortunately, the average man's stereotypical pattern of doctor avoidance can be hazardous not only to his health but to the health of his partner. Here's how:

- Untreated prostate problems can cause urinary frequency at night, eventually causing the now-awakened partner to look for other places to sleep undisturbed or leaving a bed partner sleep deprived. Like the loud snoring that accompanies obstructive sleep apnea, this untreated nocturia can destroy intimacy, drive a wedge into long-standing relationships, and eventually strain them to the breaking point.

- Untreated or poorly managed LUTS can damage a relationship by affecting the overall quality of life once shared by the couple. The symptoms, the side effects, and the change in routine can throw a curveball into what was once a normal and active life.

THE DOCTOR VISIT: DEALING WITH LUTS

Benign prostatic enlargement is one of the most common disorders in older men. Based on a thorough medical history, physical examination, and some laboratory tests, a urologist can diagnose LUTS and BPE with a high degree of confidence and suggest a variety of managements tailored to a man's condition and personal preferences.

When I see patients for LUTS complaints, I review the International Prostate Symptom Score (IPSS) questionnaire (see page 140) and the Voiding Symptoms Self-Assessment (see chart, page 138). IPSS scores of 0 to 7 are indicative of mild symptoms, 8 to 19 indicate moderate symptoms, and severe symptoms fall in the range of 20 to 35. These scores help quantify the extent and severity of filling and voiding symptoms, but they do not in any way tell a physician what is causing the symptoms.

During your doctor's visit, a careful medical history will be taken. For me, a thorough history is crucial for an accurate diagnosis. Once I am armed with all of this basic information, I can usually hone in on what is going on. If the doctor doesn't take a good history, or if you are reluctant to provide answers or give inaccurate information, there is always the risk of a misdiagnosis. Inappropriate treatment can then lead to no relief at best or a deterioration of symptoms at worst.

At the very core, we doctors are detectives, and all information, regardless of how seemingly unimportant, is vital to formulating a proper diagnosis and an effective management plan.

————————————MYTH BUSTER————————————

Even though today's doctors have access to sophisticated technology that was unimaginable one hundred years ago, information gathering is still as vitally important to the diagnostic process as it was in the past.

Doctors today are extremely busy due to increased caseloads, and some end up missing crucial clues with cursory, all-too-brief exams. As a consequence, an important diagnosis of something more serious than BPE (as well as BPE) causing LUTS can be overlooked.

The flip side of that coin is that just because you have LUTS, you should not come with the preconceived notion that you will be leaving the doctor's office with a prescription for one of the popular enlarged-prostate medications that are advertised so heavily on TV and in magazines. Many lower urinary tract symptoms are associated with what a person eats and drinks, and when; therefore, you may need only lifestyle changes to take care of a frequency issue that you thought was due to an enlarged prostate—not a prescription drug to be taken indefinitely.

I once had a busy sixty-three-year-old patient, who was also a doctor. His major complaint was that he was getting up three to five times a night to urinate, and the sleep disturbance left him fatigued during the day. Since he had no LUTS problems during the day, I asked what he drank at work. "I'm too busy," he said. "I barely drink anything."

After about ten minutes of talking to him and still trying to figure out the cause of his lower urinary tract symptoms, I finally asked him what he drank after work. "Once I'm home, I like to relax by drinking tea. I have about five to seven cups before I finally go to bed at eleven."

I almost fell off my chair! The fluid volume and the diuretic effect of the caffeine in the tea were the cause of his LUTS. Case solved.

Simple questioning like this can oftentimes reveal the source of common complaints, as it did in this case. You would be surprised to know how often patients do not connect lifestyle choices with their urinary frequency symptoms.

OTHER POSSIBLE CAUSES OF LUTS

Medications and medical conditions can also cause LUTS and it's up to the alert doctor to ask what medical conditions you may have and what drugs you are taking. Some commonly used drugs that cause LUTS include:

- Antihistamines

- Decongestants

- Diuretics

- Tricyclic antidepressants

The medical conditions that can cause LUTS are most often related to inflammation, obstruction, and problems with the nervous system. While prostate and bladder cancer can produce lower urinary tract symptoms, these conditions are less frequent causes. The most common inflammatory, obstructive, and neurological diseases that cause LUTS are listed below:

Inflammatory Causes of LUTS
Infection (bacterial and viral)

Radiation therapy

Chemotherapy

Bladder cancer

Interstitial cystitis (rare in males)

Obstructive Causes of LUTS

Benign prostatic enlargement (BPE)

Urethral strictures

Prostate cancer

Bladder stones

Bladder neck contracture or scarring after prostate surgery

Neurological Causes of LUTS

Spinal cord disease

Multiple sclerosis

Stroke

Diabetes

Parkinson's disease

Surgical injury to pelvic nerves

Other Causes of LUTS

Increased urine production

Aging bladder

A thorough doctor will also ask about any previous urinary tract or prostate infections; if your physician doesn't, be sure to mention them yourself. Also inform him or her of any prior medical procedures in the abdomen or pelvic region. Surgery can bring about pelvic nerve injury that may affect bladder storage and emptying, while a history of urinary catheterization is sometimes associated with scars within the urethra (urethral strictures), which can impede urine flow.

————————————RED FLAG————————————

If you tell your doctor about your LUTS and you simply get a prescription for a medication for treatment, get another opinion. An examination should follow a careful history taking by the physician prior to recommending management.

THE PHYSICAL EXAMINATION AND DIGITAL RECTAL EXAMINATION

To diagnose the cause of LUTS, your doctor will first take a good medical history. He may then start with an examination of the abdomen

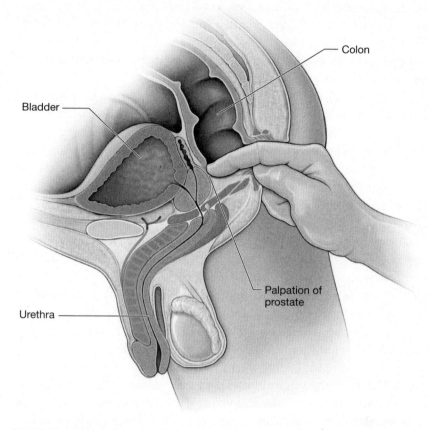

The digital rectal exam (DRE)

and genitalia if there is no history of neurological disease or symptoms. Eventually, the examination will include a prostate exam or digital rectal exam (DRE), a mildly uncomfortable but extremely valuable diagnostic tool that allows the doctor to assess the size and shape of your prostate.

I start by having a patient stand somewhat away from the examination table, spread his legs, and then bend forward until his chest is on the table, wrapping his arms under it as if giving the table a hug. This is by far the best position for a urologist to perform a DRE, especially in the overweight patient.

Your doctor will insert his gloved and heavily lubricated index finger up past the anal sphincter and then gently press against, or palpate, the prostate gland, noting both the approximate size and consistency of the prostate. Although ultrasound and magnetic resonance imaging (MRI), a noninvasive medical test that uses a powerful magnetic field and radio frequency pulses to produce detailed images, both determine prostate size and consistency more accurately than the finger, most experienced urologists are able to determine the approximate prostate size with this quicker and far less expensive exam.

During the DRE, your doctor presses the prostate to determine whether it's firm or hard in any spot, which can indicate a higher risk of prostate cancer. To get a sense of what your prostate feels like, put your thumb and pinkie finger together and use the index finger on your other hand to feel the fleshy part of the palm (thenar eminence) just below the base of your thumb. As you will see, the flesh there seems somewhat firm but compressible, which is how the prostate should feel.

Now place your thumb and index finger together and then feel the thenar eminence. It feels softer, somewhat like a marshmallow, a condition that we call "boggy." That's the feel of a prostate with chronic inflammation.

As I mentioned before, prostate size isn't always the primary issue when it comes to benign prostatic enlargement. Some men have extremely large prostates—all urologists have seen men with glands the size of apples yet without LUTS—while others can have prostates that are small and have LUTS that interfere with their quality of life.

In addition to the one-minute DRE, your doctor will also evaluate your genitals and pelvis. The abdomen will be examined and palpated for the presence of a mass, which could indicate an enlarged bladder due to retained urine.

I'll never forget the middle-aged gentleman who somehow made it to my office with abdominal discomfort after he had his appendix removed a few days earlier. He had come to see me about urination complaints. The patient had a large mass in the midline, just below his navel. When he'd called his surgeon to bring this to his attention, the doctor assured him that it was most likely nothing more than some fluid collecting near his incision and it would dissipate in a few days.

I brought him into my examination room and noticed that this mass was perfectly spherical. Upon closer examination, it turned out to be his fully distended bladder! The anesthesia plus the intravenous fluids he had been given during surgery had overstretched the hollow receptacle and caused him to go into retention. I immediately passed a catheter and removed 800 milliliters of urine—almost a quart—from his bladder.

Urinalysis is often the only laboratory test needed when symptoms are mild (International Prostate Symptom Score of 1 to 7; see page 140) and the medical history and physical examination suggest no other abnormalities.

A blood sample for a prostate-specific antigen (PSA) test to help rule out the possibility of prostate cancer will also be taken. PSA values alone are not helpful in determining whether lower urinary tract symptoms are due to benign prostatic enlargement or prostate cancer because both conditions can elevate PSA levels. However, knowing your PSA score may help predict how rapidly the prostate will increase in size over time and whether problems such as urinary retention are likely to occur. Urologists measure PSA before any treatment for BPE because the presence of prostate cancer would change management of the BPE.

———————————————RED FLAG———————————————

Do not be alarmed if your doctor orders a PSA test, because it can not only help rule out the presence of prostate cancer but also prove to be a very useful point of reference for future tests.

Another reason to measure PSA concerns possible BPE medical therapy with 5-alpha-reductase inhibitors. The two drugs in this class—dutasteride (Avodart) and finasteride (Proscar)—will reduce PSA levels by 40 percent to 50 percent after about six months of treatment, requiring you to have a second PSA taken at that time. If you don't have a baseline PSA level established before beginning therapy, it will be difficult to interpret any future PSA values. For more on the PSA test and the controversy surrounding it, go to chapter 10.

PSA LEVELS AND FUTURE PROSTATIC ENLARGEMENT

While prostate-specific antigen has served as a blood test for prostate cancer, and is the best test available for estimating the risk that prostate cancer is present, it hasn't always been clear if PSA, which is made in the epithelial cells of the prostate, could also be used to predict future cases of BPE.

At Johns Hopkins, my colleagues and I set out to find the answer, using blood samples from men enrolled in the Baltimore Longitudinal Study of Aging (BLSA). Our study, reported in the *Journal of Urology* in 2002, noted that the higher a man's PSA level when he is younger, the more likely his prostate will continue to grow abnormally, and the greater his risk for developing prostatic enlargement as he ages. Here's exactly what we found:

- The average risk of prostatic enlargement was three to eleven times higher for men aged 40 to 69 with higher PSAs compared to men with lower PSA levels.

- The twenty-year risk of prostatic enlargement was about 10 percent versus 40 percent for men aged 40 to 49.9 with PSA values below and above 0.3 nanograms per milliliter (ng/ml), respectively.

- The ten-year risk of prostatic enlargement was 10 percent versus 40 percent for men aged 50 to 59.9 with PSA levels below and above 0.8 ng/ml, respectively.

- The ten-year risk of prostatic enlargement was 20 percent versus 70 percent for men aged 60 to 69.9 with PSA levels below and above 1.7 ng/ml, respectively.

A major implication of our study was that PSA levels could be useful as one measure of risk for prostatic growth with age. And by paying closer attention to these men at an earlier age, their doctors can step in sooner in the disease process and recommend therapies that might not only prevent lower urinary tract symptoms but also reduce the risk for acute urinary retention.

FURTHER TESTING

If a man has a history of multiple diseases that could affect the lower urinary tract—for example, the presence of prostate enlargement and Parkinson's disease—further urodynamic studies may be recommended. They can include one or all of the following special tests:

Uroflowmetry: In this noninvasive test, a man urinates into an electronic device that measures the rate of his urine flow. Urine flow rates below 10 to 15 milliliters per second suggest the possibility of an obstruction. On the other hand, when the flow rate is above 15 milliliters per second, obstruction is unlikely, and therapy directed at treating prostate enlargement is less likely to be effective.

Urodynamics and Pressure-Flow Studies: Whenever there is a possibility that LUTS are related more to the bladder than to the prostate, in some cases pressure-flow studies to measure bladder pressures during storage of urine and during urination may be performed. A tiny pressure-sensing device will be inserted into the bladder via a catheter that is maneuvered through the urethra. There is little discomfort associated with passage of the catheter into the bladder. As the bladder fills with water, the device indicates the pressure inside the bladder and gives the physician a sense of how good the bladder is at storing urine.

Also, pressure can be measured during a bladder muscle contraction to assess the strength of the detrusor muscle and how effectively it squeezes. As the bladder squeezes, a high pressure accompanied by a low urine flow rate indicates obstruction that can be treated either with medication or a surgical procedure. However, a low pressure reading and a low urine flow rate suggest a primary bladder problem, *not* obstruction, and the urologist's focus then turns to coming up with an acceptable solution for emptying the bladder.

Ultrasonography: This painless imaging procedure is used when structural abnormalities in the kidneys or bladder are suspected, the amount of residual urine in the bladder needs to be measured, bladder stones are thought to be present, or the size of the prostate needs to be estimated. In an ultrasound scan, the doctor puts a gel on the skin of the lower abdomen and passes a hand-held device called a transducer over it. The sound waves it emits reflect off the internal organs, creating an image of each organ. This is the same instrument used to image a fetus during pregnancy.

Cystoscopy: This test is not always necessary for evaluation of LUTS, but whenever the urine contains any blood, cystoscopy is recommended to evaluate the inside of the bladder. After instilling an anesthetic gel into the urethra, the physician passes a cystoscope (analogous to the device used for colonoscopy) through the urethra and into the bladder, allowing him or her to view the urethra from the tip of the penis to the bladder neck and inside the bladder, including the part of the urethra that traverses the prostate. Any bladder stones, tumors, or urethral strictures can be visualized with this device. The shape and size of the prostate can also be estimated in this exam, which takes about ten to fifteen minutes to complete.

WHEN IT'S TIME TO TREAT

Prostatic enlargement, and the lower urinary tract symptoms that it can cause, primarily affects men over the age of forty. While not all men will suffer bothersome symptoms, it is estimated that 25 percent to 50 percent of those with an enlarged prostate have some degree of urinary complaints and will require some form of medical or surgical treatment. These interventions are all discussed in great detail in chapter 6.

VOIDING SYMPTOMS SELF-ASSESSMENT

The following questions are for men who have not had surgery for preexisting urinary disease. Place an *X* next to the response that best answers each query about your voiding habits.

1. **Characterize Your Symptoms**

   Irritative Symptoms

   Frequency: The most common urination symptom. The normal adult voids up to six times per day, about 250 to 300 milliliters per void. Do you void more than once every two hours or six times a day?

   Yes___ No___

   Nocturia: Nighttime urinary frequency. An adult typically wakes up no more than twice nightly to urinate. Do you wake up more than that to urinate?

   Yes___ No___

   Urgency: A strong, sudden impulse to urinate. Do you often feel the powerful, uncontrollable urge to go?

   Yes___ No___

   Dysuria: Pain with urination, usually noted at the end of the urethra. Does it hurt to urinate?

   Yes___ No___

2. **Obstruction Symptoms**

   Decreased urinary force: Is it less powerful than before?

   Yes___ No___

   Hesitancy: Delay in the start of urination. As you stand in front of the urinal, does it take many seconds before you are able to begin urinating?

   Yes___ No___

Intermittent urinary stream: Involuntary starting and stopping. Does it happen to you when you urinate?

Yes___ No___

Straining: The use of abdominal wall muscles to increase urine flow. Do you push or strain in order to urinate?

Yes___ No___

3. When Do the Symptoms Occur?

Daytime: Urinary frequency that does not occur at night is due usually to increased fluid intake during the day, the use of drugs or substances in the diet (alcohol, caffeine) that cause increased urine output (diuresis), or anxiety during the day. Daytime-only incontinence is probably due to a weak urinary sphincter or related to urgency during the day. Do you have daytime symptoms only?

Yes___ No___

Nighttime: Urinary frequency that occurs only at night (nocturnal polyuria) is usually due to one or more of the following causes: (1) consuming fluids in the late afternoon or evening, leading to increased urine output at night; (2) heart problems that result in increased urine output when lying down; (3) increased urine output at night due to alterations in the secretion of antidiuretic hormone (ADH) and the reduced ability of the kidneys to conserve water (concentrate urine); and (4) sleep apnea. Nighttime incontinence (nocturnal enuresis) may stem from an overfilled bladder that is not emptying completely. Do you have nighttime symptoms?

Yes___ No___

4. Small or Large Volume? How Often?

Use a voiding diary. (See page 194.)

5. Is There Pain or Blood with Urination?

Painful urination is usually noted at the end of the urethra or intermittently above the pubis (the front part of the pelvic ring created by the hip bones) and is typically relieved in part with urination. Pain usually implies infection or inflammation and should prompt a visit to a physician. Any bleeding with urination can signify a serious medical condition that should be evaluated by a doctor. Do you have pain or blood with urination?

Yes___ No___

6. Good Flow or Slow Flow?

Record the volume per second in a graduated container. To measure peak urinary flow, start the clock when the stream is at its peak and end before the stream begins to slow down. Convert ounces to milliliters by multiplying by 30 (1 ounce equals 30 milliliters).

Slow: Less than 10 milliliters per second	Yes___	No___
Borderline: 10 to 15 milliliters per second	Yes___	No___
Normal: Greater than 15 milliliters per second	Yes___	No___

7. Medications

A variety of medications can impact urination. Do you take any of the following drugs?

Antidepressants	Yes___	No__
Diuretics	Yes___	No___
Cold, hay fever, allergy medications containing antihistamines and/or decongestants	Yes___	No___

8. Do You Have Another Illness That Could Affect Urination?

Heart disease	Yes___	No___
Diabetes	Yes___	No___
Spinal disease	Yes___	No___
Stroke	Yes___	No___
Parkinson's disease	Yes___	No___
Sleep apnea	Yes___	No___
Enlarged prostate	Yes___	No___

THE INTERNATIONAL PROSTATE SYMPTOM SCORE (IPSS) QUESTIONNAIRE

The International Prostate Symptom Score (IPSS) questionnaire was developed to help physicians and their male patients evaluate the extent and bothersomeness of their voiding symptoms. This self-administered test can help determine the severity of your symptoms and whether treatment is needed. But the questionnaire cannot determine the underlying cause of the urinary symptoms.

Instructions: Circle the number that best answers the question. Use this key to answer each question, and then tabulate your score to assess your voiding severity.

0 = Not at all
1 = Less than one time in five
2 = Less than half the time
3 = About half the time
4 = More than half the time
5 = Almost always

1. **Incomplete emptying.** Over the past month, how often have you had the sensation of not emptying your bladder completely after you finished urinating?

   0   1   2   3   4   5

2. **Frequency.** Over the past month, how often have you had to urinate again less than two hours after you finished urinating?

   0   1   2   3   4   5

3. **Intermittency.** Over the past month, how often have you stopped and started again several times when you urinated?

   0   1   2   3   4   5

4. **Urgency.** Over the past month, how often have you found it difficult to postpone urination?

   0   1   2   3   4   5

5. **Weak stream.** Over the past month, how often have you had a weak urinary stream?

   0   1   2   3   4   5

6. **Straining.** Over the past month, how often have you had to push or strain to begin urination?

   0   1   2   3   4   5

7. **Nocturia.** Over the past month, how many times have you typically gotten up to urinate, from the time you went to bed at night until the time you got up in the morning?

   0   1   2   3   4   5

Total IPSS Score_____

Scoring of symptoms:
   Mild: 0 to 7
   Moderate: 8 to 19
   Severe: 20 to 35

   Please discuss these results with your physician. Generally, no treatment is needed if symptoms are mild, while moderate to severe symptoms typically call for some form of treatment if they are bothersome and interfering with quality of life.

Additional IPSS question
Quality of life due to urinary symptoms. If you were to spend the rest of your life with your urinary condition the way it is now, how would you feel about that? (Check one.)

   0 = Delighted
   1 = Pleased
   2 = Mostly satisfied
   3 = Mixed: about equally satisfied and dissatisfied
   4 = Mostly dissatisfied
   5 = Unhappy
   6 = Terrible

THE TAKEAWAY

- Lower urinary tract symptoms had historically been attributed to prostatism or benign prostatic hyperplasia (BPH). These imprecise terms have been replaced. The new terminology for an enlarged prostate is benign prostatic enlargement, or BPE. The associated urinary symptoms it can cause are referred to as LUTS, or lower urinary tract symptoms.

- LUTS can be categorized as irritative storage symptoms (urgency, frequency, nocturia, urge incontinence) and obstructive voiding symptoms (intermittency, weak stream, and hesitancy).

- LUTS can be present in men with and without BPE and it can be caused by bladder outlet obstruction (BOO) due to BPE. But men with a normal size prostate without BPE can also have BOO.

- BPE usually becomes a problem only when it causes LUTS. Some men with very large prostates never have LUTS, while other men with normal size prostates can experience significant LUTS from BOO due to increased smooth muscle tone in the prostate.

- Urinary retention, the inability to pass urine, can occur when men allow significant LUTS to persist for years without medical attention.

- In addition to a detailed medical history, there are a variety of urologic tests that can be performed to figure out the cause of a man's lower urinary tract symptoms.

CHAPTER SIX

TREATMENT OPTIONS FOR LUTS

A sweating ovary or a sick prostate
explains most history.

—Martin H. Fischer, MD

Too many men make compromises when it comes to their health. They put up with annoyances such as lower urinary tract symptoms, thinking wishfully that they may get better eventually. Somehow. Mysteriously. By chance, maybe. They are often too willing to wait things out and go long past the period when drug therapies can effectively work for them. For some men, it will be time for the "big guns" (surgical treatment) to help fix the problem.

Oftentimes when I am having that conversation with a patient, I find myself thinking, "Why didn't you come to see me earlier? This issue has clearly been going on for some time."

After listening to a litany of complaints ranging from interrupted sleep to bathroom mapping to seating strategies during travel and at events, one of the first questions I'm regularly asked by a new patient with lower urinary tract symptoms is, "Do you really think I need to do something about my problem?"

The short answer for most men is that treatment for LUTS is necessary only if symptoms become bothersome quality of life issues—like always having to make sure that you have an aisle seat, for quick egress to the bathroom; or getting up three times a night to use the bathroom and waking your bed partner each time in the process; or needing to know the exact location of every public toilet within a three-block radius.

If this doesn't bother you, then I suppose you might want to pass on treatment. But let's be realistic here. There is a big difference between being unaffected and being stubborn. These LUTS are not likely to go away on their own, and if you wait too long, things could get a lot worse. My advice to you is to be honest with yourself and take the necessary steps to determine the cause of the symptoms followed by the management that will improve your situation and protect against future harm.

RED FLAG

There is a distinct difference between *denying* the effect of LUTS on your daily existence and genuinely not being bothered by LUTS.

Many of my patients say that they have tried multiple herbal therapies for prostate problems, purchased from health food stores, pharmacies, and over the Internet. Do these products work? (See page 156.) The fact that these men have come to see me because of their symptoms attests to the fact that most herbal preparations—saw palmetto, stinging nettle roots, ryegrass pollen extract, pumpkin seeds, African plum tree bark—don't work that well, or if they do, their effects are modest and inconsistent at best.

If left untreated, LUTS can worsen over time and lead to more serious health problems, such as urinary retention, bladder stones, kidney damage, and urinary tract infections. LUTS are mostly a problem related to aging and there is no age cutoff or ceiling. It's estimated that 50 percent of our octogenarians will experience moderate to severe LUTS that are disturbing enough to require some form of treatment. Other studies suggest that 90 percent of men between the ages of forty-five and eighty have some type of lower urinary tract symptom. LUTS are most commonly caused by changes in the urinary tract that occur with aging and not with a specific disease. The most common identifiable causes of LUTS in males are caused by benign prostatic enlargement, overactive bladder (OAB), and nocturnal polyuria (increased urine production at night), alone or in combination. OAB and nocturnal polyuria can be caused by a number of conditions.

LUTS OPTIONS

LUTS therapy is not a one-size-fits-all solution, and the choice of management should be determined by shared decision making between a patient and a physician, considering a patient's preferences. Some men may wish to pursue the most aggressive management with the highest chance of success, even though the risks are higher than a less aggressive approach that has minimal side effects and a lower chance of success. As you will see, there are a number of management options to consider, from no treatment to surgery.

For a man who has to get out of bed to go to the bathroom two to five times a night because of voiding problems, or who has frequent urination during the day, urgency, incomplete bladder emptying, starting and stopping, or a weak stream, the traditional options have been (1) watchful waiting, (2) herbal therapies, and (3) drugs that are usually taken daily to relax smooth muscles in the prostate, shrink prostate size, relax the bladder, or (4) a combination of these strategies.

There are also several minimally invasive therapies to consider. These procedures may alter nerves within the prostate or destroy prostate tissue and reduce LUTS. Finally, there are surgical procedures, performed through the urethra, that remove prostate tissue using electrical or laser energy. Open surgeries can also remove the bulk of the prostate and ease symptoms to a great extent for those with benign prostatic enlargement (BPE) and bladder obstruction due to a very enlarged prostate. In the end, symptom relief and your satisfaction will in large part be dependent on the doctor's ability or willingness to find the cause of the lower urinary tract symptoms and present the management options in a way that leaves you with realistic expectations.

THERAPIES FOR LUTS

When the cause of LUTS is suspected to be the prostate, you have a veritable restaurant menu of possibilities:

- Watchful Waiting

- Medical Therapy

The following drugs can be used to relieve symptoms:

Alpha-blockers

    alfuzosin (UroXatral)

    doxazosin (Cardura, Cardura XL)

    tamsulosin (Flomax)

    terazosin (Hytrin)

    silodosin (Rapaflo)

5-Alpha-reductase inhibitors (5-ARIs)

    dutasteride (Avodart)

    finasteride (Proscar)

Combination Therapy

    alpha-blocker and a 5-ARI

    alpha-blocker and an anticholinergic

Anticholinergics

    oxybutynin (Ditropan)

    tolterodine (Detrol LA)

    solifenacin (Vesicare)

    darifenacin (Enablex)

    trospium (Sanctura)

- **Minimally Invasive Therapies (MIT)**

    transurethral needle ablation (TUNA)

    transurethral microwave thermotherapy (TUMT)

- **Surgical Therapies**

    transurethral incision of the prostate (TUIP)

    photoselective vaporization of the prostate (PVP)

    transurethral resection/vaporization of the prostate (TURP)

    transurethral holmium laser enuculeation of the prostate (HoLEP)

    open prostatectomy

THE LUTS TREATMENT LADDER

What to do about LUTS, and when, starts with a conversation with your physician; and possibly a urologist, depending on the severity of the symptoms and the presence of other factors such as a urinary tract infection, blood in the urine, or an elevated PSA.

The sooner you have this discussion and are able to reach some decision about management is the day that you no longer have to worry about always securing the aisle seat. You can say good-bye to a life of toilet mapping and to being roused out of bed in the middle of a dream to stumble off to the bathroom. The decision, of course, is yours to make.

RED FLAG

Like all decisions having to do with your health and well-being, take time to get the best advice and figure out what will work for you.

When I advise men seeking relief from LUTS, I refer to a treatment ladder. I explain that there are four rungs on this ladder and how far you want to climb depends on your symptoms, their cause, and your preferences. Let's review those rungs.

First Rung: Watchful Waiting: This is best for those with (1) minimal symptoms, (2) a score of less than 8 on the International Prostate Symptom Score (see page 140), and (3) those with moderate to severe symptoms that are not bothersome but with an IPSS of 8 or more.

First, I ask these men to make lifestyle changes, to see if this brings any relief. This can include reducing daily fluid intake, and avoiding alcohol and caffeinated beverages, especially in the evening if nocturia is an issue.

Second Rung: Medical Management: Prescription oral medications, just like the ones you see advertised on TV repeatedly, may be considered first-line therapy for those with bothersome symptoms due to prostate enlargement. These drugs improve bladder emptying and relieve symptoms by shrinking the prostate (5-alpha reductase inhibitors, or 5-ARIs) or by relaxing the smooth muscle fibers at the bladder neck and within the prostate (alpha-blockers). The 5-ARIs are not helpful in men without prostatic enlargement, whereas alpha-blockers can be useful in men with and without BPE that have increased smooth muscle tone within the prostate. Although there are a number of alpha-blockers from which to choose, they all have similar levels of efficacy that would be perceived by a patient as moderate symptom improvement.

Let's be clear here so that there is no misconception: to date, no medication offers a cure for LUTS, but certain drugs can alleviate the symptoms. The medications may be adequate when used either alone (as monotherapy) or in combination; many of my patients who take these drugs have reductions in LUTS that are satisfactory to them. A combination of an alpha-blocker and a 5-ARI should be considered only in men with BPE, since in those without, an alpha-blocker alone is preferable. If you stop taking the drugs, though, the symptoms will probably return.

National figures show that within a year of having started treatment, at least one-third of men discontinue medical therapy because it's costly, not effective, or brings on adverse side effects. These drugs can cause dizziness, lightheadedness, weakness, fatigue, a decrease in libido, and for some, reduced ejaculate volume or lack of seminal emission altogether. Rarely, men on 5-ARIs can experience breast enlargement and tenderness.

Third Rung: Minimally-Invasive Surgical Therapies (MIT): These therapies are best for those with moderate to severe symptoms (an IPSS score of 8 or more and BPE) that are troublesome. When medications no longer work, or their side effects can no longer be tolerated, or when a man does not want to have prostate tissue removed surgically (see the fourth rung), then it's time to consider a minimally invasive heat treatment. Researchers have developed advanced medical devices that reduce symptoms by using radiofrequency or microwave energy to heat the prostate. The actual mechanism for symptom improvement is unknown, but it could be related to changes in nerve conduction. These thermotherapy and thermal ablation (destruction of tissue) treatments create temperatures within the prostate from 70 degrees to over 150 degrees that can destroy prostate tissue. Transurethral needle ablation (TUNA) uses radiofrequency to produce heat, while transurethral microwave thermotherapy (TUMT) uses microwave energy.

Fourth Rung: Surgical Procedures: Surgery to ablate, vaporize, or remove prostate tissue is appropriate for men who have complications from an obstruction such as urinary retention, bladder stones, recurrent infections, bleeding, or renal damage. Also, men with urinary symptoms not relieved by less invasive methods and those who desire to proceed initially with the most effective approach to symptom relief might choose a surgical option.

Transurethral resection of the prostate (TURP) is considered the gold standard treatment for LUTS caused by obstruction. Laser-assisted TURP may provide similar symptom relief with lower side effects in some cases.

TREATMENT POSSIBILITIES FOR LUTS

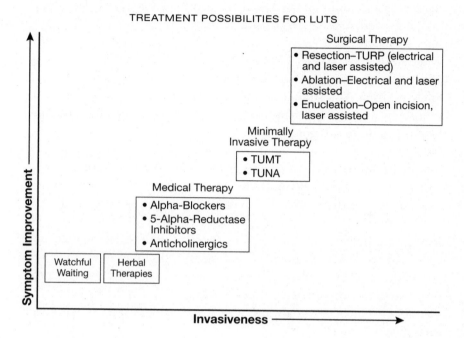

WATCHING AND WAITING

Because men differ greatly in the degree to which their symptoms cause distress, a careful discussion regarding the extent to which symptoms may interfere with daily living is important in helping patients decide on the course of treatment that's right for them. I let my patients know at our first consultation that symptoms from LUTS are unpredictable. Yet whenever I have a patient with minimal or moderate LUTS, based on his IPSS score, but the symptoms aren't particularly bothersome—I still make sure that he understands there are effective treatment options available should he eventually want to do something. On the other hand, the effects of LUTS could stay the same for years without therapy, and for one in three men who choose watchful waiting, symptoms may actually improve slightly.

For those men who are older, have a higher IPSS symptom score, a higher PSA, and a larger prostate, worsening of symptoms is likely. If that happens, it's time to consider a more aggressive intervention. Keep in mind that as long as you postpone treating the unwanted effects of LUTS, you may continue to experience those disruptive voiding symptoms.

In the meantime, I encourage annual doctor visits to monitor symptoms during watchful waiting, or more often if symptoms change. At these visits, I take an updated medical history, perform a physical exam, and, if needed, order a few basic laboratory tests.

WATCHFUL WAITING STRATEGIES

The watchful waiting strategy for LUTS does not mean that you do absolutely nothing. You should also do all that you can to help relieve the symptoms and prevent them from worsening. The following tips could help you achieve this goal.

PREVENT WEIGHT GAIN, ESPECIALLY AROUND THE ABDOMEN

Excess body weight contributes to lower urinary tract symptoms, and overweight men are more likely to develop prostatic enlargement.

In 2006 the *Journal of Clinical Endocrinology & Metabolism* published a study that was based on men enrolled in the ongoing Baltimore Longitudinal Study of Aging. According to its findings, obese men were three and a half times more likely than average to have an enlarged prostate; and diabetic men, twice as likely. Although I mentioned before that a large prostate does not always cause lower urinary tract symptoms, it does in some cases.

Other researchers have reported that LUTS is nearly five times higher among overweight men with large waists compared with men whose weight and waist measurements were normal. In a 2012 study carried out by Dr. Steven A. Kaplan, professor of urology at Weill Cornell Medical College in New York, he reported that waist size is one component of the so-called metabolic syndrome, which signifies not only an elevated risk of heart disease and diabetes but also pelvic dysfunction. The latter condition can result in LUTS and sexual dysfunction.

—MYTH BUSTER—

Not all prostates are created equal. What you eat and drink, combined with the amount of exercise you do or don't participate in, could directly affect the size of the prostate gland and whether or not you have LUTS.

Dr. Kaplan and his fellow researchers tested the idea that waist circumference may be a very useful predictor of prostate volume and the severity of LUTS. They evaluated 409 men over age forty with moderate or severe untreated voiding symptoms and divided them into three groups based on waist circumference (less than thirty-five inches, thirty-five to thirty-nine inches, greater than thirty-nine inches). A key finding was the link between waist size and lower urinary tract symptoms. Dr. Kaplan reported that the greater the waist circumference, the worse the LUTS, the larger the prostate, and the higher the PSA. Also, men with larger waists had higher rates of hypertension, heart disease, diabetes, erectile dysfunction, and problems with ejaculation.

To determine your waist circumference, wrap a tape measure around your waist at the level of the top of your hip bones until the tape feels snug without compressing your skin. Then exhale normally and take the measurement. A waist circumference greater than forty inches indicates abdominal obesity.

Abdominal obesity is particularly dangerous because it can make the body resistant to the actions of the hormone insulin, leading to unregulated blood glucose levels. Insulin resistance is associated with metabolic syndrome, a condition that significantly increases the risk of diabetes, heart attacks, and strokes, each of which dwarfs LUTS as a significant medical risk. People with metabolic syndrome have three or more of the following risk factors:

- large waist circumference (abdominal obesity),

- high blood glucose and triglyceride levels,

- low high-density lipoprotein (HDL) cholesterol level, and

- high blood pressure.

More than 40 percent of Americans over age forty have metabolic syndrome. Belly fat is associated with inflammation throughout the body, which is believed to contribute to insulin resistance as well as cardiovascular disease. Men typically deposit fat in the abdomen and develop what is commonly called a potbelly, beer belly, or simply a gut.

Men, your goal is to trim your waist size through diet and exercise. Fortunately, abdominal fat is often the first to go when you start to lose weight. Try to get at least thirty to sixty minutes of moderate intensity exercise on most days. You will also have to make alterations in your diet, perhaps by reducing your saturated fat and dietary cholesterol. You can do this by eating plenty of fresh fruits and vegetables, which are packed with fiber and antioxidant vitamins; and emphasizing whole foods over processed foods and choosing whole grains instead of refined and processed grains such as white bread and white rice. See chapter 3 for more dietary suggestions.

ENGAGE IN REGULAR PHYSICAL ACTIVITY

Studies report that regular exercise can reduce the risk of developing LUTS *and* possibly prostate cancer. The mechanisms whereby exercise might reduce LUTS are unknown. But a review of studies suggests that moderate to vigorous exercise might decrease the risk of LUTS by 25 percent when compared to the couch potato lifestyle. Aim for at least thirty minutes of moderate physical activity, such as walking, gardening, golfing, and bowling, every day or, at the very least, most days of the week.

I know that these suggestions may seem too basic for some, but when you consider that most Americans do little or nothing during the week, think of my suggestions as a good start. Adjust your schedule and then add more physical activity to your life. Your prostate, your heart, and your overall mental attitude will all benefit. For more exercise suggestions, go to chapter 2.

EAT A DIET RICH IN VEGETABLES AND LOW IN FAT

What's good for the heart is good for the prostate. Men who consume a diet high in vegetables and fruit, as opposed to a diet high in fat and red meat, are doing their hearts *and* prostates a favor. Low-fat eating significantly decreases the risk of LUTS, according to a seven-year study of 4,700 men published in the *American Journal of Epidemiology*. High-fat eating increased the risk of LUTS by 31 percent, with daily consumption of red meat boosting the risk to 38 percent. However, eating four or more servings of vegetables daily decreased the risk of LUTS by 32 percent.

Researchers believe that eating too much fat increases the body's overall inflammatory response and raises levels of estrogens and androgens. These hormones influence prostate growth and could increase LUTS. In contrast, a diet light on fat and heavy on veggies is prostate friendly and associated with lower circulating estrogens and androgens.

KEEP BLOOD SUGAR UNDER CONTROL

Poor blood sugar control exacerbates LUTS. Studies report that men with an elevated fasting glucose level of 110 mg/dl or higher tripled their risk of developing lower urinary tract symptoms. If you have diabetes, take your diabetes medication or insulin as prescribed.

**LIMIT THE AMOUNT OF FLUID CONSUMED AT ANY ONE TIME
AND DON'T DRINK ANYTHING AFTER SEVEN O'CLOCK AT NIGHT**
Excessive fluid intake, especially of alcohol or caffeine, in the hours shortly before bedtime is a major contributor to nocturia. While this may seem obvious, you would be surprised at how many patients I've counseled who failed to make this connection.

**LIMIT OR AVOID BEVERAGES THAT CONTAIN CAFFEINE
AND ALCOHOL**
Caffeine and alcohol have a diuretic effect, which can easily contribute to frequency and nocturia. In addition, caffeine, which can disrupt sleep, can also trigger the detrusor muscle of the bladder to become overactive and lead to a sense of urgency. The idea is to avoid consuming liquids that fill the bladder quickly and increase urine output.

AVOID ANTIHISTAMINES AND DECONGESTANTS
Two popular ingredients in these medications, pseudoephedrine and diphenhydramine, can worsen lower urinary tract symptoms and cause urinary retention in men with enlarged prostates by increasing smooth muscle tone or reducing detrusor contractions.

TRY DOUBLE VOIDING
After you empty your bladder, wait a few moments and try voiding again. Be careful not to push or strain to get your stream going.

DON'T DELAY URINATION
The bladder does not empty as efficiently when overdistended. Like any muscle, overdistension reduces the ability to contract. That's why men with LUTS and BOO often tell their doctors that their symptoms (slow flow, hesitancy, feeling of incomplete emptying) are worse when they get up in the morning.

Finally, if you have to go to the hospital for any elective surgical procedure, be sure to alert your doctor that you have LUTS. To avoid retention following surgery, I will often start my patients with LUTS or BPE on an alpha-blocker medication beforehand. Without the drug, the infusion of IV fluids during surgery combined with pain medications is often enough to trigger retention afterward.

Bottom line: Watchful waiting strategies may be associated with diminished lower urinary tract symptoms in some men. However, the primary disadvantage to waiting is that as long as you delay seeking more effective, definitive therapy, the longer you continue to experience annoying symptoms that stay the same or worsen in most men.

TREATING LUTS WITH HERBAL THERAPY

Most of the men I see for LUTS have already tried a variety of complementary or "natural" herbal supplements, spending hard-earned dollars on products that lack a proven record of effectiveness. While some men may have initially received benefits from one or more of the supplements they tried, their condition worsened, and that's how they ended up in my office.

Prescribed for decades in Austria, Italy, Germany, and France, where they are still highly touted and used for mild to moderate LUTS, many of these herbal products available in health food stores and pharmacies are derived from roots, seeds, fruits, or bark. Some supplements come from a single plant or a combination of plants, while others are plant extracts containing numerous ingredients, including phytosterols, plant oils, fatty acids, and phytoestrogens.

RED FLAG

Buyer beware. The Food and Drug Administration does not have jurisdiction over so-called natural products, so you are really on your own when it comes to trusting what's in each container of pills, capsules, and powders. There is no guarantee that the same ingredients will be in the same product from one bottle to the next!

SAW PALMETTO FOR LUTS

The most common supplement used for the treatment of lower urinary tract symptoms in the United States is made from the berry of the saw palmetto, a palm-like plant. A fan palm tree with razor-sharp branches that can be found all over the southern states, the saw palmetto is filled with olive-sized berries. Also known as *Serenoa repens* or *Sabal serrulatum*, this scrub plant grows wild, from my gorgeous home state of South Carolina, down south to Florida, and all the way over to Texas, and has been used for prostate and urinary tract problems for well over one hundred years. Its medicinal properties come from its blue-black berries that are harvested in August and September.

The extract of these berries, an old favorite of cowboys and people who tried natural remedies for what ailed them long before the advent of the American pharmacological industry, has been purported to be a sexual stimulant as well as a remedy for an enlarged prostate gland. Many men claim that they get relief from LUTS by taking saw palmetto pills daily.

Researchers have postulated many different reasons why men with LUTS get results from saw palmetto for LUTS. Some believe that it works through androgen signaling, but there is *no conclusive proof* of its mechanism of action or efficacy.

HERBAL LUTS PRODUCTS AND THE PLACEBO EFFECT

Some of my patients with LUTS are reluctant to take standard medications. Their symptoms are mild, they tell me, and saw palmetto works just fine for them. I'm always very happy to hear that, but, I think to myself, is it the saw palmetto or the placebo effect that's at work?

A 2006 double-blind study of 225 men, published in the *New England Journal of Medicine*, found saw palmetto to be no better than placebo in taming lower urinary tract symptoms. If you looked at changes in LUTS over time between the two groups—one took saw palmetto and the other an inactive sugar pill—there was simply no statistical difference at any point. In a 2011 study published in the *Journal of the American Medical Association*, there were no differences in LUTS between placebo and groups of men taking increasing dosages of saw palmetto.

According to the plethora of research studying the placebo effect, up to 40 percent of all people with medical problems will improve due to the placebo effect. Think about it: two in five people who receive treatment for a medical problem improve, even if the drug really does not work. They believe that whatever they're taking will make them better, and due to the placebo effect, a significant number actually do get better.

When it comes to LUTS, my take is that if men show improvement from their minor complaints after taking an herbal product such as saw palmetto, and it's inexpensive, maybe an inexpensive placebo isn't really all that bad.

THE BOTTOM LINE ON HERBAL AIDS FOR LUTS

First, check with your doctor to make sure that your LUTS complaints are not linked to a more serious ailment such as prostate cancer or untreated diabetes. If you are interested in pursuing the herbal route, I recommend that you buy the least expensive supplement purported to help with the symptoms. If you notice no improvement after thirty days, you can try another brand for another month, and, if you still have the interest, try a third brand a month after that.

After three months, if you find that your bothersome LUTS have not lessened, it's time to speak to your doctor about alternatives that are more effective. Unfortunately, it's been my experience that while extracts of twigs, herbs, and berries won't hurt, they are unlikely to help much in the long term either.

TREATING LUTS WITH MEDICATION

Until the late 1980s, the only LUTS solution available was watchful waiting or surgery—usually a transurethral resection of the prostate, or TURP, a procedure first developed and introduced in the 1920s. Then, with the introduction of effective alpha-adrenergic blocking drugs in the 1980s, the number of TURPs, the number two procedure on Medicare's payment list after cataract surgery, began to plummet. What better testament to man's desire to skip surgery and its potential complications whenever a pill is available as an alternative. From 1987 to 2000, transurethral prostate resections plummeted from 250,000 a year to barely 88,000. Even more surprisingly, this significant reduction in TURPs came in spite of the ever-increasing number of aging baby boomers enrolling in Medicare. To be fair, part of the decrease in TURPS was almost certainly related to decreased reimbursement for the procedure and not just the medical therapy.

It's been estimated that 30 percent of American men older than fifty now have moderate to severe lower urinary tract symptoms, which broadly breaks down to about nine million men who are thinking about their LUTS management options. Although no drug offers a lifetime cure, many men can be managed adequately by taking one tiny pill a day. The medications available for treating LUTS fall into the following categories:

- Alpha-adrenergic blockers, or alpha-blockers

- 5-alpha reductase inhibitors, or 5-ARIs

- PDE-5 inhibitors

- Anticholinergics

Over the years, I have found that when patients are satisfied that a particular drug helps relieve their LUTS, they are perfectly willing to stay on the medication if there are no bothersome side effects. The order of the day then becomes finding the best possible drug, or combination of drugs, for any given patient.

ALPHA-BLOCKERS: HOW THEY WORK

Years ago, alpha-blockers were originally used to treat hypertension by reducing the tension of smooth muscles in blood vessel walls. These medications, which include Hytrin (terazosin), Cardura (doxazosin), and Minipress (prazosin), lower blood pressure levels by interrupting the nerve impulses that constrict small arteries. These arteries then dilate, or expand, which enhances blood flow and reduces blood pressure.

Investigators found that these drugs worked very well for lower urinary tract symptoms, too, by blocking the receptors that mediate smooth muscle tone in the prostate and nearby bladder neck, thereby relaxing smooth muscle within the prostate and at the bladder neck. But because the drugs were not selective for alpha-blocker receptors in the prostate, they relaxed smooth muscle in other areas of the body, including blood vessels, and this resulted in side effects such as dizziness, fatigue, headaches, and heart palpitations.

The alpha-blocking drugs used today for LUTS are slightly different and more prostate specific, working to relax smooth muscle in the prostate and less so in other areas. This can lead to fairly quick improvement in LUTS in men whose symptoms are moderate to severe.

Daily use of an alpha-blocker may increase urinary flow and relieve symptoms of urinary frequency and nighttime urination. In one study of more than 6,000 men comparing the efficacy of the drugs, their symptom scores decreased as much as 40 percent while urinary flow rates increased by as much as 25 percent.

The following alpha-blockers are considered appropriate for treating lower urinary tract symptoms and appear to have equal effectiveness:

> alfuzosin (UroXatral),
> doxazosin (Cardura),
> tamsulosin (Flomax),
> terazosin (Hytrin), and
> silodosin (Rapaflo).

ALPHA-BLOCKER SIDE EFFECTS

An advantage of alpha-blockers is that they work almost immediately. They also offer the additional benefit of helping manage hypertension in men with LUTS. However, alpha-blockers alone are not optimal therapy for hypertension, and the two conditions should be treated separately. The drugs' side effects have to be considered; the most common are dizziness, a drop in blood pressure when standing (postural hypotension), headache, weakness, and sexual dysfunction. Some men may also suffer from a stuffy nose or stomach distress.

It's possible that using these drugs daily can also cause ejaculatory disturbances manifested by a decrease in ejaculate volume, probably due to a reduction in the muscle contractions that propel seminal fluid, and/or the inability of the bladder neck to close during orgasm. This leads to retrograde ejaculation of semen into the bladder. This occurrence may be more common—a rate as high as 20 percent to 30 percent—with the newer alpha-blockers such as Rapaflo. The lack of semen does not affect one's ability to achieve a hard erection, climax, and experience a pleasurable orgasm. The only thing missing from the equation is the semen itself.

RED FLAG

If you plan on having children while using alpha-blocker medications for LUTS, then you need to get busy before you start taking them or, if you are already on an alpha-blocker, stop for a while.

When discussing therapeutic options for LUTS with patients, I always warn them that both drugs and surgery can cause ejaculatory disturbance. The side effect is less likely with medication, but it's not uncommon for someone who used to ejaculate anywhere from 3 to 5 milliliters, or about a teaspoon (which is average, according to a 2010 study by the World Health Organization), to express nothing or very little after taking a pill.

Some patients just can't get over this drawback of alpha-blockers and quit the medication. Their ejaculate returns soon after—along with their lower urinary tract symptoms. Men should recognize that their side effects can vary from one alpha-blocker to another, and a different drug from the same category might cause no ejaculatory disturbance.

DRUG-DRUG INTERACTIONS

When you take multiple drugs at once, they interact with each other, either boosting or reducing the intended impact of each medication.

This is why it is vital that you tell your urologist about all the medications that you currently take, including herbal supplements. As long as your doctor is aware of all drugs and over-the-counter supplements that you use, adding a new LUTS medication to your daily routine should not cause problems.

MYTH BUSTER

Don't make the mistake of *not* telling your doctor what herbal supplements you are taking just because you believe they are "natural." Even herbs can cause drug interactions.

Here is a short list of drugs that can induce unfortunate interactions if taken with alpha-blockers.

Erection Drugs: Men taking alpha-blockers for LUTS should be aware that they may interact with the oral phosphodiesterase type-5 (PDE-5) inhibitors most often used to treat erectile dysfunction—Viagra (sildenafil), Cialis (tadalafil), and Levitra (vardenafil)—and can trigger a dangerous drop in blood pressure when these drugs are used together. This can cause you to faint if you stand up too quickly. Talk to your doctor about possible interactions between alpha-blockers and PDE-5 inhibitors so that the safest combination can be chosen at the lowest dosage that is effective.

Antihypertensive Medications: For those men already taking blood pressure medication, alpha-blocker dosages may need to be adjusted to account for the drugs' blood-pressure-lowering effects. Alpha-blockers may induce angina (chest pain resulting from an inadequate supply of oxygen to the heart) in men with coronary heart disease.

RED FLAG

Men taking alpha-blockers for LUTS who plan to have cataract surgery need to alert their doctor that they are using the medication, because not doing so can have serious consequences. Use of alpha-blockers has been found to cause intraoperative floppy iris syndrome (IFIS) during the operation, a condition that makes the iris billow out and prolapse during a cataract procedure and can significantly increase the risk for complications. You will need to go off the drug but can resume taking it following surgery.

5-ALPHA-REDUCTASE INHIBITORS (5-ARIS)

Proscar and Avodart make up another category of LUTS drugs called 5-alpha reductase inhibitors, or 5-ARIs. Like alpha-blockers, they reduce lower urinary tract symptoms in men with benign prostatic enlargement, but unlike alpha-blockers, they also help shrink the prostate over a six- to twelve-month period and can reduce the risk of urinary retention and the need for future prostate surgery. Also, unlike alpha-blockers, they work only in men with an enlarged prostate and are not recommended for men with a prostate volume below 30 to 40 cubic centimeters.

The 5-ARIs work by inhibiting an enzyme called 5-alpha-reductase that triggers the conversion of testosterone to dihydrotestosterone, the most potent androgen inside the prostate cells, and the one that's responsible for growth and maintenance of the prostate. Take the pill daily, and you can slow prostate growth, improve urinary symptoms, and lower the risk of future urinary retention and the need for surgery if the prostate enlarges. 5-ARIs can shrink the prostate by 20 percent to 30 percent in most men by interfering with this hormonal chain of events.

5-alpha-reductase inhibitors do have their limitations. The medication must be taken daily, may take as long as three to six months to work, and ultimately may reduce your LUTS only moderately. Although side effects are few, they can include decreased libido, reduced semen output, and erectile dysfunction. These side effects are reversible once the drug is stopped.

Your doctor will tell you that since 5-ARIs lower PSA levels by about 50 percent after six months of treatment, in order to best assess prostate cancer risk, a patient's PSA value must be corrected by the doctor by a factor of 2 for the first two years of use to achieve an accurate reading and by a factor of 2.5 for longer-term use of the drugs. In men on Proscar or Avodart, any rise in prostate-specific antigen should prompt the suspicion of prostate cancer.

Compliance may also be an issue with LUTS medications, as it is with most drugs that have to be taken regularly. Cost is a factor, too. Since 5-ARIs are often taken in combination with an alpha-blocker, many people can't afford the insurance copay on two drugs, and even if they can, they often refuse to fill their prescription because they don't want to take two medications. Remember, a drug can't work if you're not taking it, so if you are serious about symptom relief, take your medication as prescribed.

ALPHA-BLOCKER OR 5-ARI?

When your LUTS symptoms are moderately or severely bothersome, the best and fastest way to get relief is generally with an alpha-blocker, which is considered the first line of therapy for LUTS. There is no difference between alpha-blockers in response rates based on your age, symptom severity, flow rate, prostate volume, or PSA. Better yet, all of the drugs in this category appear to work equally well.

Some experts believe that the best option for treating LUTS and preventing the progression of symptoms in men with BPE is combination therapy with an alpha-blocker and a 5-ARI—but only if you have a prostate larger than 40 grams.

Data from the Medical Therapy of Prostatic Symptoms (MTOPS) study confirm this. Researchers looked at the results of three thousand LUTS patients who took the 5-ARI Proscar alone, the alpha-blocker Cardura alone, the combination of the two, and placebo. The result: combination therapy with Cardura and Proscar slowed the progression of LUTS, and reduced the risk of urinary retention and the need for surgery to a greater extent than with either drug used alone.

For dosing and pill-taking convenience, we now have Jalyn, approved by the FDA in 2010. It combines two LUTS drugs with different mechanisms of action, dutasteride and tamsulosin into one pill that's taken once daily. The dutasteride, the generic form of the 5-ARI Avodart, shrinks the prostate over time while the alpha-blocker tamsulosin (the active ingredient in Flomax), relaxes the muscles at the bladder neck and in the prostate. The end result for some men with LUTS and BPE is improved flow and an eventual decrease in prostate size. But in men without prostatic enlargement, an alpha-blocker alone should be used, not Jalyn.

It is estimated that 1.5 million American men are currently on a lifetime regimen of these LUTS drugs. As noted before, no medication offers a cure for LUTS due to BPE. The drugs relieve LUTS, and if they are stopped, the symptoms will recur.

ANTICHOLINERGICS FOR LUTS

Anticholinergic drugs, which block nerve transmissions to the bladder, can enhance bladder storage and relieve urination urgency problems by reducing bladder sensitivity. These drugs are often used for overactive bladder (OAB) and can be used in combination with alpha-blockers for

LUTS. They should not be prescribed to men with a reduced flow rate and urine retention. But for men who have mostly storage symptoms (frequency, urgency, nocturia) without evidence of urinary obstruction, anticholinergics can effectively reduce LUTS. For more on these drugs, go to chapter 7.

ERECTILE DYSFUNCTION (ED) DRUGS FOR LUTS: NOT THE STANDARD OF CARE BUT PERHAPS SOON TO BE

Viagra was introduced in 1998 as the first PDE-5 inhibitor, an erectile dysfunction drug that could improve the frequency of successful intercourse among men with erectile dysfunction due to multiple causes. Since Viagra's debut, two additional ED drugs, Cialis and Levitra, were approved by the Food and Drug Administration.

Shortly after Viagra was first approved, Dr. Irwin Goldstein, the urologist who was involved in the clinical trials for most of the early erection drugs, said that within ten years, Viagra's medicinal value would move well beyond simply restoring erections. It was a bold prediction at the time, but one that has, in fact, come true. Over time, as tens of millions of men used the drug, doctors noted that these erection medications did much more than improve erections.

Additional uses have been found for Viagra and other ED drugs, and there have been ongoing human trials with them to see if they can help stroke victims regain and improve movement and speech; boost memory and learning skills of people with memory complaints; improve the ability of patients with heart failure to exercise by increasing oxygen uptake; and help people get over the debilitating effects of altitude sickness.

Now there is another possible use: LUTS therapy.

In the last few years, it has become obvious to urologists that men suffering from lower urinary tract symptoms were also bothered by erectile dysfunction. We used to look at these ailments in aging men as separate problems occurring in the same people by coincidence. We are now realizing that LUTS and ED are linked in some cases, and that the causes of the two disorders may overlap.

In a 2009 erection drug study of Cialis among 581 men with both ED and moderate to severe LUTS due to BPE, both erectile function and LUTS improved significantly among men taking Cialis when compared to placebo. Other studies have reported that the magnitude of improvement in International Prostate Symptom Scores for men with moderate to severe complaints appeared to be comparable to that achieved with alpha-blockers and 5-ARIs, although without the improvement in urinary flow.

So why do PDE-5 inhibitors reduce LUTS? No one knows for sure, but there are several plausible explanations. Let's first review how PDE-5 inhibitors work for ED. The drugs block the enzyme PDE-5 that is present in the corpora cavernosa, a pair of chambers that travel the length of the penis. By blocking PDE-5, blood flow increases in the penis, and an erection can occur if there is adequate sexual stimulation.

What does this have to do with LUTS? It turns out that PDE-5 is also present in the bladder as well as in the urethra and prostate. We have already seen that smooth muscle is a key component of bladder and prostate tissues, and that alterations in smooth muscle tone can result in LUTS. One explanation for the positive effects of ED drugs on LUTS is its effects on the relaxation of smooth muscle in the bladder and prostate. Other possibilities include improved blood flow to these tissues, and yet another explanation might be that ED drugs alter faulty nerve signals that lead to LUTS.

Not only are the penile veins relaxed by the medication, but these drugs might also cause small blood vessels in the prostate and bladder to dilate, improving urinary symptoms in the process.

At this time, PDE-5 inhibitors that are routinely used to treat ED are not considered standard care for LUTS therapy. However, we know that up to 30 percent of patients discontinue alpha-blocker medications for their LUTS within the first twelve months due to adverse side effects or nonresponse. Researchers are now trying to find out if ED medications can be used as new agents for treating lower urinary tract symptoms either alone or in combination with alpha-blockers. And, of course, PDE-5 inhibitors would offer men with LUTS a nice bonus: improved erections. I have yet to meet a man who would say no to that.

Table 6.1. Drugs for Treating LUTS

Drug	Recommended Dosage	When Taken	Mode of Action	Side Effects
Alpha Blockers (Alpha-1-adrenergic blockers)				
Cardura/ Cardura XL (doxazosin)	1.0 to 8.0 milligrams	Cardura is taken once daily; Cardura XL is taken daily at breakfast.	Blocks alpha-adrenergic receptors and relaxes tissue in the prostate, prostate capsule, and bladder neck.	Dizziness, fatigue, low blood pressure, headache, nasal congestion; Rapaflo causes retrograde ejaculation.
Flomax (tamsulosin)	0.4 to 0.8 milligrams	Taken a half hour following the same daily meal.		
Hytrin (terazosin)	1.0 to 10.0 milligrams	Once daily in the morning.		
Rapaflo (silodosin)	8.0 milligrams	Once daily at mealtime.		
UroXatral (alfuzosin)	10.0 milligrams (extended release)	Following the same daily meal.		
5-Alpha-Reductase Inhibitors				
Avodart (dutasteride)	0.5 milligrams	Once daily, with or without food.	Blocks 5-alpha-reductase, an enzyme that converts testosterone to dihydrotestosterone, the hormone that causes prostate growth. This drug causes the prostate to shrink over a nine- to twelve-month span.	Erectile dysfunction (less than 5 percent), decreased ejaculate, decreased libido, breast swelling (less than 1 percent).
Proscar (finasteride)	5.0 milligrams	Once daily, with or without food		

Drug	Recommended Dosage	When Taken	Mode of Action	Side Effects
Combination Drug				
Jalyn (dutasteride/ tamsulosin)	0.5 milligrams dutasteride/ 0.4 milligrams tamsulosin	Thirty minutes following the same daily meal.	Same as dutasteride and tamsulosin.	Same as dutasteride and tamsulosin.
Anticholinergics				
Detrol (tolterodine)	2.0 to 4.0 milligrams	Twice daily; once daily.	Decreases frequency, urgency, and urge-related incontinence.	Dry mouth, constipation.
Ditropan (oxybutynin)	2 to 5 milligrams	Once or twice daily.	Same.	Same.
Oxytrol (oxybutynin transdermal patch)	3.9 milligrams (patch)	Twice a week.	Same.	Same.
Enablex (darifenacin)	7.5 milligrams 15.0 milligrams	Once daily.	Same.	Same.
Sanctura (trospium)	20.0 milligrams 60.0 milligrams	Twice daily. Once per morning.	Same.	Same.
Toviaz (fesoterodine)	4.0 milligrams 8.0 milligrams	Once daily.	Same.	Same.
Vesicare (solifenacin)	5.0 milligrams 10.0 milligrams	Once daily.	Same.	Same.

WHAT TO DO WHEN DRUGS DON'T WORK FOR LUTS

Some men will stop taking drugs for LUTS because they don't like a particular side effect such as reduced ejaculate, while for others the LUTS recur or worsen after a period of initial improvement. In general, the majority of patients experience a moderate reduction in LUTS with medical therapy. For benign prostatic enlargement, combination therapy has been shown to slow the likelihood of progression of symptoms and complications from obstruction such as urinary retention.

Despite the success of medical therapy for hundreds of thousands of men, there are some who stop medical therapy because of no symptom improvement or side effects such as sexual dysfunction. Some may go on to develop progressive worsening of LUTS and others progress to complications of BPE, such as urinary retention, even when they have followed through with all the recommended fluid management, dietary alterations, and lifestyle changes that have been outlined.

RED FLAG

Do not be discouraged if medical therapy does not work. There are other options.

When 5-ARIs and alpha-blockers lose their effectiveness, or a man is ready to try something else, I will question him about his current symptoms and compare his IPSS prior to beginning therapy to the current IPSS to see if and to what extent his LUTS have changed. A urine flow rate and postvoid residual (the amount of urine left in the bladder after urination) are also part of the evaluation. Comparing these results with those from his initial visit will give me an objective view of how he is doing right now.

At this point, it's time to review the remaining options. These include:

- **Minimally invasive therapies (MIT)**
    - TUNA (transurethral needle ablation)
    - TUMT (transurethral microwave thermotherapy)
- **Incision, resection, and electrovaporization**
    - TUIP (transurethral incision of the prostate)
    - TURP (transurethral resection of the prostate)
    - HoLRP (holmium laser resection of the prostate)
    - TUVP (transurethral electrovaporization of the prostate)
    - PVP (photoselective electrovaporization of the prostate)
- **Ablation**
    - HoLAP (transurethral holmium laser ablation of the prostate)
- **Enucleation**
    - HoLEP (transurethral holmium laser enuculeation of the prostate)
    - Open prostatectomy or laparoscopic with robotic assistance

---
MYTH BUSTER

Minimally invasive therapies and surgical treatment for LUTS do not remove the risk of prostate cancer, since the zone where most cancers arise is not affected by the LUTS treatment.

MINIMALLY INVASIVE THERAPIES FOR LUTS (MIT): TRANSURETHRAL NEEDLE ABLATION OF THE PROSTATE (TUNA) AND TRANSURETHRAL MICROWAVE THERMOTHERAPY (TUMT)

It may be time to consider minimally invasive therapies when (1) drugs are not the patient's preferred initial therapy for LUTS; (2) medications prescribed for LUTS do not work; (3) the drugs' side effects can no longer be tolerated; or (4) the patient wants to avoid a surgical procedure that could require hospitalization.

Transurethral needle ablation and transurethral microwave thermotherapy of the prostate, minimally invasive therapies used for troublesome moderate to severe LUTS, apply heat inside the prostate, destroying tissue without cutting the gland. They don't reduce the size of the prostate but improve urinary symptoms and quality of life, possibly by interfering with nerve transmission and muscle function. And it can all be done right in the doctor's office.

Transurethral needle ablation uses radiofrequency energy applied by a needle to heat prostate tissue to as much as 200 degrees, while transurethral microwave thermotherapy delivers heat through a catheter tube.

MIT ADVANTAGES AND DISADVANTAGES

The fact that TUNA and TUMT are outpatient procedures with minimal risk of sexual side effects makes them appealing to many LUTS patients. In some cases, these minimally invasive therapies offer a safe, effective, and lasting treatment that reduces lower urinary tract symptoms to a greater extent than medication and are less invasive than surgical options, which have a higher risk of causing bleeding and sexual dysfunction. Another major plus of needle ablation and microwave thermotherapy is that they don't burn any bridges, which is an important point. Neither procedure precludes a surgical solution in the future if that should become necessary.

However, there are downsides to MIT procedures, too. More convenient, less invasive, and no hospitalization does not always produce superior results; nor does it mean that TUNA and TUMT are the best therapies. Let's examine the key disadvantages of minimally invasive therapies for LUTS:

1. It takes longer for symptoms to improve.

2. The prostatic tissue in the targeted area is destroyed but not immediately removed from the prostate. Because of this, up to 40 percent of men will experience acute swelling and even urinary retention.

3. Some men will need to use a urinary catheter until the body reabsorbs the dead tissue, which may take anywhere from days to weeks.

4. More than half of all men with lower urinary tract symptoms undergoing TUNA or TUMT will need additional treatment at some point. For some, this might be within a year, while for others it might occur within five years. The durability of TUNA and TUMT is less well established than when compared with transurethral resection of the prostate.

5. It is difficult to predict in advance which men will benefit.

MAKING A CHOICE

Although a number of other minimally invasive therapies have been investigated for LUTS, including injections of alcohol and Botox, TUNA and TUMT are the two most commonly used today. Currently there isn't one procedure that stands out as being better than another. Therefore, when considering treatment, don't search for a urologist who performs a particular procedure or technique. Instead focus on the urologist and his experience in patient care. Choosing a new doctor can be a challenging task. In addition to finding someone who is qualified to handle your care, check on the doctor's years of experience and the management options that he uses for LUTS.

A well-trained urologist will be able to diagnose the problem causing the LUTS and be able to choose from a variety of options that can ease symptoms. Just because a urologist does not perform a particular procedure does not mean that your outcome won't be excellent if the doctor is experienced at treating the condition with his preferred approach. Still, the urologist should explain why he/she is using one option versus another. You should never feel uncomfortable asking your doctor about options or participating in the final decision making. Here are some key questions you may want to ask your urologist:

- What is your long-term success rate with the procedure you are recommending?

- Will I require a catheter after treatment? For how long?

- Will this procedure decrease seminal fluid or cause erectile dysfunction?

- Is this procedure durable, or will I need to have frequent follow-up procedures after this one?

BEFORE THE PROCEDURE: WHAT YOU NEED TO KNOW
Prior to initiating any minimally invasive therapy, two visits with your urologist are generally needed.

Visit 1. All patients must first undergo a thorough history and physical exam, DRE, urinalysis, and a PSA test to rule out causes of LUTS that are more serious than BPE, such as an infection or bladder or prostate cancer. Don't be alarmed by this; it's standard protocol.

The severity of symptoms is measured by the International Prostate Symptom Score (IPSS) questionnaire (see page 140), with scores of 0 to 7 indicating mild symptoms; 8 to 19, moderate symptoms; and marks of 20 to 35, severe symptoms. In addition, the IPSS includes this key question: "If you were to spend the rest of your life with your urinary condition the way it is now, how would you feel about that?" The patient's answer goes a long way toward helping the urologist guide him in deciding on management. Let's say that two men both have moderate lower urinary tract symptoms, but while one finds them only mildly disruptive, to the other man, they're intolerable. Naturally, the two patients are likely to choose different courses of management, despite having similar diagnoses. Someone who responds to the above question by circling 0 ("Delighted") or 1 ("Pleased") indicates to me that he is not ready to pursue any therapy, even if it's minimally invasive.

Visit 2. In some cases, flowmetry and an ultrasound scan to estimate postvoid residuals (PVR) will be performed. Flowmetry, a study that measures the volume and flow of urine, can indicate a high likelihood of obstruction if peak urine flow rates are below 10 milliliters per second (ml/sec). Measuring postvoid residuals is done to determine the volume of urine left in the bladder after urination. Men who have normal flow rates (above 15 ml/sec) and low PVRs with mainly storage symptoms (frequency, urgency, nocturia) are not likely to benefit from MIT or surgical management, and causes other than benign prostatic enlargement should be explored.

In patients who are considering minimally invasive therapy, cystoscopy is performed to evaluate the anatomy of the prostate and confirm that no large, obstructing median lobe is present in the prostate and growing into the bladder, which may negate the benefits of minimally invasive therapies. In this diagnostic procedure, a slender instrument with optics called a cystoscope is inserted through the opening of the urethra in the penis and into the bladder, which allows the urologist to see the urethra, prostate, and bladder. If the prostate is markedly enlarged, an ultrasound may be performed to estimate the volume of the prostate gland. Patients with glands greater than 80 cubic centimeters may not respond well to minimally invasive therapies, and a surgical option might be more appropriate.

RED FLAG

Larger prostates need special attention, and only certain BPE procedures will work effectively on the larger glands.

TRANSURETHRAL MICROWAVE THERMOTHERAPY (TUMT)

TUMT is most appropriate for men who have moderately sized prostates (30 to 60 cubic centimeters); and those with moderate (IPSS of 8 to 19) or severe (20 to 35) symptoms that are bothersome.

TUMT requires only a local anesthetic that is placed within the urethra. A special catheter inserted through the urethra then delivers microwave energy at temperatures high enough to destroy prostatic tissue, including the nerves. At the same time, a special cooling system prevents damage to the surrounding tissue, particularly the urethra and the rectum. TUMT takes anywhere from thirty to sixty minutes to complete, depending on the size of the prostate. For the first week or so after the procedure, patients must use a urinary catheter. As for relief of the lower urinary tract symptoms, that typically occurs within four to twelve weeks.

Side effects from transurethral microwave thermotherapy are usually minor and generally disappear with time. TUMT is less likely than surgical procedures to cause bleeding or sexual dysfunction, but it is associated with a higher risk of urinary tract infection. The reason for that is the catheterization, and the longer the tube is in place, the higher the risk. To reduce the risk of infection, antibiotics are often prescribed either after the procedure or after the catheter is withdrawn. Other side effects include short-term incontinence and urinary retention.

WHAT YOU CAN EXPECT FROM TUMT

Numerous clinical studies in the United States and in Europe, including several that have followed patients for more than five years, show that transurethral microwave thermotherapy satisfactorily relieves LUTS in 85 percent of patients. Research reports that TUMT typically produces a 40 percent to 70 percent reduction in IPSS scores. A comparison of TUMT and the surgical procedure TURP (transurethral resection of prostate tissue) demonstrated that TURP produced a greater decline in IPSS and a longer-lasting increase in flow rates than TUMT. However, the microwave therapy resulted in less sexual dysfunction and bleeding when compared to TURP.

TUMT: THE BOTTOM LINE

Improvements in IPSS symptom scores can be considerable for some men who opt for this office-based, minimally invasive therapy. Patients with IPSS scores typically in the range of 20 or higher preprocedure can expect scores of 10 or lower three months after treatment. Urination is easier, and peak urinary flow is increased. As with any medical procedure, individual results vary.

Numerous studies of transurethral microwave thermotherapy report that there are many men who do not derive any appreciable benefit from the therapy. Durability can be an issue with TUMT, and many patients will need retreatment within a few years. TUMT does not outperform surgery in the magnitude of symptom reduction and durability, but since it can be performed as an outpatient procedure and does have efficacy, it is well worth considering.

TRANSURETHRAL NEEDLE ABLATION OF THE PROSTATE (TUNA)

Transurethral needle ablation of the prostate, or TUNA, is an in-office procedure that involves the insertion of two microwave needle electrodes into the prostate to deliver heat that brings about tissue destruction but not a substantial reduction in prostate volume.

First, patients are administered intravenous sedation and a urethral gel to mask pain. Using a cystoscope for guidance, the urologist moves the radiofrequency needles through the urethra and then pierces the lobes of the prostate to gain entrance. Radiofrequency energy is then used to heat the tissue to well over 200 degrees and destroy sections of prostate tissue near the tip of the electrode. This leaves cavities in the tissue that are eventually replaced by scarring. The device is then maneuvered to treat different areas of the prostate, with the entire procedure generally taking less than thirty minutes.

Since urinary retention is the most common side effect and may occur in as many as 40 percent of cases and may last for two days or longer in some, patients typically wear a catheter for one to three days. Most men can return to their normal activities within twenty-four to seventy-two hours.

Voiding symptoms may take two to six weeks before they begin subsiding, and some men may continue to see improvement up to two to three months after the procedure. Therefore, the therapy should not be considered truly successful until three months have elapsed.

This heat therapy is not suitable for every man with LUTS, and it does have limitations. TUNA may not be effective in men with extremely large prostates. The American Urological Association describes the ideal candidate as a man with obstructive symptoms, a prostate volume of 60 cubic centimeters or less, and prostate enlargement mainly in the lobes on either side of the urethra.

According to the many studies that have examined the benefits of TUNA, most patients report improvements ranging from 40 percent to 70 percent after one year, increasing to 73 percent at the two-year mark. In a clinical trial that followed patients for five years, researchers reported that average IPSS scores dropped from 24 to 11, with significant boosts in peak flow rate and overall quality of life.

TUNA VERSUS TURP

In a randomized trial reported in the *Journal of Urology*, researchers compared TUNA with TURP, which is the gold standard for the surgical management of benign prostatic enlargement in patients with bothersome LUTS. They found that the benefits of both procedures were maintained at five years. TUNA, however, was associated with fewer complications such as incontinence or urethral strictures. None of the TUNA patients experienced retrograde ejaculation, while this was a complaint for 41 percent of the men who underwent resection. And although erectile dysfunction occurred in 3 percent of men who underwent TUNA procedures, that figure paled in comparison to the 21 percent of TURP patients with ED complaints.

SURGICAL PROCEDURES FOR LUTS DUE TO BPE

Transurethral resection of the prostate used to be the first line therapy for lower urinary tract symptoms attributable to benign prostatic enlargement. However, because of the availability of medications and MIT, TURP is usually not the first management option.

Understandably, men want a procedure with the highest chance of eliminating LUTS without recurrence, and surgery usually fulfills that wish. Men without LUTS but with complications of obstruction—such as urinary retention, bleeding, or infection—that cannot be treated effectively with less invasive options will most likely require surgery as well.

Surgical therapy is most appropriate for men with severe LUTS, with or without complications. These patients are often in retention and can't urinate. Most have had catheters inserted to relieve their recurrent retention. They typically have to sit down to urinate because they have to contract their abdominal muscles to get urine past the obstruction, and they never feel like their bladder is empty afterward. Men who often stand in front of the urinal for lengthy periods, with their urine stream coming out in short, weak, repetitive bursts, are also typical surgical candidates.

Other complications that make surgical therapy the procedure of choice include:

- **Anatomic abnormalities:** a large median lobe protruding into the bladder acting like a ball valve, or a high bladder neck that significantly limits outflow of urine.

- **Bladder dysfunction:** limits emptying, leading to recurrent urinary tract infections.

- **Kidney damage:** prevents the body from filtering blood

- **Bladder stones:** cause chronic inflammation in the bladder and lead to infections

- **Recurrent bleeding from an enlarged prostate:** can cause retention of urine

In the discussion that follows, I describe various surgical approaches that can all be carried out through the urethra. That means these are transurethral procedures, which don't require surgeons to make an incision in the abdomen. You should remember that the choice of one surgical approach over another depends on your prostate anatomy (shape and size), the balance between benefits and risks, and the urologist's breadth of experience with each approach.

The most favorable outcome is likely to occur with a combination of a well-informed patient who has realistic expectations, and a surgeon experienced in the most suitable option for that patient's prostate anatomy. The various approaches are an alphabet soup of acronyms that usually contain the word *transurethral*.

RESECTION, ABLATION, AND INCISION PROCEDURES
TRANSURETHRAL RESECTION OF THE PROSTATE (TURP)

Both electrical and laser energy sources can be used to remove prostate tissue that is obstructing the bladder outlet and causing lower urinary tract symptoms. Transurethral resection using electrical energy has long been the therapy against which all others are measured. Not only does it get the job done, but it's also durable. Fewer than 10 percent of patients will require a repeat procedure five to ten years later, whereas more than 70 percent of men who opted for minimally invasive therapies will need further therapy. While TURP can be performed on an outpatient basis in many cases, for some a one-night hospitalization is necessary.

Transurethral resection improves symptoms in up to 95 percent of patients, which is a major reason why it's been the go-to BPE therapy for patients with the highest IPSS scores or incomplete bladder emptying leading to complications such as urinary tract infections.

How It's Done
The inpatient procedure is performed using a flexible resectoscope through the urethra in a sixty- to ninety-minute operation under general or spinal anesthesia. The handheld scope, which is linked to a video camera, has an attached wire loop that delivers a high-energy current. The surgeon uses the device to pare away strips of prostatic tissue and then drop them into the bladder. When the operation is over, these prostate "chips" are then removed from the bladder with a suction device. Tissue samples are sent to the pathology laboratory to rule out the presence of prostate cancer.

A catheter, inserted through the urethra into the bladder as the operation is being finished, will be used for up to three days to prevent urinary retention and allow healing. When your doctor removes the catheter, you may notice a powerful urge to urinate over the span of two days. Don't be alarmed; this is common and soon disappears.

There is little or no pain associated with TURP. Improvement in LUTS is noticeable immediately after surgery, and men who had the highest IPSS scores and evidence of obstruction (low urinary flow rates) beforehand show the greatest improvements. You can expect to recover fully within three weeks.

TURP Benefits
The satisfaction rate for transurethral resection is significantly better than what can be achieved with medication, minimally invasive therapies, or the various self-help measures employed during watchful waiting. A marked improvement is seen by about 90 percent to 95 percent of men with severe symptoms and by roughly 80 percent of those with moderate symptoms.

TURP Side Effects
The most common complications immediately following transurethral resection are the need for recatheterization, bleeding, and urinary tract infection. Most TURP studies report improved erectile function following this procedure. However, reduced ejaculation, or retrograde ejaculation, is common with the surgery, as it is with laser procedures, and may affect as many as 50 percent to 60 percent of men. If you still want

to have children, be sure to speak to your doctor about banking your sperm beforehand.

In a large study comparing watchful waiting to TURP, there was a 1 percent risk of urinary incontinence with TURP, which was similar to the risk for the watchful waiting group. The decline in sexual function was also identical between the two groups. The study emphasized that foregoing treatment can eventually bring about a reduced quality of life rivaling the side effects of surgical intervention. Nevertheless, patients' desires to avoid TURP side effects, not to mention a hospital stay and several days of catheterization, has led to development of alternatives to prostate resection. Let's review them.

TRANSURETHRAL ELECTROVAPORIZATION OF THE PROSTATE (TUVP)

TUVP is very similar to TURP, but instead of a resectoscope with a wire loop to cut tissue, the loop is replaced with a device with a large surface area that is used to vaporize tissue with a higher current. Like TURP, this procedure requires general or spinal anesthesia and takes about an hour to perform. Symptom scores, urinary flow, and quality of life outcomes are similar to TURP results. When compared to resection, there may be shorter hospitalization and less blood loss with electrovaporization. However, TUVP may be associated with more irritative symptoms, urinary retention, and reoperations when compared with TURP.

TRANSURETHRAL INCISION OF THE PROSTATE (TUIP)

TUIP is an ideal procedure for the man who has bothersome symptoms and a small prostate of 30 cubic centimeters or less. Unlike TURP and TUVP, this outpatient procedure involves making several incisions in the prostate. This releases the constriction of the urethra caused by the prostate capsule. With transurethral incision, a man could expect symptom relief similar to that of resection and ablation procedures, but with a lower risk of retrograde ejaculation and scar tissue at the bladder neck.

LASER-ASSISTED RESECTION AND ABLATION

Urologists are generally drawn to innovative gadgets, and when the laser (which stands for light amplification by the stimulated emission of radiation) was introduced in the 1990s for the treatment of lower urinary tract symptoms due to BPE, there was plenty of excitement within the urological community that these devices would magically vaporize prostatic tissue, relieving symptoms in an instant.

Of course, that's not the case. As with any new technology, glitches had to be fixed to refine the capability of lasers to treat LUTS. Even so, laser therapy for benign prostatic enlargement has created a ground-swell of interest from both surgeons and patients, and it is becoming a popular alternative to medications and traditional surgical procedures. That's because lasers offer a powerful source of energy that can selectively destroy prostate tissue safely and easily. In addition, it is now a popular option for patients who have large prostates or are too ill to undergo a resection.

The commonly used lasers for prostate surgery today are the holmium laser and the potassium-titanyl-phosphate laser (KTP, or Green-Light). Holmium laser resection of the prostate (HoLRP), holmium laser ablation of the prostate (HoLAP), and photoselective vaporization (PVP) using the KTP laser are all effective and safe approaches to resect and ablate prostate tissue.

The move toward laser-assisted procedures has been driven primarily by a notable decrease in blood loss, lower transfusion rates, shorter catheterization times, and shorter hospitalizations when compared with TURP. In general, the improvement in lower urinary tract symptoms following laser-assisted procedures is comparable to that of resection, except for, according to some studies, increased reoperation rates. At some point, the laser treatment may become the first-line therapy for benign prostatic enlargement. However, we are not there yet.

Photoselective Laser Electrovaporization of the Prostate (PVP)

The most popular laser-assisted approach is photoselective laser electrovaporization of the prostate, or PVP. More popularly known as GreenLight laser electrovaporization, this procedure uses a special high-powered green wavelength of laser light that vaporizes prostatic tissue. Patients can generally expect a rapid restoration of urine flow with symptom improvement within twenty-four hours. Most are able to leave the hospital the same day and without a catheter, although some physicians advise wearing one until the next day.

PVP generally takes less than an hour to perform, but it really comes down to the size of the prostate—the larger it is, the longer you can expect your procedure to take—the vascularity of the prostate, and your doctor's skill. PVP can be offered to most patients, regardless of age, configuration of the prostate, or severity of symptoms, although men with larger prostates, especially those above 100 cubic centimeters, may be best treated with an enucleation procedure (described below). Since PVP causes minimal bleeding, patients taking warfarin (Coumadin) or other blood-thinning medications can also be treated.

Following the procedure, pain is minimal, if present at all, and excessive bleeding is unlikely, as are bladder spasms. A dose of antibiotics is usually given prior to the procedure and for several days after catheter removal.

A study analyzing more than fifteen clinical trials that compared PVP to TURP reported similar improvements in lower urinary tract symptoms based on IPSS scores and increases in maximum urinary flow rates. In addition, patients who underwent the PVP procedure had shorter hospital stays but a higher risk for urinary retention (8 percent versus 3 percent) and reoperation (5 percent versus 2 percent).

A final reminder: since the intense heat vaporizes prostatic tissue, there will be no tissue sample available to send to the pathologist to examine for the presence of prostate cancer.

ENUCLEATION PROCEDURES FOR THE LARGE PROSTATE

When prostates are small (30 cubic centimeters or below) and surgery is required, a prostate incision (TUIP) is the best approach for most men with LUTS complaints. For those with prostates in the range of 30 to 80 cubic centimeters, a transurethral resection or ablation procedure is usually performed with electrical or laser energy. But for prostates measuring 80 to 100 cubic centimeters or more, most urologists prefer an enucleation procedure because of the inability to resect or ablate large amounts of tissue through the urethra.

Enucleation means removing tissue from a surrounding capsule. When the prostate enlarges in men with benign prostatic enlargement, the growing tissue in the center compresses the periphery of the prostate into a thick capsule. Imagine an orange with the peel as the capsule of compressed tissue, and the juicy part inside as the BPE tissue that needs to be removed. Through an incision in the prostate capsule or bladder, the inner part of the prostate can be enucleated, leaving behind the capsule.

Enucleation, referred to as a simple prostatectomy, makes up less than 5 percent of BPE surgical procedures in the United States. Do not confuse it with radical prostatectomy, a mainstay of prostate cancer surgery. See chapter 13 for more information on this surgery performed through an incision in the abdomen or laparoscopically with robotic assistance.

The two most commonly performed enucleation procedures for BPE are the suprapubic and retropubic prostatectomies. Both require an incision above the pubic bone to gain access to the bladder and prostate under general or spinal anesthesia, a hospitalization of three to five days, and a recovery period of four to six weeks.

A suprapubic prostatectomy involves opening the bladder and removing the inner portion of the prostate through the bladder. Postsurgery, two catheters are left for drainage of urine—one in the bladder and one in the urethra. These are usually removed three to seven days after the procedure.

In a retropubic prostatectomy, an incision is made in the prostate capsule, and the inner prostate tissue is removed without entering the bladder. In most cases, only a urethral catheter is necessary postsurgery for about a week. As in transurethral resection of the prostate, tissue samples are sent to the pathology laboratory to be examined for the presence of cancer.

Some surgeons have been using a robot-assisted laparoscopic approach to enucleation of the prostate. With this procedure, small instruments controlled by a robotic arm are placed through portholes in the abdomen and used to perform the enucleation procedure. This approach is in its infancy but may be associated with less blood loss and shorter hospital stays when compared to the open enucleation.

Open Prostatectomy Side Effects

Like TURP, an open prostatectomy is an effective way to relieve symptoms of BPE. Complications, however, are more common with open prostatectomy as compared to TURP. These can include bleeding, reoperation for severe bleeding, and urinary tract infections. Long-term complications, including erectile dysfunction, incontinence, and retrograde ejaculation, are slightly more common with open prostatectomy than with TURP. As a result, open prostatectomy is reserved for otherwise healthy men with the largest prostates who cannot undergo a transurethral procedure.

HOLEP: THE NEW KID ON THE BLOCK

My colleague Dr. James Lingeman at Indiana University has popular-ized an innovative transurethral approach to enucleation: holmium laser enucleation of the prostate (HoLEP), in which the holmium laser is used in a knife-like fashion to cut away prostatic tissue—as if cut-ting a slice of pie—and then place it in the bladder. A special tool called a morcellator is then used to remove the tissue from the bladder. This approach avoids an abdominal incision and is associated with less blood loss, as well as shorter catheterization, hospitalization, and recovery times. Most patients leave the hospital after one day, and a urethral cath-eter is removed in one to two days after the procedure.

In a recent study in the *Journal of Urology in* 2010, Dr. Lingeman's group reported on data from more than one thousand HoLEP proce-dures performed from 1998 to 2009 at the Methodist Hospital in Indi-anapolis. Their findings over an average of seven years following the HoLEP (average age seventy-five; average prostate size, 100 cubic centi-meters) were very impressive:

- Average IPSS symptom scores of 20 dropped to 5.

- Maximum urinary flow rate of 8.4 ml/sec before HoLEP jumped to 28 ml/sec after the procedure.

- Only three patients suffered urinary retention, and only one required reoperation for bleeding six years after the procedure.

Most urologists are not yet familiar or comfortable with this special-ized approach, so if you are interested in pursuing HoLEP, be sure to find a physician who has vast experience with the technology.

WHAT I WOULD DO IF I HAD LUTS

I've had a lot of time to think about what I would do if I were the patient on the other side of my desk. If I had unwanted lower urinary tract symptoms that involved mostly storage (frequency, urgency, nocturia) and a prostate that was not enlarged, I would first look at my liquid and food intake to see if I could alter anything to reduce the symptoms.

If the symptoms still troubled me, I would start off with medical therapy—probably an alpha-blocker. If I had benign prostatic enlargement and mixed symptoms (storage and emptying) that were not relieved by one drug or combination therapy, or if it worked well for a few years and then symptoms became bothersome again, I would return to my urologist and discuss surgical options.

My reasoning for avoiding minimally invasive therapies and going to surgery would be MIT's lower chance of success and durability when compared with surgery.

Finally, I would make sure that I had the surgical procedure performed by an experienced doctor, which is something I can't stress enough. Surgical expertise, based on measurable, consistently superior results, is something I value highly. And you should too. When you take the time to find an expert, you're in good hands.

THE TAKEAWAY

- LUTS therapy is not a one-size-fits-all solution. The choice of management depends on the cause of the symptoms, and should be agreed upon mutually by the patient and the physician, taking into consideration the risks and benefits of the management options and the patient's preferences.

- Watchful waiting is a good strategy for (1) men with minimal symptoms, an IPSS score of less than 8; and (2) for those with moderate to severe symptoms that are not bothersome.

- Alpha-blocker medications are generally considered the first-line medical therapy for LUTS thought to be due to the prostate.

- Men with large prostates—greater than 40 grams—and LUTS are the best candidates for treating benign prostatic enlargement with 5-alpha-reductase inhibitor medication.

- For men with prostate enlargement and LUTS, the combination of an alpha-blocker and a 5-alpha-reductase inhibitor reduces the chance of symptom progression, urinary retention, and the need for surgery.

- There are a variety of minimally invasive therapies for bothersome LUTS related to the prostate, including microwave and radiofrequency procedures.

- Surgery to ablate, vaporize, or remove prostate tissue is appropriate for men who have benign prostate enlargement (BPE), bothersome LUTS due to obstruction, or complications from BPE due to urinary retention, bladder stones, recurrent infections, bleeding, and renal damage. In addition, men with urinary symptoms not relieved by less invasive alternatives and those who desire to proceed initially with the most effective approach to symptom relief might choose a surgical option.

- Transurethral resection of the prostate (TURP) is considered the gold standard treatment for LUTS caused by obstructing prostate tissue. Laser-assisted TURP may provide similar symptom relief with lower side effects in some cases.

CHAPTER SEVEN

THE OVERACTIVE BLADDER

The length of a film should be directly related to the
endurance of the human bladder.

—Alfred Hitchcock

In the simplest terms, overactive bladder, or OAB, is an inability to store urine efficiently. Men with OAB have a reduced capacity to store urine and can't delay urination or "hold it"—even when the bladder is still in the process of filling with an average volume of urine. For them, even small amounts of urine can trigger a desperate need to go. OAB has many of the hallmarks of urinary frequency, a predominantly lifestyle-related problem for some that was discussed in detail in chapter 4. But OAB goes beyond frequency to urgency: a sudden desire to urinate that cannot be deferred until a later time. The urgency can be extreme enough to cause embarrassing public slips and even significant incontinence.

An estimated thirty-three million Americans are affected by OAB, a condition that constitutes a significant social problem for many due to the uncontrolled contractions of the bladder and urinary leakage. And while many doctors used to think that the majority of people with OAB were women, men are afflicted as well, almost equally. The National Overactive Bladder Evaluation (NOBLE) program conducted a phone survey of almost twelve thousand people and reported that 17 percent of women and 16 percent of men interviewed had OAB.

Many people with overactive bladder mistakenly believe that it is just part of the aging process without a solution, while others are simply too embarrassed to speak to their physicians about the problem. And so years fly by, with many men just putting up with it, and about one in four suffering not only the urge and frequency, but also the associated incontinence.

Often misdiagnosed and treated as a prostate problem, OAB is a bladder condition that can result from a number of causes, including long-standing urinary obstruction caused by an enlarged prostate. In some cases, OAB can be alleviated by taking relatively simple measures such as voiding at timed intervals, restricting fluid intake, oral medication, and electrical stimulation of the bladder, to name just a few. Unfortunately, by the time men are diagnosed with overactive bladder, they have often acquired behaviors that actually exacerbate their condition and need to be reversed. The retraining phase of OAB management is vital to recovery.

There is a good deal of nuance required to diagnose OAB correctly. It must be differentiated from bladder storage symptoms—frequency, urgency, urge incontinence—that can be caused by urinary tract infections, bladder injury due to radiation, neurological disease, and benign prostatic enlargement causing urinary obstruction. The management option with the best success will depend on the cause of the OAB. There are similar overlapping symptoms regardless of the cause, and it takes a careful doctor to parse out the differences and find a solution that restores a patient's peace of mind, quality of life, and self-confidence.

Urinary symptoms can be debilitating psychologically. Afflicted men often abandon exercise, hobbies, socializing, career advancement, and even personal relationships. Too embarrassed to speak of it, too vibrant in all other ways to consider it a legitimate medical ailment—they can't claim they're sick—men endure OAB for years and become more and more reclusive, burdened by their secret. However, there are management options for OAB that can improve a man's quality of life, and that start with understanding the disease and directing the management accordingly.

CHUCK'S STORY

Chuck, forty-two, is a TV sports producer for a major network who spends so much time on the road and overseas at sporting events that he has to have friends pick up his mail regularly to keep his mailbox from overflowing. But unfortunately, mail is the least of Chuck's overflow problems. The need to urinate urgently and often is at the top of his list.

When the urge hits on city streets, Chuck rushes into a restaurant or store to ask to use the bathroom. When owners reply with "Customers only," he explains that he suffers from incontinence. Still no response, incontinence hits.

His biggest fear, however, is being airborne. Flying from one sporting event to the next kicks his urination issues up a notch, especially when the lavatories are in use and he has to wait anxiously outside the door. And then there is the stress of having the Fasten Seat Belt sign light up, ordering him to stay put.

Chuck's Roman holiday at a local trattoria is just one example of his many OAB stories: "I encountered a man standing in front of the men's room, waiting his turn to go in. Finally, I couldn't take it anymore. The 'I'm really struggling to hold it in' dance was in full effect, and I felt like I was going to lose it, so I actually paid this guy to let me go ahead of him. Ignominy coupled with embarrassment, I rushed passed him as he pocketed the cash—laughing to himself the whole time, I'm sure.

"Pathetic, I know, but that's how bad it's been for me for the past four years. I am desperate, and I need help. I can't go on like this anymore. My life is being stolen from me."

"I HAVE TO GO"

When someone urgently tells you, "I have to go," you instinctively know exactly what he means. In Chuck's case, the problem was overactive bladder. When you have OAB, the urge to urinate is so intense, so frequent, and so unpredictable that you no longer are in control of your bladder; it controls you.

TOILET MAPPING

Men with frequency problems are often thinking ahead obsessively. They know where every restroom is located from the time they make it out their front door, reach their workplace, and then come home. I call this "toilet mapping," and I have yet to find a man with OAB who is not adept at it.

It goes without saying that any shopping is done mainly in stores with accessible facilities, or else men with OAB choose to do most of their shopping online. While convenient, being able to shop from home also allows men to justify being less social. But more importantly, it keeps them from getting appropriate medical help.

Another strategy that men with OAB employ commonly is called defensive urination. They go to the bathroom repeatedly during the day, just in case they may not be near a toilet later. "This actually is used therapeutically and is also known as timed voiding," explains OAB expert Dr. Roger Dmochowski, a professor in the Department of Urologic Surgery at Vanderbilt University Medical Center in Nashville. "It can be very helpful if done in combination with other interventions."

Some people with overactive bladder accept grudgingly that they now have to wear adult diapers or sanitary napkins to catch any urine leaking. Dark and baggy clothing is often worn to hide the absorbent undergarments and mask the occasional accidental spills.

When the OAB worsens, many, like Chuck, limit their fluid consumption in order to reduce urine output. This strategy, however, can be difficult in warm weather climates where fluid intake is necessary to prevent dehydration. What's more, cutting back on liquids can concentrate the urine and, for some, increase the irritating effects of foods on the bladder, actually worsening symptoms.

Although OAB is not life threatening, it can have significant effects on a man's quality of life and mental health. In addition to avoiding social activities, intimacy and sex can take a backseat to OAB, and some men ultimately suffer from depression as a result of their situation. As with chronic pain syndromes, OAB can be a debilitating, life-altering problem.

The good news is that no matter what your age, overactive bladder can be treated. There are nondrug strategies that include behavioral modifications, medications to relax the bladder, nerve stimulation of pelvic nerves, and Botox injections.

STORING AND EMPTYING

If you're not familiar with the urination basics and would like a more detailed look at the production, storage, and emptying of urine, chapter 4 explains it in greater detail.

The function of the bladder and urinary outlet can be distilled into two major tasks: storage and emptying of urine. These phenomena are hardwired in the brain and closely coordinated. An analogy is the accelerator and brake pedals on your car.

Urine, the end product of the kidneys' filtration of the blood, is composed mostly of water, salts, and a by-product of food metabolism called urea. Normally, urine is produced and then eliminated from the body about six times a day, with about 250 milliliters (almost 8.5 ounces) at each void. Urine produced by the kidneys is transported to the bladder, the balloon-like organ located behind the pubic bone that changes size according to the state of hydration.

The bladder, an organ composed of muscle and connective tissue, is connected to the tip of the penis by a thin tube called the urethra. Urination occurs when a person recognizes that the bladder is full through signals sent from the bladder to the brain—that's the accelerator. But instead of instructing the detrusor muscle in the bladder wall to contract immediately, the brain transmits an inhibitory signal (the brake) to the bladder to put it in relax mode. This allows you time to find a restroom.

Once you're at the toilet, the inhibitory signals from the brain are shut off. Then the muscles of the pelvic floor relax. These muscles provide support to the bladder, the rectum, and the bladder outlet muscles called the sphincter. The detrusor muscle contracts, and urine flows. Once the bladder is empty, the bladder relaxes, the outlet closes, and the cycle starts all over again.

You don't think twice about this process unless there is a problem with bladder filling or the ability to empty the bladder. Overactive bladder is a filling problem that can have numerous causes. But the bottom line is that the bladder is not filling normally and the man is getting the signal too often and too soon that urination is necessary, and in some cases, it's contracting without permission.

The central nervous system and the cerebral cortex region of the brain regulate bladder filling and emptying tightly. When we're born, we are hardwired in a primitive fashion. Your model for this is the infant who voids automatically, night or day, when the bladder fills. When we become potty trained, however, we learn to control the signals with higher brain function in order to modulate the entire process and delay urination until an appropriate time.

OAB is defined by symptoms that include urgency with or without urge incontinence (incontinence that occurs after a strong desire to urinate). It's usually associated with both frequency and nocturia, or night-time urination. Men with frequency and/or nocturia alone would not be classified as having overactive bladder.

The urgency felt with OAB is presumed to be due to a bladder contraction that occurs without a person's authorization. These contractions can be generated by a neurological ailment such as Parkinson's disease, stroke, multiple sclerosis, and spinal cord disease. Changes in the bladder caused by inflammation from infections or radiation can be triggers, as can long-standing obstruction of the bladder due to prostatic enlargement. In this chapter, the focus is on the man with OAB that develops *without* an identifiable underlying cause such as neurological disease, inflammation, or obstruction of the bladder.

CAUSES OF BLADDER (DETRUSOR) OVERACTIVITY

Overactive bladder occurs when the nerves within the bladder wall and those carrying messages to the spinal cord for the trip up to the brain no longer work properly. Messages coming back from the brain through the spinal cord to inhibit a bladder contraction can also be faulty. In both instances, the bladder's detrusor muscle can become overactive, and instead of staying at rest until you give it permission to contract, the bladder squeezes inadvertently while still filling. This is known as bladder or detrusor overactivity. We call it OAB for short.

Urological experts speculate that OAB may also be related to several ongoing aging processes that involve nerve signals and chronic medical ailments that increase with age. There may also be a genetic component at work here as well. A number of different drugs, both prescription and over the counter, can complicate or worsen preexisting OAB, such as certain sedatives, diuretics, sleeping pills, and cold medications.

OAB SYMPTOMS

OAB is a distressing condition characterized by the symptoms of urinary urgency, frequency day and night, and sometimes urge incontinence. Physicians refer to these symptoms as filling symptoms in contrast to voiding symptoms. Here's what that means:

- **Urinary Urgency.** Normally the desire to urinate is termed the urge to urinate. Urgency is an abnormally strong desire to urinate, which cannot be deferred. This is the key symptom of OAB, without which the diagnosis is not made.

- **Frequency.** An increased rate (frequency) of urination, generally more than eight times a day and/or two or more times a night is known as nocturia. Different individuals may have different "normals" that can depend on fluid intake, among other factors.

- **Urge Incontinence.** If the urgency cannot be suppressed, or a bathroom cannot be found in time, an involuntary loss of urine called incontinence will occur. If incontinence occurs after urgency, it is termed urge incontinence.

WHEN TO SEEK MEDICAL CARE
FOR OVERACTIVE BLADDER

If you answer yes to one or more of the following questions, speak to your physician about the possibility of OAB:

- Do you urinate more than eight times in a twenty-four-hour period?

- Do you go to the bathroom so frequently that it interferes with things you want to do?

- Do you have to get up two or more times at night to go to the bathroom?

- Do you frequently have strong, sudden urges to urinate?

- Do you have uncontrollable urges to urinate that sometimes result in wetting yourself?

- Do you use pads to protect your clothing from wetting?

- When you go out, do you make sure that you know the location of available bathrooms?

- Do you avoid certain places if you think there won't be a bathroom available?

If you have chronic urinary problems, start by consulting your family doctor. Depending on the complexity of your case, you may then be referred to a urologist for more detailed testing and treatment.

DIAGNOSING OAB

Overactive bladder diagnosis is based primarily on the particular history of symptoms that you present to your doctor, so be honest with your health care provider. The more specific the information you provide, the more likely it is that you will come away with a proper diagnosis.

In addition to a careful history obtained by a health care provider, the evaluation will usually include an assessment of the severity of the symptoms, a digital rectal examination, a prostate-specific antigen blood test to evaluate the prostate for enlargement or cancer, an evaluation of a urine sample to rule out infection, and an assessment of the frequency and amount of urine using a frequency volume chart.

In some cases in which a neurological disease (stroke, multiple sclerosis, Parkinson's disease) is thought to be the cause, the physician will order a test called a urodynamic evaluation, to assess the bladder's ability to store urine under low pressure without unwanted contractions. After coating the urethra with lidocaine gel, a pressure sensor, which is half the diameter of a pencil, is inserted and eased into the bladder. The urodynamic test is performed by filling the bladder with fluid while the pressure sensor gives a readout of internal function. High pressure readings at low volume indicates a loss of bladder function that is often seen in neurological diseases.

DIFFERENTIATING OAB FROM BPE

There are men with OAB caused by an enlarged prostate obstructing urine flow. Benign prostatic enlargement (see chapter 5) is a noncancerous enlargement of the prostate and the most common benign tumor found in man. This prostatic growth, a part of the aging process for many men, can cause the gland to compress the urethra, making urination difficult, painful, or both. Although the exact cause of BPE is not known, the condition is very common in men over the age of fifty.

While OAB is a bladder storage problem, BPE is an emptying problem initially that can eventually affect the ability of the bladder to store urine if obstruction is present long term. So it's not surprising that the storage symptoms (frequency and urgency with or without incontinence) of overactive bladder can be present in men with benign prostatic enlargement. The tip-off that BPE may be the underlying problem is a history of the following bladder-emptying symptoms:

- difficulty starting urination or hesitancy,

- weak urine flow or slow stream,

- intermittent urine flow that starts and stops,

- feeling of being unable to completely empty the bladder, and

- straining to urinate.

A measure of the rate of the urinary stream (which is called a flow rate, or flowmetry), and the amount of urine left in the bladder after urination (postvoid residual), are sometimes used to assess bladder emptying in men thought to have BPE-related urination symptoms.

Benign prostatic enlargement is not the cause of all male urination symptoms as once thought, although it gets blamed for the vast majority of them. It's not uncommon for a man to have both OAB and BPE at the same time, and physicians are now using medical therapy to treat both with good results. But sometimes medical therapy is not enough, and the enlarged prostate may need to be treated surgically. (See chapter 6.)

—————————————MYTH BUSTER—————————————

Advertisements make it seem that drugs for OAB and BPE provide magic relief for all. Medications can play a primary role in management but are not the answer for all men.

TREATING OAB EFFECTIVELY: KEEP IT SIMPLE

When OAB is suspected, a detailed voiding diary can provide the information that is needed to begin lifestyle alterations and behavioral modifications that could improve your symptoms. Making regular entries in the diary can help reveal specific situations in which urgency, frequency, and incontinence occur, such as "having to go" immediately after coming home from work. Your physician can then use this information to help him pinpoint situations that are associated with your particular symptoms and suggest changes to prevent or reduce those symptoms.

This seemingly simple detective work also makes you an active partner in managing your condition. The knowledge of what specific triggers exist for your "bladder misbehavior" can be empowering, allowing you to gain control rather than remaining a bystander in the process. Below, you'll find a sample copy of the bladder diary.

Lifestyle alterations, behavioral therapy, and drug therapy are the main management options for overactive bladder. The simplest approach that will accomplish the goal of reducing symptoms is always the best. Let's start with lifestyle changes that are commonly recommended for an OAB patient.

SAMPLE BLADDER DIARY

Complete one form for each day for four days before your appointment with a health care provider. In order to keep the most accurate diary possible, you'll want to keep it with you at all times and write down the events as they happen. Take the completed forms with you to the doctor's office.

Time	Fluids	Foods	Urinate	Leakage	Did You Feel an Urge to Urinate?	What Were You Doing at the Time?
			How much? (small, medium, large)			
6:00 a.m. to 7:00 a.m.	• Water, 1 4-oz cup • Coffee, 2 8-oz cups • Apple juice, 1 4-oz cup • Milk, 1 6-oz cup	• Cereal, 1 bowl oatmeal	1 medium	0	yes	Getting up from chair.

Time	Fluids	Foods	Urinate	Leakage	Did You Feel an Urge to Urinate?	What Were You Doing at the Time?
7:00 a.m. to 8:00 a.m.						
8:00 a.m. to 9:00 a.m.						
9:00 a.m. to 10:00 a.m.						
10:00 a.m. to 11:00 a.m.						
11:00 a.m. to 12:00 p.m.						
12:00 p.m. to 1:00 p.m.						

Time	Fluids	Foods	Urinate	Leakage	Did You Feel an Urge to Urinate?	What Were You Doing at the Time?
1:00 p.m. to 2:00 p.m.						
2:00 p.m. to 3:00 p.m.						
3:00 p.m. to 4:00 p.m.						
4:00 p.m. to 5:00 p.m.						
5:00 p.m. to 6:00 p.m.						
6:00 p.m. to 7:00 p.m.						

Time	Fluids	Foods	Urinate	Leakage	Did You Feel an Urge to Urinate?	What Were You Doing at the Time?
7:00 p.m. to 8:00 p.m.						
8:00 p.m. to 9:00 p.m.						
9:00 p.m. to 10:00 p.m.						
10:00 p.m. to 11:00 p.m.						
11:00 p.m. to 12:00 a.m.						
12:00 a.m. to 1:00 a.m.						

Time	Fluids	Foods	Urinate	Leakage	Did You Feel an Urge to Urinate?	What Were You Doing at the Time?
1:00 a.m. to 2:00 a.m.						
2:00 a.m. to 3:00 a.m.						
3:00 a.m. to 4:00 a.m.						
4:00 a.m. to 5:00 a.m.						
5:00 a.m. to 6:00 a.m.						

"BLADDER IRRITANTS": FIND AND ELIMINATE

Simple alterations such as paying attention to fluid intake, eliminating liquids and foods that are bladder irritants, losing weight, treating constipation, and eliminating tobacco can reduce the symptoms of OAB.

For obvious reasons, liquids have traditionally been thought to be the only contributing factor to overactive bladder and frequency issues, but that is not the case. Food, and its specific acidic content, could also play a role. Animal studies show that acidic components found in diet beverages and soft drinks can stimulate bladder activity. While there is some speculation that certain dietary components can cause OAB, there is little human data to positively identify the primary offenders. That said, I still recommend that a patient bothered by overactive bladder evaluate different foods and beverages that might be exacerbating symptoms.

Be forewarned that supermarket shelves are full of potential bladder triggers that may cause an increase in OAB symptoms. Bladder irritants are very subjective. Chocolate, for example, may lead to increased urinary symptoms for some, while others are not affected. In order to reduce your OAB symptoms, you should first identify the specific foods and drinks that are particularly troublesome. Nearly 50 percent of people suffering from OAB will find that eliminating just one "trigger" food or beverage greatly eases their distress.

RED FLAG

Caffeine and alcohol are two of the most common examples of liquids that will make you void more frequently; but any liquid in large quantity that is consumed quickly can increase urine production and urinary frequency.

For example, reducing the consumption of caffeine or alcohol can reduce urinary symptoms in men with overactive bladder. Since caffeine and alcohol bring about increased production of urine and faster bladder filling, it is not surprising that both can cause urgency. In addition to coffee and tea, caffeine is also found in cola, chocolate, and certain nonprescription headache medications.

Anything that leads to rapid bladder filling, such as drinking a large amount of fluid at any one time, can increase symptoms. Therefore, spacing out your fluid intake over the day tends to reduce symptoms.

Nicotine in tobacco can also increase urinary symptoms in those with OAB. There are data to suggest that nicotine can increase bladder overactivity and exacerbate OAB symptoms, and that men who stop smoking can reduce their symptoms. Smoking is one of the worst things that you can do for your overall health, and since it may contribute to OAB, it's a good idea to quit.

There are many other consumables that could increase OAB symptoms. Concentrated citrus products such as orange or grapefruit juice sometimes cause problems and should be eliminated from the diet if drinking them appears to increase OAB symptoms. Other products that could potentially exacerbate OAB are listed below.

Do your best to eliminate problem foods, beverages, and medications from your diet. First try taking out one item that you think might be the troublemaker. After a week or so, you can gradually reintroduce one of these foods or beverages back into your diet and see if the urinary frequency or urgency recurs. Chart your progress in your bladder diary. Surprisingly, you may find that just reducing the amount that you consume will greatly help improve your bladder symptoms without your having to give up some of your favorite foods.

"Understand, too, that this is simply a laundry list of foods and beverages," Dr. Dmochowski points out, "and it's certainly not definitive. We are all individuals, and while many items on this list may have a universal effect, there are some irritants that pose no problems whatsoever."

Apples/apple juice
Applesauce
Apricots
Artichoke hearts
Aspirin
Bananas
Beer
Beets
Bell peppers
Blackberries
Buttermilk
Cantaloupe
Capers
Carbonated
   beverages
Chili
Chocolate
Coffee
Cottage cheese
Cranberries/
   cranberry juice
Cream cheese

Cucumbers
Fruit cocktail
Grape juice
Grapefruit
Grapes
Honey
Horseradish
Ibuprofen
Jalapeños
Ketchup
Lemons
Lemonade
Limes
Molasses
Mustard
Nectarines
Olives
Onions
Oranges/
   orange juice
Pineapple/
   pineapple juice

Plums
Prunes
Raisins
Red cabbage
Red peppers
Sauerkraut
Seltzer
Soy sauce
Sports drinks
Strawberries
Tabasco sauce
Tea (black)
Tomatoes/tomato-
   based products
Tuna
Vinegar
Wine (red
   and white)
Worcestershire
   sauce
Yogurt

———————————RED FLAG———————————

When it comes to uncovering bladder irritants, there is a certain level of tweaking and healthy trial-and-error that comes into play. Finding what works for you is not an exact science.

OBESITY AND CONSTIPATION: LOSE WEIGHT, GET REGULAR!

According to a study published in 2010, obese men were more likely to have severe OAB symptoms when compared to their thinner counterparts. Men with a body mass index over 30 were significantly more likely to have more voids per day, more urge incontinence episodes, and more severe urgency than those with a BMI of 30 or less.

The exact cause for the relationship between obesity and urinary symptoms is unknown, but like many of the diseases discussed in this book, being overweight or obese seems to exacerbate male health issues, from cardiovascular disease, to sexual function, to urination symptoms.

For unclear reasons, there is an association between constipation and overactive bladder in both men and women, especially in the elderly. Increasing dietary fiber can reduce constipation and help establish regular bowel movements, which may possibly reduce OAB symptoms. Men with OAB should not delay the urge to eliminate but rather empty their bowel immediately when there is the sensation of fullness.

BEHAVIORAL THERAPY

Another OAB management strategy is changing particular urination habits that may be worsening OAB symptoms. Bladder training involves working with a health care professional to learn how to resist the feeling of urgency and postpone voiding. This approach, timed voiding, means urinating according to a timetable rather than in response to a feeling of urgency.

Your program will entail the use of special exercises and a bladder diary. Be patient: a bladder training program can take two months or longer to result in improvement. This training is often recommended in addition to taking prescription OAB medications. (See next section.)

STARTING THE BLADDER RETRAINING PROGRAM

Dr. Patricia Goode has been medical director of the Continence Clinic at the University of Alabama at Birmingham for twenty years and has directed the Continence Clinic at the Birmingham Veterans Affairs

Medical Center for the past decade. She's very familiar with OAB and treats it effectively with a multistep plan that begins below. "After an extended period of frequent urination, the bladder 'thermostat' that controls the amount of urine the bladder holds is set at a very low volume and needs to be 'reset' to a higher volume," explains Dr. Goode.

"Surprisingly, in treating OAB, you may be asked to drink more water. Since many people significantly restrict the intake of water and other beverages in the mistaken belief that this will eliminate their OAB symptoms, in actuality the now highly concentrated and dark yellow urine can irritate the bladder and result in the need to urinate even when the bladder is far from full.

"Therefore, in order to encourage your bladder to hold a larger volume, the urine going into your bladder should be as dilute and nonirritating as possible. This happens when you drink plenty of water."

Dr. Goode warns that when you first start drinking more water, you may find that the urinary frequency actually increases, but that will change when your bladder gradually adapts. Progress should be monitored with your voiding diary. Over time, you will gradually see an increase in the volume of urine that you void.

Dr. Goode uses the following bladder retraining program with her OAB patients and has had a great deal of success with it:

Step 1: Change old habits.

1. **Cut back or eliminate all caffeinated and alcoholic beverages.** Caffeine has a diuretic effect and increases urine production, and alcohol decreases the production of antidiuretic hormone (ADH), leading to increased urine production. See what happens when you scale back or stop drinking these beverages.

2. **Drink at least one quart of water per day, gradually increasing to two quarts per day.** If you are already consuming more than two quarts of water daily, your urgency and frequency may improve a good bit by cutting back to just two quarts. However, don't drink less fluid if you perspire considerably or if you must drink lots of water to prevent kidney stones.

3. **When you get the urge to urinate, try to hold it for five minutes before going to the bathroom.** Each week, add five min-

utes to the length of time that you hold the urine after you have the urge. Initially, you might want to try this in the safety of your own home until you build skill and confidence.

4. **Your goal is to hold between 300 and 400 milliliters (about a third of a quart) of urine in your bladder and urinate every two to four hours during the day.** Once you have your bladder capacity at a larger volume, you can gradually decrease your fluid intake and decrease the frequency of urination. However, you will want to continue drinking enough fluids to keep your urine pale yellow and prevent the concentrated urine from irritating the bladder and causing urgency.

Step 2: Perform Pelvic Floor Muscle Training Exercises.

The pelvic floor muscles are an important component of the urination process, and these exercises can be a vital part of a bladder retraining program. Commonly called Kegel (*Kay*-gull) exercises (after Arnold H. Kegel, MD, a gynecologist who developed them), these simple exercises can help restore a more normal urination pattern.

Pelvic exercises can be effective because the neural system is "plastic," meaning that it can be molded and reprogrammed. Just think about it: a young child is toilet trained, learns to feed himself, hold a pencil, ride a tricycle. As each new skill is mastered, it is imprinted within the brain. In addition, stimulation of the sphincteric muscles with a pelvic floor contraction can lead to bladder muscle (detrusor) relaxation. With pelvic floor exercises, we try to reprogram the entire urinary process, teaching the bladder to respond as it once did.

Here's how to perform pelvic floor muscle training exercises:

Get started by locating the muscle to be exercised. As you begin urinating, try to stop or slow the urine stream *without* tensing the muscles of your legs, buttocks, or abdomen. The muscles that you want to contract are those that are used to keep from passing gas. When contracting the appropriate muscles, you should feel a lifting sensation, like the penis is being elevated.

Now you are ready to exercise regularly. Set aside two times each day for exercising and performing the following contractions while standing:

Quick contractions (QC). Tighten and relax the pelvic floor as rapidly as you can.

Slow contractions (SC). Contract the pelvic floor and hold to a count of three (gradually increasing to a count of ten per exercise), and then *relax* completely before the next contraction. Relax for as long as you contracted, in order to allow the muscle to build strength optimally.

In the beginning, check yourself frequently by placing one hand on your abdomen and buttocks to ensure that you do not feel your belly, thigh, or buttock muscles move. If there is movement, continue to experiment until you have isolated the muscles of the pelvic floor. See page 208 for the specific eight-week OAB pelvic floor program.

Step 3: Use your pelvic floor muscles to prevent urgency and leakage.

1. **Although you may think that you need to rush to make it to the toilet, doing so can make urgency worse.** You may have noticed that the closer you get to the toilet, the more likely you are to experience leakage. You can get control of your urgency before you start walking to the bathroom. Here's how: Standing still, do repeated quick contractions of your pelvic floor muscles until the urgent sensation calms. Try this at home first with minor urgency so that you develop skill and confidence. Remember: don't rush. "Freeze and squeeze."

2. **If urgency comes back on the way to the bathroom, freeze and squeeze again** until the urgency is under control. If in public, look at your cell phone or wristwatch, and no one will know what you are doing.

3. **Contractions of the pelvic floor muscles can prevent sudden urgency and incontinence.** Contract your pelvic floor muscles as you get out of the car or golf cart; when you stand up from the bed or a chair; or when you sneeze, cough, or laugh. This will help prevent accidental urine loss. If you forget, and the

urgency comes on, freeze and squeeze until you are in control. Don't rush to the bathroom.

TREATING OAB WITH MEDICATION

A review of thirteen trials with a total of more than 1,700 patients enrolled found that those taking OAB drugs were more likely to see their symptoms improve than were those treated only with bladder training. But combined drug treatment and simultaneous bladder training appeared to be more effective than drug therapy alone. Given the potential side effects of medications, it makes sense to begin managing overactive bladder through lifestyle and behavioral changes first, adding medication only if a nondrug approach fails to reduce symptoms.

There are safe and effective prescription drugs for OAB that can enhance the storage of urine, acting locally in the bladder and centrally within the brain. But the main class of drugs used to relieve OAB symptoms are called antimuscarinics—so named because of the bladder receptors they block. While once thought to relieve symptoms by blocking bladder contractions, the latest evidence suggests that antimuscarinics also improve the receptacle's ability to store urine by decreasing the sensation of bladder filling. The patient taking one of these drugs might get the "message" that the bladder is full less often, and avoid an embarrassing accident.

While antimuscarinics are the standard medical therapy for OAB, they are not without some adverse side effects, including dry mouth, dry eyes, and constipation. Drug companies are working to develop more bladder-specific medicines that will not affect other organs, thereby reducing the risk of side effects.

Here are the most commonly used drugs for alleviating symptoms from overactive bladder:

Detrol/Detrol LA (tolterodine)
Ditropan/Ditropan XL (oxybutynin)
Enablex (darifenacin)
Gelnique gel (oxybutynin)
Oxytrol (a transdermal, or skin, patch) (oxybutynin)
Sanctura/Sanctura XR (trospium)
Toviaz (fesoterodine)
Vesicare (solifenacin)

Patients often find if one medication doesn't work satisfactorily, another one might. It's not uncommon for a physician to take a trial-and-error approach to finding the drug that works best for a particular patient.

OAB DRUGS AND THE BRAIN

Some patients taking an antimuscarinic drug, particularly the elderly, can show a decline in cognitive function such as memory loss, confusion, or hallucinations. This occurs because the receptors that the drug blocks to improve OAB symptoms are present in the brain as well as the bladder. While most patients taking these drugs will not experience symptoms related to brain function, if you do, you should discontinue the medication immediately and contact the physician who prescribed it.

WHEN NOTHING SEEMS TO WORK

For some men, even the combination of lifestyle changes and antimuscarinic drugs does not relieve overactive bladder symptoms. At that point, it's time to consider more detailed studies of the bladder (if they haven't been done already) to characterize its ability to fill properly and the extent to which the organ contracts abnormally. Armed with this information, the alternatives can then include Botox injections into the bladder and the use of a special nerve-stimulation device.

BOTOX: IT'S NOT JUST FOR WRINKLES

Small injected amounts of Botox (botulinum toxin type A) can be used to temporarily paralyze overactive muscles causing spasticity from cerebral palsy or strokes, spasms of the vocal cords, torticollis (twisted neck), writer's cramp, bladder dysfunction, and facial wrinkles. Treatment effects are temporary, usually lasting about three months or more, at which time it needs to be repeated.

Many clinical trials evaluating Botox injections have reported that they were more effective than both no treatment and other forms of management such as antimuscarinic drugs, in improving the quality of life of patients with overactive bladder. Botox also reduced urgency and incontinence episodes, and increased bladder storage capacity.

The powerful neurotoxin is injected into the bladder muscle at multiple sites, and works by blocking the release of acetylcholine, the chemical that signals the bladder muscle to contract. Botox, considered experimental in the US for treating OAB, recently received FDA approval to treat the spasticity that occurs in muscles of the elbow, wrist, and fingers after strokes, brain injuries, and with neurological disease such as multiple sclerosis. It is approved for other disorders that lead to spasticity of muscles as well.

Botox has not yet been approved by the FDA for use in treating overactive bladder. However, in the off-label treatment of the ailment, that is, in treating a condition other than the one for which it received FDA approval, many doctors report that office-based injections twice a year are often all that's needed to keep patients with even severe OAB symptom free. But Botox should be used only when less invasive options such as lifestyle and behavioral changes—with or without antimuscarinics—don't work. As with any invasive procedure, Botox injections used to treat OAB can cause side effects, including urinary retention and urinary tract infections.

A PACEMAKER FOR THE BLADDER

Another option for OAB patients when symptoms do not respond to nonsurgical approaches is the implantation of a tiny electrical generator under the skin in the upper buttock area to stimulate the sacral nerves with mild electrical impulses, which influences the pelvic floor muscles and sphincters that control urination. The device is implanted in a minimally invasive surgical procedure that is typically performed under local anesthesia as an outpatient. Sacral nerve stimulation was approved by the FDA in 1997 for patients who are unresponsive to all other treatment options. This is termed refractory overactive bladder.

It might seem counterintuitive that stimulation of the pelvic floor muscles could reduce OAB symptoms, when the problem is bladder overactivity. But the fact that it works, even though we don't know how, is further evidence that we still have a lot to learn about what causes OAB. Sacral nerve stimulation, in some patients, affects nerve signals that have gone awry, allowing appropriate filling and storage of urine within the bladder.

In a review of trials evaluating sacral nerve stimulation, some patients experienced a reduction in symptoms, but not without a risk of chronic pain and the need to have the device removed. About two in three patients achieved a 50 percent improvement in frequency or incontinence episodes.

THE EIGHT-WEEK PELVIC FLOOR
MUSCLE REHABILITATION SCHEDULE

Example: During week 1, perform five quick contractions *twice* daily, ten slow contractions and relaxations to a count of three, and five quick contractions.

Week 1
5 Quick Contractions, 10-3 sec Short Contractions, 5 Quick Contractions

Date	Day	A.M.	P.M.
_____	Monday	___	___
_____	Tuesday	___	___
_____	Wednesday	___	___
_____	Thursday	___	___
_____	Friday	___	___
_____	Saturday	___	___
_____	Sunday	___	___

Week 2
10 Quick Contractions, 15 4-sec Short Contractions, 10 Quick Contractions

Date	Day	A.M.	P.M.
_____	Monday	___	___
_____	Tuesday	___	___
_____	Wednesday	___	___
_____	Thursday	___	___
_____	Friday	___	___
_____	Saturday	___	___
_____	Sunday	___	___

Week 3

15 Quick Contractions, 20 5-sec Short Contractions, 15 Quick Contractions

Date	Day	A.M.	P.M.
_____	Monday	____	____
_____	Tuesday	____	____
_____	Wednesday	____	____
_____	Thursday	____	____
_____	Friday	____	____
_____	Saturday	____	____
_____	Sunday	____	____

Week 4

15 Quick Contractions, 20 6-sec Short Contractions, 15 Quick Contractions

Date	Day	A.M.	P.M.
_____	Monday	____	____
_____	Tuesday	____	____
_____	Wednesday	____	____
_____	Thursday	____	____
_____	Friday	____	____
_____	Saturday	____	____
_____	Sunday	____	____

Week 5

20 Quick Contractions, 20 7-sec Short Contractions, 20 Quick Contractions

Date	Day	A.M.	P.M.
_____	Monday	____	____
_____	Tuesday	____	____
_____	Wednesday	____	____
_____	Thursday	____	____
_____	Friday	____	____
_____	Saturday	____	____
_____	Sunday	____	____

Week 6

30 Quick Contractions, 25 8-sec Short Contractions, 30 Quick Contractions

Date	Day	A.M.	P.M.
_____	Monday	___	___
_____	Tuesday	___	___
_____	Wednesday	___	___
_____	Thursday	___	___
_____	Friday	___	___
_____	Saturday	___	___
_____	Sunday	___	___

Week 7

40 Quick Contractions, 25 9-sec Short Contractions, 40 Quick Contractions

Date	Day	A.M.	P.M.
_____	Monday	___	___
_____	Tuesday	___	___
_____	Wednesday	___	___
_____	Thursday	___	___
_____	Friday	___	___
_____	Saturday	___	___
_____	Sunday	___	___

Week 8

50 Quick Contractions, 25 10-sec Short Contractions, 50 Quick Contractions

Date	Day	A.M.	P.M.
_____	Monday	___	___
_____	Tuesday	___	___
_____	Wednesday	___	___
_____	Thursday	___	___
_____	Friday	___	___
_____	Saturday	___	___
_____	Sunday	___	___

Continue performing sets of fifty. Increase if desired. The total number can be divided up during the course of the entire day.

VOIDING DIARY RECORD

Record the date and time and answer every question each time you go to the toilet and/or have a leakage episode. This chart should be maintained for at least seventy-two consecutive hours.

Date	Time	Volume: Void (in Milliliters or Ounces)	Leakage Episode (Urge/Stress)	Severity: S=Slight; M=Moderate; H=Heavy

Date	Time	Volume: Void (in Milliliters or Ounces)	Leakage Episode (Urge/Stress)	Severity: S=Slight; M=Moderate; H=Heavy

THE TAKEAWAY

- The major symptom of overactive bladder is urgency: a sudden desire to urinate that cannot be deferred.

- OAB symptoms can also include urinary frequency and incontinence associated with urgency.

- OAB symptoms result from an inability to store urine, without the frequent sensation of the need to void, and associated urges that can be accompanied by incontinence.

- OAB is often misdiagnosed as a prostate problem in males.

- Many people mistakenly think that nothing can be done to treat overactive bladder and their untreated symptoms can lead to diminished quality of life. But most cases can be managed successfully with a combination of lifestyle changes and drug therapy.

- When less invasive approaches do not relieve OAB symptoms, Botox injections into the bladder or sacral nerve stimulation with an implantable device can improve bladder storage and alleviate symptoms.

PART THREE

INFLAMMATION OF THE PROSTATE

If you have tears,
prepare to shed them now.

—William Shakespeare

PROSTATITIS: IF YOU DON'T UNDERSTAND IT, RECLASSIFY IT

Prostatitis is defined as an inflammatory disease of the prostate. You have to understand that inflammation is not equal to an infection, but inflammation can be caused by an infection. And that's where the problem begins with prostatitis: with the terminology.

Imagine going to a major league baseball game, sitting in a great seat along the third baseline, and then getting hit in your arm by a foul ball. You will have intense inflammation at the site of injury, and it will be red, warm, and swollen. This inflammation is not caused by an infection. On the other hand, if you nick your finger with pruning shears while working in your rose garden, you may develop an infection under the skin, and there will be an intense inflammatory reaction due to the infection. If an infection had not occurred, you might never have noticed the inflammation from the simple nick of the skin.

Similarly, inflammation of the prostate can result from infections, but not always. And it gets more complicated because the symptoms that are associated with prostatic inflammation may be present without any inflammation or evidence of an infection.

Confused yet? Don't worry. Physicians were confused for decades—and many still are, but less so today thanks to a number of clinical scientists who have taken on the mission of understanding one of the most misunderstood diseases in all of medicine: prostatitis.

Prostatitis that is caused by a bacterial infection is easy to diagnose, and the treatment is straightforward: a course of antibiotics. This is not so for the 90 percent of men that have prostatitis-like symptoms, which often consist of debilitating pain, no evidence of a bacterial cause, and no obvious reason whatsoever for the symptoms. This enigmatic nonbacterial disorder is now referred to as chronic prostatitis/chronic pelvic pain syndrome. We call it CP/CPPS for short.

REEXAMINING PROSTATITIS

There is an old adage in medicine: if you don't understand it, reclassify it. And that is just what has happened with prostatitis. Looking back, we have been through four distinct periods with the diagnosis and treatment of this disease. In the early 1900s, the first period, men who came to the doctor's office with symptoms suggestive of prostatitis—including pelvic and genital pain, back pain, fatigue, and post-ejaculatory pain—were most often treated by prostatic massage in an effort to clear the prostate and its passages from the buildup of retained secretions. A finger was inserted into the anus and pressed against the rectal wall to put pressure on the prostate. This was the only treatment available, and it worked well for some.

During the second period in the mid 1900s, antibiotics were the mainstay of treatment for virtually everyone suspected of having prostatitis. Of course, the antibiotics didn't work well when no infection was present, but they were prescribed nonetheless because nothing else was available. Many doctors simply hoped that the placebo effect would take over and help those who were in such obvious pain. It obviously didn't, since many men with excruciating pain went on to see numerous doctors in their pursuit of a cure.

The next era in prostatitis treatment began in the 1960s with a method for identifying an infection within the prostate, based on the laboratory analysis of prostatic secretions in the urine after a digital rectal examination. Armed with this information, many urologists began to prescribe antibiotics only to those with a prostate-specific infection.

But that left the vast majority of men with prostatitis symptoms and no evidence of infection in limbo, with no cause for their disorder and no viable treatment options. Enter the National Institutes of Health, the efforts of which marked the beginning of the fourth distinct prostatitis era in 1995. Leading prostatitis experts convened for a workshop to better understand and treat prostatitis. Out of this brainstorming session came the NIH classification of prostatitis that now emphasizes that pain is the characteristic and distinguishing feature of nonbacterial chronic prostatitis. This is called chronic prostatitis/chronic pelvic pain syndrome, or CP/CPPS. Perhaps more importantly, the NIH workshop led to the formation of a collaborative research network comprised of urologists, psychiatrists, pain specialists, and physical therapists that has conducted many of the landmark studies to further our understanding of the extent of the disease among men. These medical experts have attempted to describe who gets CPPS, how costly it is, what happens over time to men who have it, how we quantify the associated symptoms, how we can track symptom changes with and without treatment, and how best to treat it. Due to their efforts, we have learned more about CP/CPPS in the last ten years than in the entire previous century.

In the upcoming chapter, I will explore the basics of the different types of prostatitis and review the latest thinking on diagnosing and treating CPPS. I will also detail some of the most recent discoveries that finally give hope to men with this painful, debilitating, and baffling inflammatory prostate condition.

CHAPTER EIGHT

CHRONIC PROSTATITIS/CHRONIC PELVIC PAIN SYNDROME

A Painful Condition with a New Name and Revolutionary New Ways to Treat It

Pain is such an uncomfortable feeling that even a tiny
amount of it is enough to ruin every enjoyment.

—Will Rogers

Years ago, Trevor had been diagnosed with prostatitis, an infection of his prostate gland, and even though he had seen several doctors, they had told him there was nothing they could do to help him.

The pain was typically a deep, dull ache in his perineum, that soft, smooth area between his anus and scrotum. On a scale of 0 to 10, with 10 being teeth-gritting unbearable, his personal pain meter usually fluctuated between 2 and 8, shooting to 10 after every ejaculation.

"At the peak of orgasm, it feels as if someone were pinching me behind my testicle, tugging it back toward my anus," he told me during his first visit to my office. "It is unbearable. It feels like fire shooting through my penis. At first I tried to ignore it and tried to concentrate on the sex, which is supposed to be one of life's great pleasures. I kept telling myself that it would probably get better on its own. But it didn't. After a while, sex became something that I avoided."

No over-the-counter pain medication seemed to bring Trevor prolonged relief. After talking with a clerk at a health food store, he started drinking cranberry juice and decaffeinated coffee, and this seemed to help for a week and then stopped. One doctor he went to see said that he had prostatodynia. When Trevor asked what it was, the doctor said it was another name for a painful prostate. He gave him a prescription for ciprofloxacin (Cipro). This powerful antibiotic seemed to take the pain level down several notches, although it never knocked it out completely. Then, for no apparent reason, the drug quit working after just five weeks.

Once his pain resumed, Trevor's depression, which by now had become an everyday part of his life, returned in full force too. "I knew that I wasn't crazy," he reflected. "I knew that there was something very real going on with me, despite the fact that no one had any answers. I was back in my living hell."

WHAT'S THIS LEADING TO?
IT MUST BE SOMETHING VERY BAD

In the back of Trevor's mind was an even bigger fear: that one day this pain would lead to prostate or testicular cancer. Adding to his daily unease was the fact that he was totally convinced this pain would be with him for the rest of his life.

Of the eight doctors Trevor had seen, all had ruled out testicular cancer. Three told him that he had benign prostatic enlargement, or BPE, and treated him with medication designed to ease his urinary flow. But after a new urologist examined him and diagnosed him with kidney stones, not BPE, this soon led to a urogram, a detailed x-ray of his urinary system. Trevor waited with baited breath for the results of the test.

"Good news!" his urologist finally told him over the phone. "Your urinary system is okay."

Plunged back into a deep funk, Trevor rallied several weeks later and went to another urologist, who suspected a possible problem with his bowels. "It could be a tumor in the colon that is causing the pain," he told Trevor, and directed him to a colorectal specialist.

When Trevor awakened shortly after his colonoscopy exam was finished, the smiling medical expert informed him, "You have no tumor, inflammatory bowel disease, or polyps in your colon. You get a clean bill of health." For most people, of course, that would be great news, but not for Trevor, who once again was left without an explanation for his excruciating pain.

Several months of his medical odyssey were also marked by numerous visits to a psychologist and then to a psychiatrist. Both suspected that Trevor was depressed (he was), which was causing him to "overexpress"—in other words, exaggerate—the pain in his pelvic region. Find a way to lift that "darkness" from his life, the psychiatrist counseled him, and the prostatitis would ease up, if not disappear.

Trevor then started and stopped four different antidepressants during an eighteen-month span. The terrible physical pain remained, the depression never really lifted, and he marked his fiftieth birthday alienated from his teenage daughter and wife, sitting in front of the TV watching a football game. When asked to describe his life at the half-century mark, he had one word: miserable.

PROSTATITIS: FORGET THAT
YOU EVER HEARD THE TERM

As unsettling and bizarre as it may seem, Trevor's medical odyssey is not all that unique. For men with pelvic pain who have been diagnosed with prostatitis, the search for relief—from the pain between the scrotum and rectum that typically radiates to the testes—is continual. Unfortunately, many never get any help. That's because they have been misdiagnosed with a condition that doctors call *prostatitis*.

Prostatitis is a medical term that is used too often to describe a constellation of symptoms for which there is no easy explanation. Physicians are beginning to replace it with chronic prostatitis/chronic pelvic pain syndrome: CP/CPPS, or CPPS for short. Granted, it's a mouthful but a better term because it more clearly defines the medical syndrome from which millions of men in the United States actually suffer. No longer do we consider this to be a stand-alone medical problem caused by an infection within the prostate (prostatitis); instead we recognize that the symptoms are probably the result of a combination of inflammation and/or dysfunction of pelvic organs, including nerves and muscles. Not surprisingly, after months, oftentimes years with this untreated problem, patients frequently develop psychosocial issues

With this name change from prostatitis to CPPS comes better management, because it alerts patients and doctors that this is a syndrome, not an infection of the prostate meant to be treated with antibiotics. The name change also helps steer patients to a team of medical experts— urologists, physical therapists, psychiatrists, psychologists, pain specialists—who can help provide the care that they may need.

We now define CPPS as chronic pelvic pain lasting three months or more, with no signs of bacterial infection. In most cases, CPPS patients have experienced an inciting event, such as trauma to or inflammation of the prostate or urinary tract. Although the inciting event has subsided, it brought about changes in the urinary tract and surrounding muscles and nerves, generating chronic diffuse pain throughout the area just outside of the prostate. This, in turn, can cause the pelvic floor muscles to tighten. CPPS does not usually respond to anti-inflammatory medications or long-term antibiotics, which had been the common course of treatment offered for the past few decades.

THE PATIENT PROFILE

Patients who suffer CPPS tend to be very similar in their disposition. The symptoms that they present with and their levels of pain and discomfort vary, but they are easily recognized, and Trevor was no exception.

First and foremost, many CPPS sufferers are supremely frustrated. Can you blame them? Their desperate search for answers and relief, an undertaking that has spanned many years, tends to end consistently in bitter disappointment. As you saw with Trevor, it is not uncommon for patients to visit dozens of doctors, covering the full spectrum of disciplines. Along the way, they shed the comforts of a stable life; their priority is to limit the pain.

Anxiety plays a huge role in the life of a patient with CPPS. This may be a direct result of the CPPS itself or its cause, but that remains to be seen. Many of these men believe that they must have a life-threatening ailment, such as prostate cancer. Not only do many assume that they are near death, they believe it is a foregone conclusion and that there is simply no way to alter that dire scenario.

Another very common source of intense anxiety is the unshakable thought of having contracted some obscure sexually transmitted disease. Some men will even recall the exact date and time that they had unprotected sex, with this being the moment that everything changed for the worse. Furthermore, they keep replaying the event over and over again in their minds, each time beating themselves up for not wearing a condom. This feeling of guilt becomes overwhelming.

It doesn't help a person's stress level if he's convinced that he is dying of cancer or suffering from some type of STD, and he keeps being referred to medical specialists in these fields. Many have lost faith in the profession's ability to make their lives better. Traditionally, physicians are perceived as the problem solvers, as the folks with answers, and when that perception is betrayed, these men feel that they have no one to turn to anymore. Their sense of hope evaporates.

Many patients with CPPS are very melancholic. It then becomes the doctor's job to coach them back to life and to let them know that as dismal as it may seem, they are not alone.

CP/CPPS: MISDIAGNOSED, INAPPROPRIATELY TREATED

Of the three prostate-related conditions that this book covers in great detail (the others being lower urinary tract symptoms and prostate cancer), chronic prostatitis/chronic pelvic pain syndrome is the least understood and the most inappropriately treated of all. Not only is CP/CPPS the most common urologic diagnosis in men younger than fifty, it is the third most common urologic diagnosis in men older than fifty (after LUTS and prostate cancer). Some experts estimate that there are more than 270,000 new cases of CP/CPPS each year. According to the National Institutes of Health, as many as 35 percent of all men over age fifty have this perplexing condition, which sends them to urologists' offices in record numbers. It's estimated that 3 percent to 12 percent of all visits to the urologist are for CP/CPPS complaints. Due to high levels of misdiagnosis and subsequent multiple visits to doctors' offices, the cost to the health care system is now more than $84 million annually. In a study of the cost of CPPS, investigators found that the average annual total cost of almost $4,500 per patient was higher than that for rheumatoid arthritis and low back pain.

What follows is an explanation of the differences between (1) acute and chronic bacterial prostatitis, both of which are caused by an infection and can be successfully treated with medication; and (2) CPPS, which has no known cause but is treatable. Multiple therapies are available that may help relieve symptoms, oftentimes permanently.

CLASSIFYING PROSTATITIS

Based on a 1995 consensus workshop of the National Institutes of Health (NIH), there are now four major categories of prostatitis:

1. **Acute bacterial prostatitis.** This acute bacterial infection of the prostate gland accounts for 2 percent to 5 percent of cases of prostatitis and responds to antibiotics.

2. **Chronic bacterial prostatitis.** This recurrent bacterial infection of the prostate accounts for another 2 percent to 5 percent of cases and responds to antibiotics given for a longer duration.

3. **Chronic nonbacterial prostatitis/chronic pelvic pain syndrome (CP/CPPS).** CP/CPPS, defined by pelvic pain lasting at least three months, is the most common type and accounts for 90 percent to 95 percent of all cases. No infectious cause can be found.

   It may be either inflammatory (classified as IIIA) or noninflammatory (IIIB), based on the presence or absence of white blood cells in the prostatic fluid. White blood cells serve as our personal bodyguards. Whenever a germ appears or an infection starts, white blood cells increase in number and go into attack mode to battle the infection.

4. **Asymptomatic inflammatory prostatitis.** In this particular ailment, the prevalence of which is unknown, the patient does not have any symptoms, but white blood cells, which are signs of infection, are observed in prostatic secretions or prostate tissue.

CATEGORY 1: ACUTE BACTERIAL PROSTATITIS

Acute bacterial prostatitis, which is caused by a bacterial infection that has worked its way into ducts within the prostate from the urethra, can be triggered by urinary retention, unprotected anal sex, and a variety of immune disorders. Also, the commonly performed prostate biopsy to rule out prostate cancer in men with an abnormality on prostate examination or a suspicious PSA test can result in acute prostatitis.

As with any other infection, the body's immune system sends chemicals to the area to attack the foreign invader. A high fever with a temperature over 100 degrees, muscle aches, chills, and pain in the lower back and perineum are not uncommon with the ailment.

Urinary frequency, urgency, and burning (dysuria) upon urination are also common, as is difficulty urinating due to the infection (stranguary). I liken the latter symptom to having a throat infection. When your throat is infected, you try not to swallow due to the pain. The same thing happens when the lining of the urinary tract (prostate, urethra, and bladder) are infected. When it comes time to urinate, you'll naturally hesitate on account of the swelling and pain, and you will void very little urine as a consequence.

EFFECTIVE TREATMENT FOR ACUTE BACTERIAL PROSTATITIS

While CP/CPPS is common and difficult to manage, acute bacterial prostatitis is relatively easy to identify. Urinary complaints are common and, in addition to a high fever, many men have lower abdominal symptoms as well. While performing a digital rectal exam (DRE), the doctor finds that the prostate is tender.

Once a urine culture has been taken to attempt to culture the organisms causing the infection, antibiotics will be used to kill the offending bacteria. The most common drugs used are fluoroquinolones, a class of agents that includes levofloxacin (Levaquin) and ciprofloxacin (Cipro). They zero in on prostatic tissue and are able to kill most bacteria within a few days.

While pain, fever, and chills may disappear within forty-eight to seventy-two hours, drug treatment typically extends from two to six weeks to ensure that all bacteria are eradicated. If there are accompanying urinary difficulties, I will oftentimes prescribe Flomax (tamsulosin), Cardura (doxazosin), Hytrin (terazosin), or UroXatral (alfuzosin), to be taken along with the antibiotics.

In some cases, men who have developed urinary retention will use a catheter to allow urine to pass until the swelling in the prostate or urethra finally resolves. If the symptoms do not improve, then it could be that the bacteria in question are not sensitive to that particular antibiotic and another should be tried.

A more serious scenario is when the acute infection is not adequately treated and an abscess forms within the prostate. This is diagnosed by ultrasound or a computed tomography (CT) scan, a machine that combines a series of X-ray views taken from many different angles to produce cross-sectional images of the body's soft tissues. The prostate must be drained to rid the body of infection. Drainage can be performed through the urethra with endoscopic instruments.

The good news is that once the infection has been eradicated, prostate pain disappears, and the problem is often resolved forever. Even so, there are many men who are often frightened by the increase in PSA that can occur with acute prostatitis; levels above 20 to 30 nanograms per milliliter (ng/ml) are not uncommon. There is no reason to measure PSA during an episode of prostatitis, since it will be elevated from inflammation and leakage of prostate-specific antigen into the blood. With antibiotics, the PSA will usually return to baseline values, but this often takes months.

CATEGORY 2: CHRONIC BACTERIAL PROSTATITIS

Chronic bacterial prostatitis typically develops because the original acute bacterial prostatitis was inadequately treated: either for too short a duration or with the wrong antibiotic. The infection may also stem from prostatic calculi, tiny stones found within the prostate in which the bacteria can "hide" and remain untreated. Symptoms of this chronic variant are similar to acute prostatitis (without the fever and chills, however) and include urinary symptoms and pain.

While a relatively rare ailment (comprising about 5 percent of all cases), men with bacterial prostatitis need a follow-up urine culture. Based on the bacteria that are present, fluoroquinolones will typically be prescribed for an additional six weeks or longer. Cure rates generally approach 70 percent, but follow-up evaluations are needed to ensure that the drugs have, in fact, worked. Patients whose symptoms have recurred after initial treatment will eventually be cured following long-term antibiotic therapy.

CATEGORY 3: CHRONIC NONBACTERIAL PROSTATITIS/ CHRONIC PELVIC PAIN SYNDROME

Nine in ten men diagnosed with "prostatitis" today do not have an infection within the prostate, and treatment with antibiotics does not help in most cases. These men with chronic nonbacterial prostatitis have chronic pelvic pain syndrome, or CP/CPPS. Sadly, they represent one of the most difficult management problems in urology because the underlying cause of this disorder is unknown. And while there is no evidence of a bacterial infection in men with nonbacterial CP/CPPS, some of these men may have developed the chronic pain disorder due to a *prior* infection within the prostate or urinary tract.

The term *prostatitis* comes from decades of misunderstanding the disease entity CPPS and attributing the cause of all prostatitis syndromes to bacteria. Even so, when most men complain to their doctor about pelvic pain that may or may not be combined with urinary symptoms, most doctors immediately think prostate infection. Out comes the prescription pad for an antibiotic—oftentimes without any testing whatsoever for a bacterial infection. A study conducted by a group of prostatitis investigators found that when compared to men on placebo, those treated with antibiotics did not exhibit any greater improvement in CPPS symptoms.

A kneejerk diagnosis and treatment with antibiotics made without indications of infection puts patients at risk for side effects from an antibiotic that can include diarrhea and allergic reactions. And then there is the real possibility of developing antibiotic resistance, making it more likely that a microorganism will be able to withstand the effects of this antibiotic in the future.

In many instances, the patient is urged to come back in a few weeks. But in reality, many doctors understand that the antibiotics won't work and that they have nothing else in their armamentarium to offer. And so they secretly hope that the patient will not return.

Unfortunately, men with CPPS have a reputation for being difficult to work with because of the chronic nature of their pain and their seemingly endless complaints. Many physicians view them as needy, demanding, and carrying lots of "psychological baggage," while others simply don't believe the patients' complaints.

However, CPPS patients' complaints are just as real as complaints from those with arthritis, fibromyalgia, or a broken ankle. Some of these men simply have the volume turned up too loud in the pain processing areas of their brains. They often need specialized physical therapy to rehabilitate their pelvic floor muscles, which have shortened, tightened, and gone into spasm, causing pain in the groin, abdominal area, back, and hips.

CATEGORY 4: ASYMPTOMATIC PROSTATITIS

It's estimated that about one-third of adult males are affected by asymptomatic prostatitis. However, most men never realize that they have this condition until a urologist, concerned about a rising PSA level, performs a rectal examination and massage of the prostate and discovers signs of inflammation after a microscopic exam of prostatic secretions that exit the urethra after the massage. Aymptomatic prostatitis may also be uncovered during an evaluation for infertility, a microscopic examination of surgically removed prostate tissue as treatment of bladder overflow obstruction, or examination of prostate biopsy tissue usually done for an elevated PSA.

In the case of elevated PSA and asymptomatic prostatitis, a two- to four-week course of antibiotics may eliminate an infection if present. If the PSA does not normalize, a biopsy may then be recommended to detect the presence of possible prostate cancer.

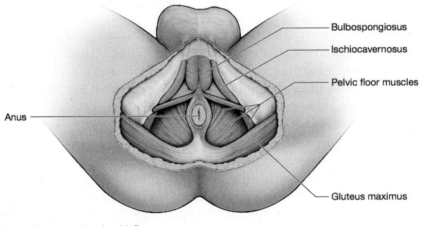

Muscles that support the male pelvic floor

THE PELVIC FLOOR

Many men are unaware of the pelvic floor, where it's located, what it consists of, what it does, and how things can go wrong with the various muscles there.

"The best way to describe the pelvis is to think about it as a bony ring," says Dr. Mary McVearry, a doctor of physical therapy at the Walter Reed National Military Medical Center in Bethesda, Maryland, and an expert in pelvic floor dysfunction. "On the bottom of it are a bowl of muscles that attach to the front, back, and sides of the pelvic bones and sacrum. They are used for postural support to help hold us erect, forming the basement of the well-known 'core.' Additionally, the pelvic floor muscles contract to help stop the flow of urination as well as relax appropriately to allow us to urinate and defecate. And lastly, the pelvic floor plays a role in sexual function by facilitating increased blood flow for erections and arousal."

Like a sling or hammock, the pelvic floor muscles support the organs of the pelvis, including the bladder, prostate, and rectum. These same muscles also wrap around the urethra and rectum, forming part of the sphincters that control urine and stool, respectively. There are also various blood vessels and nerves that innervate the pelvic floor, allowing for normal function. And just like anywhere else in your body, you can hold a lot of tension in these pelvic muscles—whether it be due to chronic inflammation, infection, trauma, postural deficits, or stress. Any surgery in the area, including a radical prostatectomy, can also affect the pelvic floor muscles.

"Many people with CPPS have problems with this specific group of muscles," Dr. McVearry says, "and it's usually related to too much pelvic floor tension. These muscles may spasm and remain in spasm, resulting in diffuse pelvic pain, pain with intercourse or sexual stimulation, and a variety of urination or bowel problems."

THE GOOD NEWS: YOUR AILMENT IS REAL— AND THERE IS HELP

CPPS produces pain in the pelvic region that lasts more than three months. Some men also experience urinary symptoms and pain during or after ejaculation. Studies have found that pain associated with ejaculation is one of the symptoms most characteristic of CPPS. Others have pains elsewhere in the abdomen and low back. Many patients have told me that it hurts when they sit down, as if they were sitting on a peach pit. Some say the pain is so unremitting that they feel like their lives are over.

Although the perineum is the most common site of pain, chronic pelvic pain syndrome can also be painful in the testes, the entire penis, the shaft or the tip of the penis, the mid to lower abdomen, and the lower back. The pain can occur in one or several of these sites.

The discomfort of CPPS tends to wax and wane, and some days it is much worse than others. For some men, the pain suddenly disappears, only to reappear weeks, sometimes months, later. There's no good explanation as to why that is. We do know that ejaculation is the activity that most exacerbates the pain. Not surprisingly, the frequency of a man's sexual encounters often plummets after he develops CPPS. It's tough to get in the mood when you know beforehand the pain that awaits at climax.

According to urologic researchers, the decline in quality of life due to CPPS is on a par with Crohn's disease (intestinal inflammation), heart pain (angina), and type 2 diabetes. The unrelenting discomfort men feel is often so severe that some take extended leave from their jobs, while others simply quit because their work output has been compromised.

Surprisingly, for all the difficulty that the ailment causes, chronic pelvic pain syndrome is not life threatening. Unfortunately, it is not highly responsive to any one type of therapy. Since there are no known cures for it, the ailment tends to be ignored or minimized by doctors. However, a urologist with an understanding of this malady can find the best combination of therapies to suit your individual situation. There are many things we can now do to help manage CPPS symptoms and significantly improve your quality of life. Read on!

UPOINT

A major recent breakthrough in the understanding of chronic pelvic pain syndrome is the UPOINT system for conceptualizing the syndrome. Thanks to the breakthrough work of two urologists who have spent more than two decades collectively researching CPPS, doctors are now slowly coming to understand that effective treatment must be individualized, with the symptoms noted and placed into specific phenotypes (characteristics), or domains. We realize now that CPPS is a syndrome, not one specific disease with one specific therapy.

In 2009 Daniel A. Shoskes, MD, a urologist at Cleveland Clinic's Glickman Urological and Kidney Institute, and J. Curtis Nickel, professor of urology at Queens University in Kingston, Ontario, described their hypothesis at the annual scientific meeting of the American Urological Association in Chicago. Their UPOINT (a mnemonic for urinary, psychosocial, organ specific, infection, neurologic/systemic, tenderness of skeletal muscles) system is used by physicians to assess the whole patient with CPPS, noting and then categorizing his specific complaints after a careful history has been taken and a physical examination performed.

"We don't have any validated disease markers for CPPS," notes Dr. Shoskes. "Nor do we have any blood or urine tests for this disorder. So I came up with a list of domains I knew from my own clinical experience to be discriminative.

"Men with CPPS all have different symptoms, but they can all be placed into certain categories based on their particular complaints," he continues. "And each of these categories has therapies that are proven to work for those specific symptoms. By phenotyping each patient, this allows for customized treatment plans and, most of all, validates all those patients who have long complained of more than just 'prostate problems' when seeking help from their doctors."

THE UPOINT EXAM: A UNIQUE MANAGEMENT STRATEGY

"It all starts with your doctor," says Dr. Shoskes. "If a patient is suspected of having CPPS, instead of registering complaints to his doctor and simply receiving a prescription for an antibiotic when he has no infection, or getting a bladder drug when he mainly has abdominal complaints, the savvy doctor knows that CPPS is heterogeneous and that categorizing a patient based on his underlying complaints and then treating those symptoms is the way to go."

This is how Dr. Shoskes conducts a CPPS exam utilizing UPOINT: A complete history is taken and a physical examination performed. The doctor documents pain location, frequency, and severity. Questions about urination are asked, as are questions about sexual functioning, recurrent urinary tract infections, sexually transmitted disease, genitourinary surgeries, and neurological conditions and symptoms.

The history also includes questions about irritable bowel syndrome, a common disorder of the large intestine that leads to abdominal pain and cramping, and changes in bowel movements. The doctor will also ask about nonurological and unexplained clinical conditions such as fibromyalgia, a common disorder characterized by long-term, body-wide pain and tenderness in the joints, muscles, tendons, and other soft tissues that's accompanied by fatigue, mood and memory issue; chronic fatigue syndrome, a complicated disorder characterized by severe and continued fatigue that's not relieved by rest and isn't directly caused by any other medical condition; low back pain; and migraine headaches.

Levels of depression, anxiety, stress, and incidences of catastrophizing are also reviewed.

Patients should arrive with a fairly full bladder so that a urine analysis and culture can be performed. Urine flow will be measured while urinating into a Uroflow device, a special urinal that allows the urologist to also determine such parameters as average flow and total voided volume. An ultrasound of the bladder will then be conducted to assess bladder emptying.

A two-glass urine test may also be obtained. Culture results of a midstream urine specimen will reflect cells and organisms from the bladder (first glass), and this specimen is compared to a urine sample collected after a prostatic massage (second glass) that will reflect cells and bacteria from the prostate shed into the urine.

"In addition, I ask that the NIH Chronic Prostatitis Symptom Index be completed," Dr. Shoskes says. (See below.) "I don't use this nine-question review as a diagnostic tool but simply to measure the degree of symptoms that the patient has."

NIH CHRONIC PROSTATITIS SYMPTOM INDEX

The National Institutes of Health Chronic Prostatitis Symptom Index, or CPSI, is a tool that provides an effective method to measure the extent of chronic pelvic pain. The beauty of the CPSI is that it is specifically designed to assess a man's current level of pain. It gets precise answers in four key domains: pain or discomfort, urination complaints, impact of symptoms, and quality of life impact.

This gives men an objective and extremely helpful evaluation of their current level of pain and discomfort. To be honest and fair to yourself, answer these questions truthfully. The object of the questionnaire is not to "pass" or "fail" but rather to give you the answers you need to procure the best solution to your problem and to track the success of treatments.

After circling the appropriate numbers, rate yourself with the accompanying scale. The CPSI will allow you and your doctor to identify the key areas of concern. In subsequent doctor visits, or after taking medication or undergoing physical therapy to treat your pelvic pain, you can chart your progress by filling out the questionnaire again and comparing your current responses to the previous results. Chances are good that your answers following treatment will reflect improvements both physically and psychologically. (Photocopy these pages so that you'll have a clean copy of the questionnaire when you want to reassess yourself.)

Note: For each question, please circle only one number.

Pain or Discomfort

1. In the last week, have you experienced any pain or discomfort in the following areas?

	Yes	No
a. Perineum (area between rectum and testicles)	1	0
b. Testicles	1	0
c. Tip of the penis (not related to urination)	1	0
d. Below your waist, in your pubic or bladder area	1	0

2. In the last week, have you experienced:

	Yes	No
a. Pain or burning during urination?	1	0
b. Pain or discomfort during or after sexual climax (ejaculation)	1	0

3. How often have you had pain or discomfort in any of these areas over the last week?

0 Never
1 Rarely
2 Sometimes
3 Often
4 Usually
5 Always

4. Which number best describes your *average* pain or discomfort on the days that you had it over the last week?

0   1   2   3   4   5   6   7   8   9   10
No pain   Pain as bad as you can imagine

Urinary Symptoms

5. How often have you had a sensation of not emptying your bladder completely after you finished urinating, over the last week?

0 Not at all
1 Less than one time in five
2 Less than half the time
3 About half the time
4 More than half the time
5 Almost always

6. How often have you had to urinate again less than two hours after you finished urinating, over the last week?

   0 Not at all

   1 Less than one time in five

   2 Less than half the time

   3 About half the time

   4 More than half the time

   5 Almost always

Impact of Symptoms

7. How much have your symptoms kept you from doing the kinds of things you would usually do, over the last week?

   0 None

   1 Only a little

   2 Some

   3 A lot

8. How much did you think about your symptoms over the last week?

   0 None

   1 Only a little

   2 Some

   3 A lot

Quality of Life

9. If you were to spend the rest of your life with your symptoms just the way they have been during the last week, how would you feel about that?

   0 Delighted

   1 Pleased

   2 Mostly satisfied

   3 Mixed (about equally satisfied and dissatisfied)

   4 Mostly dissatisfied

   5 Unhappy

   6 Terrible

What the Scores Mean

All the queries break down into four specific areas, or domains, as follows. Add your scores to the appropriate column on the right.

Pain or Discomfort: Total of items 1a, 1b, 1c, 1d, 2a, 2b, 3, and 4 =   _____

Urinary Symptoms: Total of items 5 and 6 =   _____

Impact of Symptoms and Quality of Life: Total of items 7, 8, and 9 =   _____

Total: _____

Mild = 0 to 9

Moderate = 10 to 18

Severe = 19 to 31

Adapted from M. S. Litwin, et al., "The National Institutes of Health Chronic Prostatitis Symptom Index: Development and Validation of a New Outcome Measure—Chronic Prostatitis Collaborative Research Network," *Journal of Urology* 162, no. 2 (August 1999): 369–75.

THE NEXT STEP

Answering the questionnaire and assessing your results will give you an honest indication of the extent and bother of your CPPS. But keep in mind that while the CPSI is a helpful aid, it should not be used as a diagnostic tool. Most importantly, it should not replace a visit to your doctor. Use the CPSI as a supporting document at the physician visit. With answers in hand, it will be easier for you to approach your physician for help. And, in turn, it will help simplify treatment options for the doctor as well. Filling out the questionnaire is a big step toward dealing with your CPPS. Knowing the extent of your problem can lead you toward a solution.

PHYSICAL EXAMINATION

A thorough examination of the pelvic region will be performed, which includes a full rectal and prostate exam. The pelvis not only contains the prostate and bladder but also the pelvic floor muscles. In addition to having you tense and relax specific pelvic floor muscles, your doctor will examine your back, abdomen, and legs. Your posture will also be evaluated.

"An assessment of pain and tenderness will be made during the abdominal, perineal, pelvic floor, rectal, and penile examination," explains Dr. Shoskes. "I emphasize to all my residents that CPPS pain is not a subtle finding." In documenting pain, the quality, location, frequency, and severity will also be noted.

CPPS: THE DOMINO EFFECT

Dr. Shoskes believes that there may be a domino effect related to CPPS, with the original cause of the problem not actually linked to symptoms but rather setting up the pelvic region for increasing levels of distress. Here's how it happens:

1. **Prostatic Injury**

   The prostate may be injured from an infection or a traumatic injury—an overly vigorous spinning class, for example. In addition, the ejaculatory ducts leading from the prostate gland into the urethra may have become obstructed, or urine may have backed up into the prostatic ducts. "It's not this initial insult or injury that produces the symptoms," notes Dr. Shoskes, but it is the precipitator.

2. **Inflammation**

   In response to the injury, two chemical messengers, chemokines and cytokines, are released to assist in the healing process, and inflammation may soon develop. A side effect of this healing process is swelling and pain, not only at the injury site— the prostate—but also in the penis, scrotum, and lower back because of the interconnection of the pelvic floor nerves.

3. **Neuromuscular Pain**

   In response to the injury and subsequent inflammation and pain, the pelvic floor muscles, nerves, and the bladder neck can then be affected, which can lead to significant urinary and sexual complaints. These can include reduced stream, urinary frequency, urgency, and nocturia.

The dominoes keep falling, with chronic pain developing over time due to a change in the nervous system's response to pain. This can then lead to depression, catastrophizing, increased stress, and inability to cope, all of which can negatively impact quality of life.

UPOINT: CATEGORIZING AND TREATING CPPS

Pain is the most prevalent feature of chronic pelvic pain syndrome, but there are other symptoms as well. After conducting a medical history, physical examination, and other investigations, the doctor can then clinically categorize (phenotype) the patient as having one or more of the UPOINT domains based on these symptoms:

URINARY SYMPTOMS

The man with this urinary phenotype has one or more of the following findings:

- Bothersome urinary frequency

- Urgency and/or nocturia

- Residual urine (more than 100 milliliters) measured by ultra-sound equipment

- CPSI score greater than 4

TREATMENT

Patients with a urinary phenotype may be prescribed alpha-blockers such as alfuzosin (UroXatral) and tamsulosin (Flomax), drugs that can help relax smooth muscle in the prostate, relieving tension at the urinary outlet and allowing easier urinary flow. Lifestyle changes are also recommended to help improve urinary symptoms. These can include:

- avoiding over-the-counter antihistamines or decongestants,

- not delaying urination,

- limiting the amount of fluid consumed at any one time and not drinking anything after seven o'clock at night,

- avoiding beverages that contain caffeine, and limiting alcohol intake,

- cutting back on spicy or salty foods,

- engaging in regular physical activity, and

- keeping blood sugar under control.

PSYCHOSOCIAL SYMPTOMS

Some CPPS patients have difficulty coping with pain and often suffer from depression, anxiety, and stress. Catastrophizing, the tendency to believe something is worse than it actually is, is common in pain syndromes, and patients will be asked if chronic pelvic pain syndrome makes them feel hopeless and leaves them with a feeling of helplessness.

"Catastrophizing is a very well-established phenomenon, especially in people with chronic illness," notes Dr. Shoskes. "It's the adult analogy of taking away a toddler's favorite blanket. Although we all recognize that we have not done them direct harm, the psychological reaction is excessive, as if their world has come to an end.

"When you have CPPS and you catastrophize, things that normally wouldn't set you off, do set you off. There is definitely a discrepancy between how much pain a person feels and how much his condition is actually producing. Interestingly enough, in every study we have done in UPOINT, catastrophizing has been the biggest driver of severity of symptoms and has had the most negative impact on quality of life."

TREATMENT

The all-important mind-body interaction cannot be overlooked. Stress management and psychological support and counseling are recommended for men with psychological complaints. Patients are encouraged to seek counseling with a social worker, psychologist, or psychiatrist. Antidepressant medication may be prescribed, if needed, by a psychiatrist.

ORGAN SPECIFIC (BLADDER AND/OR PROSTATE) SYMPTOMS

Trauma, infection, and inflammation of the bladder and prostate are common triggers of CPPS, and long-standing pain stemming from nerves and muscles near these organs is not unusual. "I will also check for interstitial cystitis," says Dr. Shoskes. "This ailment, also known as IC and painful bladder syndrome, is a chronic disorder characterized by an irritated or inflamed bladder wall and decreased bladder capacity." Although most of the seven hundred thousand people in the United States who have interstitial cystitis are women, it's estimated that men now comprise 10 percent of cases.

TREATMENT

Organ-specific therapies are reserved for those whose pain is localized to the prostate or bladder on physical examination. These can include the use of quercetin and bee pollen. Quercetin is a flavonol, a plant-derived compound that is used as a nutritional supplement. Bee pollen, which comes from pollen collected on the bodies of bees, contains rutin, quercetin, and other flavonoids. "These natural products have clinical trial data that suggest that they reduce inflammation in the prostate," says Dr. Shoskes.

"If you use quercetin," he cautions, "be aware that many quercetin supplements found in health food stores have vitamin C in them, and this is not recommended, because vitamin C can worsen urinary symptoms."

The Prosta-Q brand, sold by Farr Labs (www.farrlabs.com; 877-284-3976), does not contain vitamin C and is one that Dr. Shoskes recommends to his patients. He suggests that quercetin be taken two to three times a day with meals. Some users notice improvement in their prostate or bladder complaints after the first few doses, although others find that they must take it for at least three months to see any changes. "If there is no symptom improvement after eight to twelve weeks, the product is unlikely to help," says Dr. Shoskes.

INFECTION SYMPTOMS

Although antibiotic therapy is overused and ineffective in treating CPPS, when an infection within the prostate or urethra is documented in a man with urinary symptoms, antibiotics can lead to complete resolution of symptoms.

TREATMENT

Urine cultures will be examined for evidence of bacteria. Antibiotics will be prescribed when needed. Infections generally respond well to these medications following a first occurrence of CPPS. About 75 percent of men who have not previously been treated with an antibiotic will improve.

NEUROLOGICAL/SYSTEMIC CONDITION SYMPTOMS

Is there pain outside of the pelvic region? Oftentimes patients with chronic pelvic pain syndrome also have other pain-related medical conditions; most notably fibromyalgia, irritable bowel syndrome, migraine headache, and pain in the low back or legs. If so, they are phenotyped in this category.

TREATMENT

In addition to making sure that these related ailments are treated effectively, CPPS patients may also benefit from the use of epilepsy drugs, including gabapentin (Neurontin) and pregabalin (Lyrica). Two members of the tricyclic family of antidepressants, amitriptyline (Elavil) and nortriptyline (Aventyl), can also be used to help inhibit pain impulses by increasing the ability of descending nerves to mute the pain messages. Some doctors are also trying acupuncture, physical therapy (see page 244), Viagra, and pentosan polysulfate (Elmiron), a drug typically prescribed for men and women with interstitial cystitis, to relieve chronic pain symptoms. Referral to a pain center can also be made if these therapies do not bring adequate relief.

TENDERNESS OF MUSCLES SYMPTOMS

Many men have abnormal findings when the muscles of the pelvic floor and abdomen are examined. This can range from spasming and tenderness to muscle knotting and fatigue. It's quite common for this pain to radiate to other parts of the body as well, and when you try to move, it hurts. This pain can be in your lower back, thighs, and hips. When the pain radiates out to the rectum and bladder, it often becomes difficult to defecate and urinate.

TREATMENT

Therapy includes regular sessions of pelvic muscle therapy with a physical therapist who understands how the muscles of the pelvic floor work in unison to support the pelvic organs. Therapy focuses on the underlying causes of your pain. A combination of heat therapy, physical therapy, progressive relaxation exercises, and yoga exercises may also be tried to relieve the spasming, weakness, or debilitating pain. Biofeedback, a technique that trains you to improve bodily functions such as heart rate and blood pressure by using your mind, may also be tried.

CENTRAL SENSITIZATION: A POSSIBLE CAUSE OF CPPS

Some researchers think that people with chronic pelvic pain syndrome have certain chemical abnormalities that cause the central nervous system to become oversensitive and magnify pain sensations. This is known as the theory of central sensitization, and here is how it works.

Let's suppose that you accidentally slammed your perineal area between your anus and your scrotum on the crossbar of your mountain bike. Pain receptors in your perineum detect the injury and send a message in the form of electrical impulses through a nerve to your spinal cord to indicate that you have hurt yourself. The impulses enter the spinal cord and ascend to the brain, including those regions linked with both the emotional and physical experiences of pain.

Researchers now believe that some people with CPPS may have abnormalities in these central brain structures, as well as high levels of a neurotransmitter called substance P, which increases the pain experience; and glutamate, which excites brain cells, causing them to generate even more electrical signals. This leads to a major discrepancy between how much pain the condition actually produces and how much pain a person actually feels.

Your brain also generates electrical impulses that stimulate the body's production of pain-suppressing chemicals called endorphins, which help modify or inhibit pain messages. These descending nerve impulses travel down from the brain to the spinal cord and back to the injury site. But people with chronic pelvic pain syndrome have a number of factors in common, such as stress and depression, which interferes with these important nerve impulses, making the pain seem more intense than it should.

Repeated activation of this complex chain of events—as often occurs in people with chronic pain—can permanently lower the point at which the body's pain-response system is triggered. As a result, people with CPPS feel pain at lowered levels of stimulation than do their healthy counterparts, and it takes relatively little sensory input for the pain to remain constant.

A 2011 study published in the *Journal of Urology* uniquely characterized for the first time with magnetic resonance imaging (MRI) the brain function and anatomy of patients with chronic pelvic pain syndrome. The investigators evaluated male CPPS sufferers and age-matched men without the disorder. This intriguing work found that the pain in men with CPPS was associated with specific pain activation patterns. An unanswered question is to what extent these findings are responsible for the symptoms experienced by CPPS patients.

HOW YOUR DOCTOR CAN USE UPOINT

Based on this basic in-office exam, patients can be classified into one or more of the UPOINT categories. Dr. Shoskes recommends that therapy can then be selected as indicated by the features experienced by the patient. For example, a patient with urinary symptoms, prostate tenderness, and spasming of the pelvic side wall may be prescribed alfuzosin, an alpha-blocker, to relax the smooth muscle of the prostate and bladder neck; a quercetin–bee pollen combination; and pelvic physical therapy sessions to reduce his symptoms.

On the other hand, another patient with severe urinary symptoms linked to bladder filling, fibromyalgia, and depression may be prescribed pentosan polysulfate, nortriptyline, bladder medications, and psychological counseling.

Dr. Shoskes acknowledges that UPOINT can easily be misused. "A patient can go to a doctor with complaints of pelvic pain, and the doctor immediately says, 'Hah! You have CPPS and I will start UPOINT,' when in reality," he says, "the patient could have a kidney stone, bladder cancer, or a hernia.

The starting point for Dr. Shoskes has to be the diagnosis. Once a diagnosis of CPPS has been established, then UPOINT can be used.

USING UPOINT TO GUIDE THERAPY:
THE SIX DOMAINS AND RECOMMENDED THERAPIES

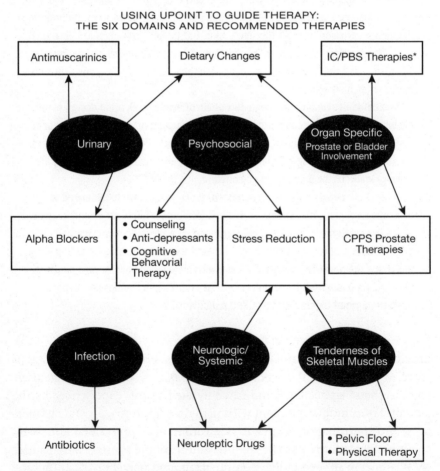

*IC: interstitial cystitis; PBS: painful bladder syndrome.
Adapted from Nickel, J. C., and Shoskes, D., *Current Urology Reports* 2009; 10:307–312.

HOW DO YOU KNOW IF CPPS TREATMENT IS WORKING?

Unfortunately, the success of therapy for chronic pelvic pain syndrome is not yet measured by cure. But patients frequently see a reduction in symptom severity, improved quality of life, and less disability.

People with CPPS have to understand that, in most cases, no pill is going to give them immediate and complete relief. Rather, it's up to them to participate in management that might include exercise, stress reduction, and physical therapy designed to relieve pelvic floor distress. A willingness to be proactive and to learn ways to take better control over one's symptoms is a critical factor in managing CPPS.

"Most people do get better," emphasizes Dr. Shoskes. "The average age of the patient with this disease is forty. If nobody got better, my waiting room would be filled with seventy-year-old patients who'd had the disease for thirty years, and that is not the case."

HOW TO FIND A DOCTOR

Even when doctors do recognize and diagnose chronic pelvic pain syndrome, they often feel that they don't have the proper resources to help patients. Moreover, they may be loath to identify a disorder that leaves them feeling helpless in their ability to care for it.

To achieve the best outcome, doctors and patients both need to adopt a positive and practical attitude toward CPPS. Clinicians must be prepared to accept the syndrome as a real illness that causes genuine pain and acknowledge that it has a tremendous impact on patients' lives. Patients must appreciate that their physician treats many other conditions, that CPPS symptoms can closely mimic these other disorders, and that some forms of CPPS treatment are still experimental.

If you suspect that you have chronic pelvic pain syndrome, consult a doctor who has experience with treating it. Some physicians are still not familiar with the diagnostic criteria for CPPS. A urologist is usually the medical specialist with the most experience diagnosing the syndrome.

Once you have been diagnosed with CPPS, a good way to work with your urologist is to use the UPOINT System Web site (www.upointmd .com) created by Dr. Shoskes specifically to help doctors and patients make the best treatment decisions. Together with your physician, enter the requested information. Click the button, and you will then be given some direction as to what treatment strategies can be suggested for your particular case.

TREATING CPPS WITH PHYSICAL THERAPY

"Does your burning pelvic pain only come with orgasm, or do you feel that pain at other times?"

This is the kind of frank question that Dr. Mary McVearry typically asks her CPPS patients during their first office visit. Dr. McVearry treats scores of men—a majority of them active-duty soldiers, as well as retirees—for chronic pelvic pain syndrome, and presently she is the only pelvic floor specialist working for the entire U.S. Department of Defense. All of her patients, and they range in age from nineteen to seventy, are referred to her by urologists, pain specialists, colorectal physicians, and gastroenterologists at Walter Reed to help alleviate their unremitting pelvic pain.

Most of the men who see Dr. McVearry had never thought about physical therapy for their pelvic region. The entire time they have had CPPS, they were told that an infection in their prostate was the trouble spot—the epicenter of their dull, aching pain—or that there was simply no explanation. So Dr. McVearry spends a good portion of first one-hour visits with new patients explaining why CPPS may have nothing to do with the prostate and more to do with pelvic floor anatomy, including nearby musculature, organs, connective tissues, blood supply, and nerves.

Here is a multiweek hands-on program without prescription pills or surgery. Rather, it's a daily program of letting the body heal itself with specific relaxation, stretching, and strengthening exercises, both done one-on-one in her office during each appointment and then in the home setting every day by her patients.

Pelvic rehabilitation may entail manual techniques to massage certain muscles, heat therapy, and, in some cases, using biofeedback. In the latter therapy, either a special computerized probe is inserted into the rectum or electrodes are placed on the skin between the anus and scrotum, to sense muscle activity. The patient learns how to relax certain groups of muscles until the discomfort level drops. The equipment may have a visual graphic on the monitor or else make a beeping sound to assure the patient that he is making progress in releasing the muscle tension in the pelvic floor. Making use of this technology allows a person to learn how to change or control his own pelvic floor muscle tone.

TREATING A SPASMING MUSCLE WITH PELVIC FLOOR THERAPY

Pelvic floor therapy is a little-known treatment that has been overlooked by doctors because so many think of chronic pelvic pain syndrome as a prostate problem and fail to recognize it as a multifaceted condition that may involve muscle-related problems.

Why physical therapy for CPPS? For starters, it can be due in part to spasming of the pelvic floor muscles that was caused by some inciting event such as infection or trauma. "If you develop shoulder pain and it doesn't get better, you may eventually get it checked out and treated with physical therapy, so it shouldn't be any different for musculoskeletal causes of pelvic pain," explains Dr. McVearry.

Although this is a relatively new way of thinking about CPPS, specialized physical therapy is now being used for the muscles of the pelvic floor and surrounding areas, which can relieve the tight muscles and soothe the tender areas called trigger points: painful, sensitive spots consisting of a tight band of muscle and connective tissue. Trigger points are typically found in the pelvic floor muscles as well as in the surrounding muscles.

Many doctors don't know much about pelvic floor problems or choose not to believe that a man's pelvic complaints are often muscle related. "The word has to get out to doctors and their patients that we now have a variety of therapies that can help relieve a man's pelvic discomfort," Dr. McVearry says.

THE GOALS OF PHYSICAL THERAPY FOR CPPS

The goals of physical therapy for chronic pelvic pain syndrome vary from patient to patient. "My goal is to be very realistic with my patients," says Dr. McVearry. She gauges success by first asking each patient, "What would make you happy?"

"Usually, they have been in pain for so long, that having no pain isn't their primary goal from therapy," she explains. "Rather, they want to have a normal life and get back to doing the things they used to do, like exercising and having sex.

"I usually tell patients, 'I don't know if I will be able to reduce your pain completely, but I hope I increase the number of good days and decrease your bad days.' If a man ends up with a baseline pain level of one or two out of ten, and he came to me with a seven or eight, I'm happy with that, and he is, too. Granted, there will be those people whose goal is to be totally free of pain. I don't know if I will be able to get them there, although I will try really hard. In the end, though, most of my patients are just happy that they found someone who cares and wants to work with them."

Physical therapy can work wonders for many men with chronic pelvic pain syndrome. The stronger the pelvic floor muscles, the more efficiently the body works. Just as a firm infrastructure supports a building and prevents it from breaking down inside, a reinforced core developed through physical therapy becomes the basis of a strong, supported, pain-free body.

DAWN OF A NEW DAY

Treating CPPS with physical therapy may be very helpful in reducing symptoms and pain of CPPS. During the course of working with a patient, a physical therapist trained to treat CPPS may insert a finger into the rectum and massage the pelvic muscles and tissues directly. There may be a brief increase in symptoms following treatment, as the problem regions are being exposed. However, this is brief, with most patients realizing significant improvement after several weeks of therapy.

"By helping the pelvic floor and surrounding areas to get out of spasm, symptoms should diminish greatly. It happens with most of my patients," says Dr. McVearry.

FINDING A PHYSICAL THERAPIST FOR CPPS TREATMENT

Physical therapists, or PTs, are uniquely qualified to help patients reduce pain, restore function, prevent disability, and improve mobility in order to move forward with life. These health care professionals diagnose and treat individuals of all ages who have medical problems such as chronic pelvic pain syndrome or other conditions that limit their abilities to move and be active.

To find a physical therapist in your area who is qualified to treat CPPS, contact the American Physical Therapy Association: 1111 North Fairfax Street, Alexandria, VA 22314-1488, 703-684-APTA (2782) or 800-999-2782, or go to its Web site at www.apta.org.

THE TAKEAWAY

- Prostatitis syndromes are classified as bacterial and nonbacterial. The majority of men with a prostatitis syndrome have the nonbacterial type, which is more accurately referred to as chronic prostatitis/chronic pelvic pain syndrome (CP/CPPS), or CPPS for short.

- Chronic pelvic pain syndrome is characterized by pain in the genitourinary tract lasting three months or more, without the presence of bacteria that cause infections. The pain may radiate to other areas.

- There is no known cause of CPPS, which affects as many as 10 percent to 15 percent of men, and shares common traits with other syndromes such as irritable bowel syndrome, chronic fatigue syndrome, and fibromyalgia.

- Pain associated with ejaculation, one characteristic of CPPS, can cause a reduction in a man's quality of life similar to that associated with other chronic diseases such as Crohn's disease, heart pain (angina), and type 2 diabetes.

- Men with CPPS are often misdiagnosed and mistreated based on the assumption that they have a prostate infection.

- A careful evaluation that includes a history and quantification of symptoms, physical examination, and urinalysis, is the cornerstone of a correct CPPS diagnosis.

- Treatment is tailored to each patient based on his specific symptoms and physical findings, and may include lifestyle and behavioral alterations, medication, counseling, physical therapy, or combinations of these.

PART FOUR

CANCER

We cannot direct the wind,
but we can adjust the sails.

—Anonymous

INTRODUCTION

"You have prostate cancer."

Those four words can knock you off your feet. For most, a cancer diagnosis is a traumatic experience. The simple knowledge of it can cause depression, and then anxiety, worry, and great uncertainty. A 2009 Swedish study of seventeen thousand men diagnosed with prostate cancer reported that they were about eleven times more likely to suffer a cardiovascular event during the first week after their diagnosis than men without cancer. The researchers, whose study was published in the medical journal *PLoS Medicine*, also reported that men with a cancer diagnosis were eight times more likely to commit suicide in the week after they received the news.

Everyone fears cancer. Many seemingly healthy men who are given the news begin to envision rogue cells running amok in their bodies, spreading and outnumbering healthy tissue at a fast clip. Their first instinct is to do whatever is necessary to rid their bodies of the prostate cancer as quickly as possible.

For most men diagnosed with prostate cancer today, the immediate panic is no longer necessary.

For years, the word *cancer* was synonymous with death, and men had a right to be terrified by a cancer diagnosis. While prostate cancers can be lethal, most cases of prostate cancer today are diagnosed at an early stage, when the tumor is still confined to the gland. And most prostate cancers grow slowly when compared to other forms of cancer. We now know that many men have prostate cancer for years without ever realizing it, and they typically die of something else—oftentimes from heart disease, the number one killer of men in the United States.

Unfortunately, most men's perception of cancer is of one disease—their impression formed by those who have died of a cancer. Many hear the six-letter word and immediately think treatment must be carried out

ASAP. Men with less aggressive prostate cancer rush to urologists and radiation oncologists for consultation and receive surgery or radiation for low-grade disease even though many of these men needed no treatment at all.

While many men achieve peace of mind after undergoing these potentially unnecessary interventions, they may also suffer negative, life-altering consequences such as urinary incontinence, sexual dysfunction, and rectal injury.

Although I have performed more than three thousand radical prostatectomy surgeries to remove cancerous prostates, I have since come to believe that prostate cancer in the United States is overtreated to a great extent. In other words, people who don't need treatment are undergoing treatment, and at staggering rates. Let me explain.

Because U.S. doctors have been screening for prostate cancer with the prostate-specific-antigen test since the late 1980s, one in six men are now diagnosed with prostate cancer. However, many of the cancers that are being discovered are small and indolent—that is, slow growing—and will never cause harm during life.

Some physicians are now calling this an overdiagnosis of prostate cancer and recommending an end to the use of the PSA test for diagnosis. However, in my opinion, the issue is about what follows a diagnosis and not about whether the PSA test should be used to detect the disease early. The PSA screening dilemma is covered in chapter 10, where I offer the pros and cons in this contentious debate.

We have no perfect method to identify which prostate cancers will remain quiescent and which will ultimately be lethal during a lifetime. But we have very good methods for assessing whether a cancer will cause harm without treatment for a decade or more. Still, most men regardless of risk are strongly urged to do something about their cancer. While this seems like reasonable behavior, since we fear the potential ramifications of cancer, this approach has led to overtreatment of prostate cancer.

By not being completely informed, men often unwittingly undergo unnecessary cancer treatments. This overtreatment will rise dramatically in the future, since prostate cancer is a disease of aging men, and over the next decade, there will be an 18 percent increase in the number of men over age seventy.

Understanding the significance of overdiagnosis and overtreatment, sixteen years ago I helped establish and continue to direct the Johns Hopkins active surveillance program, the longest continuously running program in the world using strict criteria for entry. More than one thousand carefully selected men diagnosed with prostate cancer have been enrolled in this program. Instead of surgery or radiation therapy for their cancer, these men are monitored in our program—but do not have surgery or irradiation immediately—for their cancer. Therapy is only recommended if a man's cancer changes.

The program has been a success and a model for other surveillance programs in the U.S. and Europe. Almost 60 percent of our enrollees are still undergoing active surveillance and have received no treatment. No men in the program have died from prostate cancer.

Going forward, more than two hundred thousand men in the United States will be diagnosed with prostate cancer each year. No longer should prostate cancer be lumped into one big "fear" category, with men being advised to hastily undergo invasive treatment in all cases.

In the following chapters, I will discuss why the PSA test is valuable for some and not for others, and if performed, how often the testing should be done. If a prostate biopsy is needed and cancer is discovered, the all-important question of whether your cancer calls for treatment will also be addressed. I will present four criteria that I use in helping my patients assess the severity of their disease. Finally, I will review the pros and cons of the major management options used today, including active surveillance, radical prostatectomy, external-beam radiotherapy, and interstitial radiotherapy.

CHAPTER NINE

PROSTATE CANCER

I do not wish to achieve immortality through my works.
I wish to achieve immortality by not dying.

—Woody Allen

Cancer of the prostate is the most commonly diagnosed life-threatening cancer in men, and after lung cancer, it holds the second highest mortality rate, accounting for 9 percent of all male cancer deaths. Boys born in the United States today have a one-in-six risk of being diagnosed with prostate cancer during their lifetime—thanks to the genes they inherit, their diet, and other lifestyle choices—and a one-in-thirty-five chance of dying from it.

The American Cancer Society estimated that there were 241,890 new cases of prostate cancer diagnosed in the United States in 2012 and that 28,170 men died from it. That's one new case of prostate cancer about every two to three minutes and a death from prostate cancer about every twenty minutes. But these dramatic numbers need to be considered in the context of the years of quality life that are lost each year due to the unnecessary treatment of prostate cancer.

This is what is meant when cancer experts talk about weighing the benefits versus the risks of prostate cancer screening with the PSA test; in other words, the benefit of detecting a cancer and preventing a possible death versus the risk of treating a cancer that might very well have remained asymptomatic—or even gone undetected—during a man's lifetime.

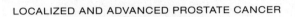

LOCALIZED AND ADVANCED PROSTATE CANCER

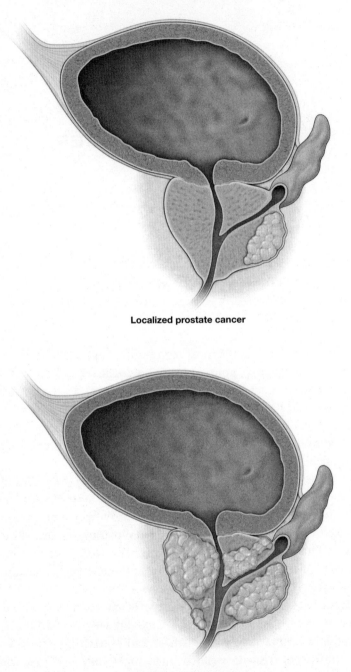

Localized prostate cancer

Advanced prostate cancer

According to autopsy studies of men in their eighties who died of other ailments, as many as two in three—or more—had some level of prostate cancer but were never bothered by it. If many of the men who would otherwise not have known about their cancer get treated—and in the United States they usually do—then it is easy to see how unnecessary treatment often occurs.

The great paradox is that at the same time, prostate cancer is without question one of the most devastating cancers among men. How to solve this dilemma of detecting and treating only those cancers destined to cause harm is the focus of many scientific laboratories and science-based companies around the world. And progress is being made. In the meantime, there are many patients who can live safely with what we call low-risk early stage prostate cancers. After weighing all of their management options, I contend that active surveillance with careful annual monitoring makes the most sense for many men today who are choosing invasive treatments.

These early cancers will be a primary focus of the upcoming chapters because they are diagnosed so frequently these days with PSA screening in the United States.

HOW PROSTATE CANCER GROWS

Most cells in the body are constantly dividing, reaching maturity, and then dying in a precisely controlled process called apoptosis, or programmed cell death. Apoptosis is a means of regulating cell growth and disposing of cells that have been injured or altered. But unlike normal cells, cancer cells are no longer regulated by programmed cell death. Apoptosis may be blocked, and cells that should have died continue to divide uncontrolled. This process increases the likelihood that a tumor will eventually develop that has acquired the features allowing invasion and spread to other sites in the body.

When it comes to most prostate cancers, cellular proliferation progresses slowly over decades, and this, together with the fact that most of these cancers probably don't begin developing until later in life, may explain why prostate cancer affects primarily older men.

Prostate cancers typically begin in the part of the prostate closest to the rectum: the peripheral zone. Cancer cells divide to form a tumor that must evade the immune system in order to continue to grow. A tumor that reaches a size of 1 centimeter—about the size of a pencil eraser tip—contains 1 billion microscopic cells and can be felt on a digital rectal examination if located close enough to the rectal surface and if it forms a nodule. It takes thirty doublings from a single cancer cell for a cancer to grow to 1 centimeter.

Before the advent of the PSA test in 1986, most prostate cancers were found by a doctor's detecting a nodule of cancerous tissue on a digital rectal examination (DRE). The next step was to biopsy tissue from the gland to prove the presence of cancer. Nowadays, an elevated level of prostate-specific antigen in the blood triggers a biopsy, typically well before the tumor grows to a size that could be felt during a DRE. So how much earlier are prostate cancers detected today, as compared with, say 40 years ago?

In a 1993 Johns Hopkins study published in the *Journal of Urology* that predated the PSA test, 185 men who were diagnosed with cancer after nodules were discovered on DRE, underwent surgery to remove the cancerous prostate. Of those men, 18, or 10 percent, had tumors that were 0.5 cubic centimeters or less, while about half had tumors above 2 cubic centimeters. Compare this with a modern PSA screening program in Scandinavia, where about half of the men had tumor volumes below 0.2 cubic centimeters. That is a tenfold difference in the average tumor volume. Investigators have calculated that with PSA testing, prostate cancers are detected about a decade earlier than would be possible without the PSA test.

In what is considered a landmark investigation more than twenty years ago, Dr. Thomas Stamey and his colleagues at Stanford University evaluated the prostates of men following prostate removal. They found that metastases—cancer cells that have migrated from the original site to other organs and formed new tumors—were associated only with primary tumors that were larger than 4 cubic centimeters and had developed aggressive microscopic features referred to as poorly differentiated or high grade. These secondary cancers, which tend to be more resistant to treatment, were far less common in men with smaller, less aggressive tumors. The experiences of men with prostate cancer and subsequent scientific studies suggest that Dr. Stamey was right on the mark.

CANCER GROWTH AND THE CLINICAL TRIAL EVIDENCE

With elevated PSAs triggering most prostate biopsies today, around 40 percent of prostate cancers are detected while still small and low grade. For a patient with a small, low-grade prostate cancer, it could be anticipated that even without treatment, an older man foregoing treatment might do just as well as the man who undergoes treatment.

In a study that will be discussed in more detail later, a large group of men with cancer detected the "old-fashioned" way (mostly by digital rectal exam) was divided into two groups. One group underwent surgery, while the other had no treatment. Fifteen years later, for those men over the age of sixty-five, there was no difference between the two groups when comparing their rates of developing metastatic disease, as well as their rates of dying from their cancer. The results of this landmark study—the Scandinavian Prostate Cancer Group Study Number 4—is one of the strongest pieces of evidence we have to empower the older man to move slowly when diagnosed with low-grade cancer instead of jumping immediately to radiation therapy or surgery.

CAUSES OF PROSTATE CANCER

No one is certain what causes prostate cancer, but other than having X and Y chromosomes, the critical risk factors for influencing whether or not you will develop the disease include age, race, and family history. As you already read in chapters 2 and 3, a poor diet and a lack of physical activity may also play an important role in the development of the cancer by causing oxidative DNA damage.

AGE AND PROSTATE CANCER

Age is a strong risk factor because the chance of developing prostate cancer rises exponentially as a man ages—faster than for any other cancer. The older you are, the more likely you are to be diagnosed with prostate cancer. Although about 5 in 10,000 men between the ages of forty and forty-nine will be diagnosed with prostate cancer, the rate jumps to 47 in 10,000 for those aged fifty to fifty-nine, and 147 in 10,000 for men aged sixty to sixty-nine. More than 65 percent of all prostate cancers are now diagnosed in men over sixty-five.

Why the drastic increase in the incidence of prostate cancer according to age as compared with other cancers? Here are a few ideas:

1. The cumulative damage from oxidative stress takes decades to bring about development and promotion of a cancer that progresses slowly but relentlessly.

2. Hormone levels that may promote cancer development change with age.

3. The immune system becomes less effective with age.

4. A combination of all of the above.

In addition, nearly seventy-seven million Americans were born between 1946 and 1964, the years of the postwar baby boom. And that massive bulge in the US population is just hitting prime time as far as prostate cancer is concerned. Four-fifths of men newly diagnosed with prostate cancer are ages sixty-five and older. What's more, the number of American males ages sixty-five and older is projected to increase by 40 percent between 2010 and 2020, and then increase another 33 percent between 2020 and 2030. It's evident that our health care system will be inundated with prostate cancer patients.

Table 9.1. Percentage of U.S. Men Diagnosed with Prostate Cancer, by Age

Age (Years)	Percentage of All Diagnosed Prostate Cancers
Younger than 50	1 percent
50 to 54	3 percent
55 to 59	6 percent
60 to 64	11 percent

SEER Cancer Statistics Review, 1975–2008, National Cancer Institute.
SEER web site: http://seer.cancer.gov/statistics/.

RACE AND PROSTATE CANCER

Although Asians residing in some Asian countries have a tenfold lower likelihood of being diagnosed with prostate cancer and a four- to five-times lower likelihood of dying of prostate cancer compared with men in the United States, there are striking differences in the rates of diagnosis and death from prostate cancer between different races in America.

African American and Caribbean men have the highest rates of prostate cancer diagnosis and death of any group of men in the world. Many studies demonstrate higher PSA levels, more aggressive and more advanced disease upon diagnosis, and higher recurrence rates after treatment for blacks with prostate cancer compared with whites— either because they have a more aggressive variant of prostate cancer or because a delay in diagnosis resulted in a more advanced cancer at the time of treatment. Other, unknown factors probably play a role in explaining the discrepancy.

IMPLICATIONS OF THE CANCER COLORING BOOK

African Americans are 50 percent more likely than non-Hispanic white men to be diagnosed with prostate cancer, and two times more likely to die of the disease. I believe that an interaction between our genes and the environment best explains many of the differences in the rates of cancer diagnosis and death between races. I think of this interaction using a coloring book and crayon analogy. The coloring book represents our genes, the crayons the environment, and the resulting picture is a health outcome such as the presence or absence of a disease such as prostate cancer.

We all inherit a set of genes from both parents. The coloring books differ from one individual to the next, and between races, whether white, yellow, tan, or black. But because of mixture among races, a white person and a black person could have coloring books that are more similar than would appear based on skin color alone. People adopt (or because of socioeconomic conditions beyond their control) have different lifestyles (crayons). The picture, or health outcome, results from the combination of coloring book and crayons, not either one alone.

For example, genes that prevent or repair DNA damage vary from one individual to another. Due to heredity, two people may have reduced abilities to fend off DNA damage from cancer-causing agents or carcinogens—and therefore a higher likelihood of developing cancer. But the first man might sidestep cancer because he eats a diet rich in foods that "turn on" similar genes that protect DNA, while the second man gorges on many of the foods that increase inflammation in tissues. That inflammation, along with his body's impaired ability to prevent genetic damage, may be enough to trigger the development or progression of a cancer.

It is likely that both genetic and environmental factors play a role in the higher rates of prostate cancers among those of African descent compared to Caucasians or those of European descent, and higher rates of prostate cancers among Caucasians when compared to those of Asian descent. In addition, socioeconomic circumstances and differences in access to health care in the United States could also explain some differences in the more advanced cancers found in African Americans when compared to whites.

Table 9.2. Prostate Cancer Incidence Rates by Race

Race/Ethnicity	Incidence
All races	156.0 per 100,000 men
White	149.5 per 100,000 men
Black	233.8 per 100,000 men
Asian/Pacific islander	88.3 per 100,000 men
American Indian/Alaska native	75.3 per 100,000 men
Hispanic	107.4 per 100,000 men

SEER Cancer Statistics Review, 1975–2008, National Cancer Institute.
SEER web site: http://seer.cancer.gov/statistics/.

FAMILY HISTORY AND INHERITANCE
OF PROSTATE CANCER GENES

Many people believe that if they develop prostate cancer, they must have inherited a "faulty" gene from one or both of their parents that caused the disease. However, inheriting a single genetic mutation that substantially increases a person's risk of prostate cancer is considered relatively rare and probably explains less than 10 percent of the lifetime risk of prostate cancer. An inherited gene mutation that causes prostate cancer is more likely among men who developed prostate cancer at an early age—less than fifty-five years old—and if there were multiple first-degree relatives with prostate cancer in multiple generations.

The greater susceptibility to prostate cancer in one individual compared to another is thought to occur most commonly because of the inheritance of multiple genes (not any one gene) that together predispose a person to cancer. These genes are not "abnormal," but rather they vary a bit from person to person and raise a person's risk of cancer a small amount. Referred to as SNPs (pronounced snips)—an acronym for single-nucleotide polymorphisms—these gene variants acting together probably explain most of the heritable risk of prostate cancer. And men of African descent appear to harbor a greater number of these SNPs when compared to those of European descent.

As of this writing, more than thirty single-nucleotide polymorphisms have been associated with a heightened susceptibility to prostate cancer. This combined-gene effect, together with lifestyle, is thought to be the most likely cause of the majority of prostate cancers. But the story is not yet complete, because when investigators evaluate the SNPs that elevate prostate cancer risk, this appears to explain less than one in five cases of prostate cancer. Further research in larger populations will undoubtedly uncover more genetic patterns associated with prostate cancer. But together with age and race, a family history of the disease is an important risk factor.

If you have several close blood relatives with prostate cancer, you have to put yourself in the at-risk category. Having a grandfather or uncle with prostate cancer increases your odds of developing cancer only slightly. However, if your father or brother had the disease, your risk doubles. Some studies show an *elevenfold* increase in cancer susceptibility for men who have two or more first-degree relatives with prostate cancer.

THE LETHAL PROSTATE CANCER: A TRIATHLETE

A great deal of research is focused on identifying the genetic alterations that are responsible for a cancer metastasizing and ending a person's life. The normal prostate cancer cell is not equipped to live outside the gland. In order to leave the prostate and begin to grow elsewhere in the body, the cancer cells have to either invade surrounding tissues or travel through the bloodstream or lymphatic system to another organ or tissue. Common sites include the pelvic lymph nodes beside the bladder and prostate, and the bones. Furthermore, it must elude the immune system, and then, once it takes up residence elsewhere, the new, secondary tumor has to establish a blood supply to survive. You can think of metastatic cancer as a tumor that has acquired powers that don't exist in most prostate cancers and certainly not in the normal cell—it's the true triathlete. (The lymphatic system, a major part of the immune system, is a complex and interconnected network comprised of organs, vessels, nodes, ducts, and capillaries that transport lymph, a fluid that traps and filters foreign substances and microbes in the body.)

A recent article in the journal *Nature* demonstrated that prostate cancer is very complex from a genetic perspective, with a wide variety of genetic alterations within each cancer cell—alterations that a scientist might liken to the disarray in the university fraternity house after an all-night party. There are pieces of DNA that have come apart and reattached themselves to neighboring DNA where they do not belong— a process called gene fusion. These gene fusions can activate tumor-promoting genes called oncogenes and deactivate tumor-suppressing genes. This complexity of genetic changes would be required for a prostate cancer to become a lethal disease. In the near future, discovery of the genetic alterations that lead to a lethal cancer may lead to new methods for treating prostate cancers.

In the meantime, adopting a healthy lifestyle or choosing your "crayons" carefully is an important strategy for lowering your risk of dying of prostate cancer, since men who adopt unhealthy lifestyles appear to be at greater risk of dying of the disease when compared to those who maintain healthy lifestyles.

WHAT YOU EAT AFFECTS PROSTATE CANCER RISK

Diet is under suspicion as a factor that could contribute to prostate cancer risk. There's growing evidence that diets high in calories, fat, dairy products, and grilled or processed meats are associated with metabolic disturbances that lead to an increased risk of fatal prostate cancer. And there is evidence that African Americans consume diets higher in fats and charred meats than their white counterparts do.

As mentioned in chapter 3, since there is a fourfold to fivefold higher rate of prostate cancer death between men in Western and Asian societies, scientists believe that what you eat and how much you eat influence prostate cancer development and progression. No foods come with a 100 percent guarantee to protect men from prostate cancer. But in countries where the diet revolves around fish, whole grains, colorful fruits and vegetables, and legumes, the men and women there have much lower rates of both prostate cancer and breast cancer.

What can you do to reduce your risk of developing prostate cancer? Granted, there are no large clinical trials assigning healthful and unhealthful foods between two groups and then tracking the rates of prostate cancer development going forward, nor will there likely ever be. But there is growing evidence for an association between diet and prostate cancer. This evidence is based on the dietary intake of large groups of men who consumed different diets and populations with differing diets, and evaluation of their rates of being diagnosed with prostate cancer and dying of the disease. For more on the important role of diet and prostate cancer, go to chapter 3.

THE SKINNY ON OBESITY AND PROSTATE CANCER

A huge percentage of the boomer population is overweight or obese. Researchers from the Beth Israel Deaconess Medical Center and the Harvard School of Medicine compared the rates of obesity among baby boomers with the obesity rates of the previous generation between 1926 and 1945. Up to 32 percent of the boomers were obese by age forty-four, whereas fewer than 18 percent of the "Greatest Generation" were obese at that age. In other words, boomers are spending more years of their lives obese, so the excess weight has a longer period during which to exert its destructive effects. It's no secret that obesity has already reached epidemic proportions in the United States.

It is becoming increasingly apparent that obesity and prostate cancer are linked in an unholy alliance. Obese men are more likely to be diagnosed with aggressive forms of prostate cancer and to have the cancer recur after treatment. Investigators from the Fred Hutchinson Cancer Research Center studied the effects of obesity on prostate cancer deaths in the United States, reviewing data from a number of well-regarded studies. Publishing in the journal *Cancer Epidemiology Biomarkers and Prevention*, the authors estimated that from 1980 to 2002, the rise in obesity increased the rate of aggressive prostate cancers by 16 percent, and the rates of prostate cancer death by as much as 23 percent.

The high prevalence of prostate cancer among aging men, the increase in the proportion of men over age sixty-five over the next decade, and rising obesity rates taken together indicate that prostate cancer will be one of the most important health challenges that men face in the next decade.

According to several studies, obese men diagnosed with prostate cancer have more than two and a half times the risk of dying from the disease as compared with men of healthy weight at the time of diagnosis.

In one recent report on obesity and prostate cancer from the Louisiana State University School of Public Health, researchers studied over a thousand men of African descent and over a thousand men of European descent. There was a strong relationship between obesity and the development of aggressive prostate cancers. When compared with men of healthy weight, obese men from both groups were one and a half to two times more likely to be diagnosed with aggressive prostate cancers that kill.

The link between obesity and prostate cancer death is probably related to many factors, including metabolic disturbances that increase tissue inflammation, which may promote more virulent tumors in some men. Alterations in the production of the sex hormones testosterone and estrogen, as well as insulin and growth factors, may also be involved in the development of more aggressive prostate cancers in obese men. Don't forget that body fat is not an inert substance. Although commonly thought of as a mass of tissue taking up volume in the body, it is now recognized that fat is active metabolically, releasing substances into the system, including those that spur inflammation. This increases the risk not only of aggressive prostate cancer but also of cardiovascular disease.

Since the evidence suggests that maintaining a healthy weight will reduce the chances of being diagnosed with a type of prostate cancer that is more likely to spread beyond the prostate, be ever mindful of what and how much you eat.

DO YOU NEED TO LOSE WEIGHT?

Probably the best measure of whether your weight is in the healthy range is to calculate your body mass index. BMI gives an estimate of body composition, which is just as important as your overall weight. Studies show that health risks increase moderately for overweight people with a body mass index of 25 to 29, but once their BMI hits 30, the threshold for obesity, the risks escalate dramatically.

If you're in the 25 to 29 BMI category, there is not enough evidence at this point to say with certainty that losing weight can lower your risk of death from prostate cancer—that is, unless you have other risk factors. The combination of being overweight with more than one additional risk factor is a warning signal that you should try to lose weight. These include:

- high blood pressure (hypertension),

- high LDL (bad) cholesterol,

- low HDL (good) cholesterol,

- high triglycerides,

- high blood glucose (sugar),

- family history of premature heart disease,

- lack of physical activity, and

- smoking tobacco.

HOW TO DETERMINE YOUR BODY MASS INDEX (BMI)

Body mass index measures the relationship of your weight to your height. Determining your BMI is easy. You can let your computer do the math for you by going to the Web site for the NIH National Heart, Lung, and Blood Institute (NHLBI) and entering your vital statistics into its BMI calculator (www.nhlbisupport.com/bmi). You also can use a calculator for the math and follow these steps:

Step 1: Weigh yourself without clothing and divide the pounds by 2.2. This will give you your weight in kilograms.

Step 2: Measure your height in stocking feet and divide the inches by 39.4. This will give you your height in meters. Multiply the number you get by itself.

Step 3: Divide the results of step 1 by the results of step 2. The result you get is your BMI.

Here is how experts at the US Centers for Disease Control and Prevention (CDC) categorize BMI results:

- Underweight = less than 18.5

- Normal weight = 18.5 to 24.9

- Overweight = 25 to 29.9

- Obesity = 30 or greater

Accordingly, for someone five feet eight inches tall, a normal weight would be 122 to 164 pounds; overweight, 165 to 196; and obese, 197 and over.

THE TAKEAWAY

- Prostate cancer is the most commonly diagnosed life-threatening cancer in American men.

- Most prostate cancers grow slowly and will never develop into a life-threatening disease. More men will die *with* prostate cancer than *from* it.

- The lifetime risk of a prostate cancer diagnosis is one in six, with a one-in-thirty risk of dying from prostate cancer.

- Age, family history, ethnicity, and lifestyle choices—especially obesity—are risk factors for developing prostate cancer.

- The chance of being diagnosed with prostate cancer rises faster with age than for any other cancer.

- Men of African descent are more likely to be diagnosed with and die from prostate cancer than men of European descent. Asians, especially those living in the East, are the least likely to develop and die from prostate cancer.

- Prostate cancers that are small and microscopically indolent in appearance pose minimal risk, and are present in about one in three men in their sixties, and two in three men aged eighty to ninety. These cancers are found at similar rates throughout the world among different races and cultures, but progress to a lethal state at different rates throughout the world.

- The interaction of genes inherited from our parents and life-style choices that we make influence the progression from small, harmless prostate cancers to those that become life threatening.

- Consuming fewer calories, reducing the fat content of your diet, eating more fruits and vegetables, and exercising regularly may help lower your risk of prostate cancer and of dying from it.

CHAPTER TEN

SCREENING AND DIAGNOSING PROSTATE CANCER

Hope is the physician of each misery.

—Irish proverb

Before the late 1980s, it was not uncommon for a physician to suspect that an older male patient might have prostate cancer if the man complained about pain in his hip or low back, or of bothersome urinary symptoms. Subsequent evaluation with a digital rectal examination (DRE), prostate biopsy, and x-rays often revealed that a prostate cancer had metastasized from the gland to the bony areas of the lower spine and pelvis. Sometimes the source of urinary symptoms was a large tumor in the prostate that was now intruding upon the urethra or the bladder.

At that time, the only way to detect prostate cancer was through a DRE. Since the prostate gland is located in front of the rectum, a doctor would slip on a lubricated rubber glove, insert a finger in the anus, and feel the prostate through the rectal wall, assessing the softness or hardness of the gland. For decades, this "educated finger" was all that we had. When used alone, digital rectal exams could uncover some cancers before they were advanced, but more than half were incurable by the time they were detected. In the second half of the 1980s, nearly one in three men died within ten years of a prostate cancer diagnosis.

This was the usual course for many men who were diagnosed with prostate cancer. Long past the time when surgery or radiation could offer a potential cure, and without any effective chemotherapy available to stop the disease's relentless progression, patients with advanced prostate cancer were destined to undergo months of hormone therapy to slow tumor growth, and narcotic analgesics to ease their pain and maintain some quality of life for whatever time they had remaining.

But beginning the late 1980s, the ten-year survival rates started to climb from 70 percent to 97 percent and prostate cancer deaths fell by 40 percent. This was due in large part to earlier detection of prostate cancers through screening with the prostate-specific antigen test.

THE PSA TEST: SHEDDING LIGHT ON PROSTATE CANCER

It used to be that over 50 percent of prostate cancers were incurable by the time they were discovered. Urologists knew that some sort of cancer screening test was needed that didn't rely on touch (palpation) alone but could detect the presence of prostate cancer in asymptomatic men long before it ever reached the lethal stage. If the tumor were diagnosed while it was still within the confines of the prostate, it could then be treated, saving countless lives.

Enter the prostate-specific-antigen test, approved by the FDA in 1994 for the early detection of prostate cancer and now widely used for this purpose. But the road to understanding how to use PSA has been a long journey, and one that continues today.

Prostate-specific antigen was first discovered in the seminal fluid—which comes in part from the prostate—in the 1960s. But it wasn't detected in the bloodstream until 1979. Once investigators described a method for measuring PSA in the circulation, the race began to determine whether or not it could be a useful prostate cancer marker. In clinical trials between 1987 and 1991, PSA was proven to be:

1. elevated in men with benign prostatic enlargement (BPE) and prostate cancer,

2. higher in men with advanced cancer compared to men with early stage prostate cancer,

3. useful for monitoring the success of treatment of prostate cancer, and

4. the single best test for detecting early prostate cancer.

Many scientists deserve credit for both the discovery of the marker in the seminal fluid and bloodstream and the science behind how to best measure it, but three urologists especially deserve kudos: Dr. Thomas Stamey, then chairman of urology at Stanford University; Dr. William Catalona, who was chairman of urology at Washington University in St. Louis; and Dr. William Cooner, a private practitioner in Mobile, Alabama. The combined efforts of these men moved PSA beyond an intriguing protein that could be measured in the bloodstream to the most useful marker in the cancer field today. Imagine the excitement if breast, ovarian, pancreatic, and lung cancer could be detected early with a simple blood test like PSA.

--------------------------------MYTH BUSTER--------------------------------

Although the prostate-specific-antigen test has been disparaged for not being specific to prostate cancer—in other words, the marker also turns up in the blood due to other health conditions such as benign prostatic enlargement and prostatitis—it is well known today that PSA is the best test available for assessing the risk that prostate cancer is present and its use is in large part responsible for reducing prostate cancer deaths in the United States.

PSA BACKGROUNDER

Secreted during ejaculation into the prostatic ducts that empty into the urethra, the primary job of PSA is to liquefy semen following ejaculation, which then promotes the movement of sperm. One of the earliest applications of this novel test in the 1970s was as a diagnostic tool that police detectives could use in sexual assault investigations. By sampling the vaginal contents and testing them for PSA, it was possible to prove that a sexual assault had taken place since females don't make PSA.

Seminal fluid is much richer in PSA than is blood. In semen, PSA is found in the range of milligrams per milliliter (mg/ml). A milligram is one-thousandth of a gram (gm), and a milliliter is one-thousandth of a liter (l). By comparison, a grain of sand might weigh a milligram. But in the blood, PSA is measured in nanograms per milliliter (ng/ml), or one billionth of a gram per milliliter. PSA is believed to enter the bloodstream when prostate disease or injury disrupts the normal pathways for secretion into the seminal fluid.

A small amount of PSA (less than 1 ng/ml) can be measured in males after puberty. With age, the level of PSA in the bloodstream rises minimally in the absence of prostate disease but elevates when disease is present. In the 1980s, Dr. Stamey established that PSA levels were higher than normal both in men with prostate enlargement *and* in those with prostate cancer, and higher still in men with advanced cancer. Because benign prostate enlargement is so prevalent in aging males, and occurs more commonly than prostate cancer, measurement of PSA to detect prostate cancer is far from the "perfect" test.

Most intriguing was the finding that after surgical removal of the entire prostate, PSA levels were undetectable; and after radiation therapy and hormonal therapy for prostate cancer, levels dropped dramatically even though the prostate was not removed. In 1986, the Food and Drug Administration approved the use of the PSA test for monitoring men who'd already been diagnosed with prostate cancer. PSA is the most accurate measure available for assessing the success of therapy for prostate cancer. After any treatment of prostate cancer, a rising level indicates that the cancer has not been eradicated completely.

PSA FOR EARLY DETECTION OF PROSTATE CANCER

The FDA withheld approval for using the PSA test to detect early stage cancer; the assumption was that it would not be useful for screening because both benign and malignant prostate disease elevated prostate-specific antigen. Eight years later, though, the test did receive the green light for that purpose. A great debate ensued: At what PSA level should a prostate biopsy be ordered? When should PSA testing begin? How often should we test? At what age should testing be discontinued—if ever? All these years later, such questions have not yet been answered in full, and we are still learning how to use the PSA test.

Even without proof that PSA testing saved lives by detecting prostate cancer when it was most treatable, most physicians enthusiastically endorsed its use in conjunction with a digital rectal exam. Doctors recommended that men over fifty undergo annual PSA screening, and that an abnormality on the DRE or PSA levels above 4.0 ng/ml called for a prostate biopsy to evaluate further whether or not cancer was present. This level was thought to balance the trade-off between missing cancers when they were still curable and avoiding unnecessary prostate biopsies. However, we now know that men with PSA levels below 4.0 ng/ml can have aggressive cancers, while those with higher levels may not have the disease at all.

About the time that early research on the PSA test was beginning in the 1980s, the ability to perform a prostate biopsy using a special rapid-firing spring-loaded needle device with ultrasound guidance was introduced to the urological community. Now it was possible to perform a prostate biopsy through the rectum into the prostate with relative ease and without sedation. The transrectal ultrasound scan enabled the physician to visualize the prostate as he or she placed the needles. Coupled with the PSA test, a prostate biopsy under ultrasound guidance quickly became the norm rather than the exception for men with elevated PSA levels.

RED FLAG

There is no PSA level below which a man can be guaranteed that prostate cancer does not exist. But the risk that prostate cancer is present increases as the PSA goes up. In one carefully designed study, biopsies performed on men aged sixty-two to ninety-one years old showed that about 7 percent of those with a PSA between 3.0 and 4.0 ng/ml harbored prostate cancer.

THE IMPACT OF THE FIRST PSA TESTS

Prostate cancer diagnoses reached historic levels by 1992 due to PSA testing and prostate biopsies, increasing more than 80 percent from just four years earlier. This could be attributed to many men going to be tested for the first time. After this "low-hanging fruit" was all "picked" and treated by urologists, new cases of prostate cancer began to decline steadily in subsequent years. Still, the age-adjusted new cases per year are much higher today than in the pre-PSA era.

PROSTATE SURGERIES BEGIN TO INCREASE

Coincidentally, prior to the widespread use of PSA in the late 1980s, the rates of radical prostatectomy surgery for prostate cancer were increasing after the discovery of an improved approach to prostate removal in the early 1980s. This anatomic approach to prostate cancer removal, which was first described by Dr. Patrick Walsh at Johns Hopkins, was associated with less blood loss and fewer side effects.

Patients and physicians greater acceptance of surgery to remove the prostate, coupled with the ability to detect prostate cancer early through PSA screening, led eventually to the initial decline in deaths from prostate cancer reported in 1994. When compared to the era prior to PSA testing, prostate cancer deaths today are down 40 percent, and the likelihood of surviving ten years after diagnosis has increased 40 percent, both in large part due to the ability to detect prostate cancer at a curable stage.

SAVING LIVES WITH PSA TESTING

Since the noncancerous conditions that cause PSA elevation are more common than cancer, most men—about 70 percent—undergo a prostate biopsy when their prostate-specific antigen level has risen for reasons other than cancer. Furthermore, PSA elevations don't indicate which men have a cancer that will cause harm versus one that would not.

It's best to think of PSA as a measure of risk: the higher the PSA, the greater *the risk* that cancer is present. But only a prostate biopsy that removes prostate tissue for laboratory analysis can confirm the presence of a malignancy. Other measures of risk commonly used with PSA to assess the likelihood that a prostate cancer is present are the findings on DRE, a family history of prostate cancer, and being of African American heritage.

The PSA is a good test—the best that we have—but it's far from perfect. Yes, with the help of PSA testing, prostate cancer is being detected earlier, at a time when it can be treated more effectively with a variety of options. And carefully conducted studies from Europe, published in leading journals such as the *New England Journal of Medicine* and the *Lancet*, have reported that men between the ages of fifty and sixty-nine who are screened with the PSA test are from 20 to 40 percent less likely to die from prostate cancer than men who are not screened.

But there are important caveats. A fifteen-year study published recently in the *New England Journal of Medicine* demonstrated the doubled-edged sword of PSA testing. Investigators compared surgery and watchful waiting for men who were detected with prostate cancer the "old-fashioned" way: with a digital rectal exam only and no PSA test. Consequently, most of the subjects had been diagnosed when their disease was more advanced than compared to a diagnosis triggered by a PSA test. Nevertheless, among men over age sixty-five, surgery did not reduce deaths from prostate cancer or the rates of metastasis when compared to watchful waiting for more than fifteen years.

How can it be that screening saves lives by reducing the number of deaths from prostate cancer, but treatment does not? The answer is that prostate cancer is most often a slow-growing disease that can take decades to spread and bring about death. Because of this slow growth rate, when cancers are detected in men over the age of sixty-five, these older men are more likely to die eventually of another cause rather than prostate cancer.

The number needed to treat (NNT) is a popular measure of the effectiveness of surgical or drug interventions. It estimates how many people need to receive a treatment before one person would experience a beneficial outcome. When the statisticians turned their attention to prostate cancer therapy, it was determined that more than thirty men would need to be treated to prevent one prostate cancer death for men over the age of sixty-five. Even with such a high NNT, virtually all men who are diagnosed in our country undergo immediate treatment of some sort.

In a recent study using National Cancer Institute data to evaluate US treatment rates of prostate cancer by age, 80 percent of men seventy-five and older receive some form of active treatment (surgery, radiation, among others) for prostate cancer after a diagnosis. Yet scientific data prove that the overwhelming majority of these men being treated will gain no benefit whatsoever and will only suffer the associated side effects of treatment.

The potential for overtreating a disease that would never cause harm is truly great because, as noted before, four in five men diagnosed today are sixty-five and older—the age at which treatment has been proven to most likely not benefit patients. And the side effects of treatment can most certainly reduce a man's quality of life. In the opinion of most men, a risk of side effects is worth it if you gain extra years of life, but not if the treatment, in fact, doesn't extend life.

Because PSA screening uncovers prostate cancers that are harmless, and because our health care system generously rewards the treatment of cancer, overtreatment is now common, especially among older men. This has led to hot debates in medical circles about the extent of harm and benefit of prostate cancer screening. However, our focus should be not on the PSA test but rather the rush to initiate treatment if cancer is confirmed with a prostate biopsy.

In the upcoming chapter, I will discuss the concept of active surveillance, a common practice in Europe but not in the United States. This approach to individualizing the management of newly diagnosed prostate cancer would dramatically reduce overtreatment. Another approach to reducing overtreatment of prostate cancer is targeted, risk-based PSA screening of those men most likely to benefit from a diagnosis.

TARGETED, RISK-BASED PSA SCREENING

In the early PSA era, investigators were focusing on how best to use the PSA test in conjunction with digital rectal examination and a biopsy with transrectal ultrasound guidance to diagnose prostate cancer. The many questions that remained unanswered, and the excitement of discovery, attracted me to Johns Hopkins as a young faculty member in the late 1980s.

In reading about screening for breast cancer and cervical cancer, I learned that investigators in other fields were using the results from prior tests to predict whether or not cancer would be diagnosed later on. For example, the standard recommendation for women is to go for an annual Pap smear, a simple office procedure to test for evidence of cervical cancer. But as I discovered, gynecologists were beginning to advise their female patients whose PAP smears had consistently tested negative that less frequent screening was sufficient.

I began to wonder if all men really needed a yearly PSA test. Could it be that maintaining a low PSA level year after year was predictive of the future risk of prostate cancer? Could men who had a history of low PSA levels be screened less frequently? If PSA were a predictor of future risk, would it be reasonable to perform a baseline PSA test at age forty and repeat it infrequently, depending upon the result?

Through the Baltimore Longitudinal Study of Aging (BLSA), I was fortunate to have forged relationships with many great clinical investigators who allowed me to address these questions. The BLSA, America's longest-running scientific study of human aging, was initiated in 1958 by the National Institute on Aging (NIA) to study what happens as people age. Male participants usually entered the study in midlife and were followed for decades until death.

Just fifteen minutes away from the Johns Hopkins campus where I worked, the BLSA had been storing blood of test volunteers in freezers since 1958. Understanding that the stored blood could provide us a "picture" of prostate-specific antigen as men aged—with some developing and some dodging prostate disease—the scientists at the BLSA agreed to measure PSA in stored samples. Over five thousand repeated measures in almost one thousand men over the span of three to four decades proved to be a gold mine in the early years of PSA discovery.

Together with my colleagues at the BLSA, we sought to answer the question of whether or not all men needed to have their PSA levels tested annually in order to detect curable prostate cancer. First, we evaluated the repeated PSA readings of participants in the longitudinal study, to determine how often men with low PSA would see their levels rise to a point that would trigger a prostate biopsy over two years and four years. We found that if a man had a PSA level below 2.0 ng/ml, it was very unlikely that over two years it would be in the range of 3.0 to 4.0 ng/ml and trigger a prostate biopsy. But if the PSA were above 2 ng/ml, at the start of the study it was not uncommon two years later for a man to have a level that would call for a prostate biopsy.

Combining these data with surgical data from Johns Hopkins allowed us to recommend in the *Journal of the American Medical Association* in 1997 that missing a curable prostate cancer would be unlikely if men with PSA readings below 2.0 ng/ml were to undergo testing every other year.

This finding has now been confirmed over a decade later in large screening trials from Europe. Reducing the frequency of PSA testing among men who don't need it will lower the numbers of false-positive test results, unnecessary biopsies, and the discovery of cancers picked up serendipitously, for which treatment is not beneficial.

WHEN TO BEGIN PSA TESTING

To further develop PSA screening recommendations and determine the age at which PSA screening should begin, I worked with Harry Guess and Kevin Ross, two epidemiologists at the University of North Carolina with expertise in computer simulations. There were reasons to suspect that PSA testing of men younger than fifty would save lives, including evidence that younger men were more likely to have curable cancers when compared with older men.

We borrowed a technique that had been used to develop cervical cancer screening recommendations, called Monte Carlo simulations. This approach involved building a model of prostate cancer development in a simulated population of men and then testing different screening strategies for preventing prostate cancer death. An important input into the model was what happened to PSA over men's lifetimes, and this information was available from our BLSA frozen blood bank.

Based on this computer simulation, we compared annual PSA screening beginning at age fifty—the prevailing recommendation at that time—with PSA testing at age forty, once again at age forty-five, and then every other year beginning at age fifty. As we reported in the *Journal of the American Medical Association*, testing PSA intermittently beginning at age forty not only reduced prostate cancer deaths but also reduced the resources utilized (PSA tests and prostate biopsies) to diagnose a prostate cancer.

PSA AND FURTHER RISK OF PROSTATE CANCER

Using the BLSA resources, it was then time to learn more about what PSA levels in men in their forties and fifties were telling us about the future risk of prostate cancer later in life. It turned out that a single PSA level among men in their forties and fifties predicted future risk more accurately than a family history of prostate cancer. For men with PSA levels above the median value (the PSA level that separates the higher half from the lower half of the population)—0.6 ng/ml for men in their forties and 0.7 ng/ml for men in their fifties—we noted a threefold to fourfold greater risk of being diagnosed with prostate cancer over the next two decades when compared with patients whose PSA values fell below the median.

This result, published in 2001, together with our previous findings, now forms the basis for many of the recommendations from the National Comprehensive Cancer Network (NCCN), an organization that develops PSA screening guidelines in the United States. Studies from Europe and data from observational groups in Scandinavia are confirming the value of targeted screening based on a PSA level in midlife rather than the one-size-fits-all approach of annual screening for all men. With targeted screening that reduces the downstream effects of unnecessary biopsies and treatments, the ratio of benefit to harm can be increased.

PROSTATE CANCER SCREENING AMONG THE ELDERLY: GREAT EXPENSE, UNLIKELY BENEFIT

By the time men reach their seventies and eighties, as many as two in three harbor small prostate cancers not destined to cause harm. About half of these are detectable by prostate biopsy. In studies of men enrolled in Medicare, about one in five prostate biopsies are performed in men with limited life expectancies. Cancer is found in about one in three, and about two in five of those with a negative biopsy undergo a repeat biopsy within five years.

Detecting these cancers in older men often leads to unnecessary treatments that will not extend life but only reduce its quality. But some older men harbor prostate cancers that can cause harm without treatment—cancers that would be missed if screening were discontinued in all older men. Some guidelines have recommended that men over the age of seventy-five no longer have PSA tests.

An alternative approach comes from a study using frozen blood samples from men in the Baltimore Longitudinal Study of Aging. Dr. Edward Schaeffer, a colleague from Johns Hopkins, wondered if a certain PSA level would help identify a group of older men with no risk of developing a life-threatening prostate cancer who therefore could safely discontinue screening. Data from the BLSA had already shown that low PSA levels in younger men were predictive of a low risk of prostate cancer in the future, so why not in older men?

Writing in the *Journal of Urology* in 2009, Dr. Schaeffer and investigators from the BLSA reported that no men in the study who had a PSA below 3.0 ng/ml in their mid seventies developed lethal prostate cancer during their remaining years of life. Since two in three men at age seventy-five have PSA levels below 3.0 ng/ml, for the first time, it was now possible to present an alternative recommendation to older men.

Instead of advising all of these men that they are too old for PSA testing, we had the scientific evidence to say, "Based on your low PSA, you are at zero-to-minimal risk of dying of prostate cancer, and you needn't worry about PSA tests anymore." I have found that most older men are relieved to hear that news.

The concept of targeted screening for those at the greatest risk of harboring prostate cancer and less frequent or no screening for those at lower risk started with the collaboration between the Department of Urology at Johns Hopkins and the BLSA. This concept is now ready for prime time and can reduce the harms of screening that include the diagnosis of cancers that otherwise would not have been detected, and the subsequent overtreatment of prostate cancer.

BECOME INFORMED ABOUT YOUR PSA OPTIONS

Many health organizations now recommend that patients and their physicians discuss the drawbacks and benefits of PSA testing before the recommended time to begin screening arrives. The evidence suggests that this discussion rarely takes place. Oftentimes a physician will simply check off the box to order a PSA test at some arbitrary age, along with other standard blood tests. My recommendation is that you become informed about PSA testing and decide whether or not it is right for you.

PSA TESTING OVER THE YEARS

If You Are in Your Forties

Prostate-specific-antigen screening for cancer can detect malignancies earlier than not screening. Prostate cancer is unlikely in men in their forties, but those younger men who do develop the disease are more likely to benefit from treatment when compared with older men. We don't know for sure if screening men in their forties will reduce prostate cancer deaths, compared with starting at age fifty. Some guidelines recommend a baseline PSA test at age forty for all men, while others advise testing only those of African American descent and/or who have a family history of prostate cancer.

If you choose to be screened, baseline PSA levels prior to age fifty can be used to compare levels at age fifty and beyond. An assessment of changes in PSA is believed by most urologists to be an important measure of prostate cancer risk.

If You Are Fifty to Sixty-nine Years Old

PSA testing at two- to four-year intervals can reduce the risk of prostate cancer death by 20 percent to 40 percent. The benefits of screening can include a reduction in the adverse health consequences that occur with advanced disease, and/or a reduction in the rate of death from prostate cancer.

The negative aspects of screening can include concerns about PSA levels; complications from a prostate biopsy or repeated prostate biopsies; and side effects of prostate cancer treatments, including urinary, bowel, and sexual dysfunction.

PSA testing in men of this age group will detect some cancers that never would have caused adverse health consequences; and treatment of these cancers causes more harm than benefit.

The younger and healthier you are, the more likely that the benefits of screening will outweigh the disadvantages. If you have serious health problems such as diabetes or heart disease, the likelihood of your benefiting from screening are lower, and you may want to consider not screening.

If You Are Seventy or Older

There is strong evidence that PSA testing beyond age seventy will not improve health outcomes for most men and that PSA testing beyond age seventy-five will result in more harm than benefit.

Men at age seventy with any serious health problems should not undergo routine PSA testing. Men without any serious health problems may want to consider PSA testing after age seventy, and for them the decision to continue can be based on a PSA level, which, if still low, is a strong predictor of a low risk of developing a lethal cancer.

These guidelines don't apply to men undergoing an evaluation for urinary symptoms in which a PSA level is an important part of the evaluation to determine the cause.

TARGETED SCREENING: WHAT I RECOMMEND
BASED ON THE AVAILABLE EVIDENCE

Because no scientific trials have proven (1) the value of PSA testing for men younger than fifty and older than sixty-nine, (2) the value of annual screening versus less frequent screening, (3) the value of a diagnosis at one PSA level versus another, the guidelines below are based on personal opinion and my experience caring for patients.

Age Forty: Have Your First PSA Test

- If your PSA is 0.6 ng/ml or lower, schedule your next PSA test when you are forty-five and then again at fifty.

- If your PSA is greater than 0.6 ng/ml but 1.0 ng/ml or less, have your next test in two years and continue with that schedule.

- If your PSA is greater than 1.0 ng/ml, retest annually.

- If your PSA is continuously rising regardless of the level, or if it reaches 2.0 ng/ml or above, see a urologist for advice.

Ages Fifty to Sixty-nine: Screen Regularly If in Good Health

- If your PSA is below 2.0 ng/ml, have a PSA test every other year.

- If your PSA is 2.0 ng/ml or above, have a PSA test annually.

- If your PSA is continuously rising or reaches a level above 3.0 ng/ml, see a urologist for advice.

Ages Seventy to Seventy-five: Consider That PSA Screening Is More Likely to Cause Harm Than Benefit for Most, and Screen Only If in Excellent Health

- If your PSA is below 1.0 ng/ml, repeat the test in four years.

- If your PSA is 1.0 to 2.0 ng/ml, repeat PSA testing at two-year intervals.

- If your PSA is 2.0 ng/ml or more, repeat PSA testing annually.

- If your PSA is continuously rising or reaches a level above 4.0 ng/ml, see a urologist for advice.

Above Age Seventy-five: Consider That PSA Screening Is Not Likely to Be Beneficial Regardless of Health If You Decide On Screening

- Consider discontinuing screening if PSA is below 3.0 ng/ml.

- If your PSA is 3.0 ng/ml or above, repeat the test annually.

- If your PSA is rising at a rate of 1.0 ng/ml every year or more than that for two consecutive years, or reaches 10.0 ng/ml or above, see a urologist for advice.

Understand that short-term fluctuations in PSA are common. Therefore, repeat any PSA test after two to four weeks before considering it abnormal. If you have any new onset of irritating urinary symptoms (frequency, urgency, pain with urination), consider a course of antibiotics before repeating the PSA test. A continuously rising PSA could be a sign of cancer in some men.

Table 10.1. The Percentage of Men with a Given PSA Level by Age*

PSA Level (ng/ml)	Aged 50 to 59	Aged 60 to 69	Aged 70 or Older	Total
2.5 or below	88 percent	75 percent	61 percent	78 percent
2.6 to 4.0	8 percent	14 percent	18 percent	12 percent
4.1 to 9.9	3 percent	9 percent	16 percent	8 percent
10.0 or above	1 percent	2 percent	5 percent	2 percent

*Based on 10,248 men and adapted from Deborah S. Smith, et al., "Longitudinal Screening for Prostate Cancer with Prostate-Specific Antigen," *Journal of the American Medical Association* 276, no. 16 (October 23, 1996): 1309–15.

PSA RECOMMENDATIONS FROM LEADING MEDICAL ORGANIZATIONS

The leading US medical organizations all encourage men to consult with their doctors about PSA testing and then make an informed decision about what they want to do. These guidelines will change as more information becomes available about the benefits and drawbacks of screening. Here are the recommendations from some leading organizations that develop guidelines for screening.

- **American Cancer Society.** Talk to your doctor about the pros and cons of testing starting at age fifty so that you can decide if screening is the right choice for you. African American men and men with a father or brother who had prostate cancer before age sixty-five should discuss with their doctor about starting testing at age forty-five. If you decide to be screened, you should have the PSA test with or without a rectal exam.

- **American Urological Association (AUA).** The AUA published a "Best Practice Statement" on PSA in 2009 recommending that the test should be offered to all men with a life expectancy of at least ten years, starting at age forty. The decision regarding whether or not to perform a prostate biopsy should be based not on a single PSA level but rather on a combination of factors that include the results of the PSA and DRE, age, family history, ethnicity, prior biopsy results, overall health and life expectancy, free PSA, PSA velocity (rate of change from year to year), and PSA density (PSA score divided by the volume of the prostate).

- **National Comprehensive Cancer Network (NCCN).** This alliance of twenty-one leading cancer centers develops guidelines for practicing physicians on early cancer detection. The NCCN recommends starting a risk-versus-benefit discussion at age forty and offering a baseline DRE and PSA at age forty. It also suggests individual decisions regarding screening men over the age of seventy-five. Like the AUA, the NCCN recommends taking into account multiple factors when considering a prostate biopsy.

- **US Preventive Services Task Force (USPSTF).** The USPSTF is an independent panel of experts in prevention and evidence-based medicine and is composed of primary care providers such as internists, pediatricians, family physicians, obstetrician-gynecologists, nurses, and health behavior specialists. These experts conduct scientific evidence reviews of a broad range of clinical preventive health care services and make recommendations for primary care clinicians and health systems.

    In October 2011, the task force issued a draft statement suggesting that routine use of PSA testing be abandoned. This controversial recommendation was based on its review of the available data from prostate cancer clinical trials, and it applies to all symptom-free men regardless of age, family history, or race. Final recommendations from the USPSTF are still pending.

PSA: PLAYING THE ODDS

The likelihood of having prostate cancer and the likelihood of its being aggressive, or a high-grade type of tumor, varies by the PSA level and whether or not the digital rectal exam is suspicious for cancer. The risk increases incrementally as PSA rises and, within any given PSA range, is higher if the DRE is abnormal. The percentage risks of finding prostate cancer on a biopsy and finding high-grade cancer in men with and without a suspicious DRE are shown in the table below:

Table 10.2. Prostate Cancer Detection by the PSA Level and the Results of the DRE (from Published Series Reporting Results of Prostate Biopsies)

PSA Level (ng/ml)	DRE Findings*	Any Cancer on Biopsy (percentage)+	Rate of High-Grade Cancer on Biopsy (percentage)†
0.0 to 1.0	–	9 percent	1 percent
1.0 to 2.0	–	17 percent	2 percent
0.0 to 2.0	–	12 percent	1 percent
		8 percent	
2.0 to 4.0	–	15 percent to 25 percent	5 percent
		21 percent	
4.0 to 10.0	+	17 percent to 32 percent	4 percent
		45 percent to 51 percent	12 percent
Above 10.0	–	43 percent to 65 percent	19 percent
	+	70 percent to 90 percent	51 percent
Below 4.0	–	15 percent	2 percent
	+	13 percent to 17 percent	
Above 4.0	–	23 percent to 38 percent	6 percent
	+	55 percent to 63 percent	21 percent

Adapted from H. Ballentine Carter, et al., "Diagnosis and Staging of Prostate Cancer," in *Campbell-Walsh Urology* (9th ed.), ed. Alan J. Wein, Louis R. Kavoussi, Alan W. Partin, and Craig A. Peters (Philadelphia: W. B. Saunders Co., 2007), 2912–31.
*DRE nonsuspicious for cancer (–); DRE suspicious for cancer (+)
†The number of cancers detected divided by the total number of men undergoing a biopsy.

FACTORS THAT CAN AFFECT YOUR PSA LEVEL

PSA elevations occur most commonly because of the presence of prostate disease such as inflammation, benign or noncancerous enlargement, and cancer. PSA elevations may indicate the presence of prostate disease, but not all men with prostate disease have elevated PSA levels. And remember, PSA elevations are not specific for cancer.

Other factors that can affect PSA levels besides prostate disease that your doctor should consider when interpreting the level are discussed below.

- **Prostate trauma.** This can occur with prostate massage, prostate biopsy, and transurethral resection of the prostate (TURP). A digital rectal exam can lead to slight increases in blood PSA, causing leakage of the protein into the blood, but these are rarely significant enough to cause a false elevation. After a prostate biopsy, the PSA usually returns to baseline in one to two months, but not always. After a TURP that removes prostate tissue, the PSA level is set at a new, lower baseline; the more tissue removed, the lower the level. A rising PSA after a new baseline has been reached after TURP should prompt suspicion of prostate cancer and may warrant further evaluation.

- **Prostate treatment.** Treatments for prostate enlargement and cancer can lower blood PSA by decreasing the amount of tissue that produces PSA and by decreasing the amount of PSA produced per cell. Examples of common treatments that lower PSA levels are (1) drug therapies to reduce or block androgen production for treatment of prostate cancer, (2) radiation therapy for cancer, and (3) surgical removal of prostate tissue for BPE and cancer.

  Drugs such as 5-alpha reductase inhibitors, used for both the treatment of prostate enlargement and male hair loss (finasteride, or Proscar; dutasteride, or Avodart; and finasteride, or Propecia), lower PSA levels by about 50 percent after twelve months of treatment. If you have been on one of these drugs for twelve to thirty months, multiplying your PSA level by the number 2 will give you the approximate "true" PSA level; for thirty months or longer, multiply your PSA level by 2.5.

  If your PSA does not decrease by 50 percent while using one of these drugs, or if it rises, your physician may suspect the presence of prostate cancer. Finasteride is marketed as Propecia for treatment of male pattern hair loss, and this 1-milligram formulation causes the same decline in blood PSA levels as the 5-milligram dosage marketed as Proscar for prostate enlargement.

- **Ejaculation.** Among men fifty years of age and older for whom PSA is primarily used to detect early stage prostate cancer, ejaculation can lead to an increase in prostate-specific antigen that could result in a false-positive elevation. This is especially true for men with a higher baseline level. You should abstain from sexual activity for forty-eight hours prior to your PSA test.

- **Acute urinary retention.** PSA levels may be elevated in men who have a sudden inability to urinate, but they will usually return to baseline within weeks after the obstruction is relieved.

- **Prostatitis.** An infection of the prostate can dramatically increase PSA. But the level will usually return to baseline one to two months after ending antibiotic treatment.

INTERPRETING YOUR PSA TEST: TO BIOPSY OR NOT?

When prostate cancer is suspected based on the results of the PSA test, determining the need for and the timing of a biopsy based solely on PSA results is not always a clear-cut process. In about 70 percent to 80 percent of cases, a biopsy triggered by an elevated PSA uncovers no cancer. Think about it: only one in four men who undergo a prostate biopsy are found to have prostate cancer; the other three have endured an unnecessary biopsy that is invasive and costly, not to mention anxiety provoking.

My advice to you is that an absolute PSA level should not automatically prompt a prostate biopsy in most cases. When PSA levels are less than 10.0 ng/ml and cancer is suspected, a physician should consider a number of additional factors before recommending a biopsy.

In general, urologists are more suspicious of prostate cancer at any given PSA level if a man is young—especially below age sixty—or is of African descent, or has never previously undergone a prostate biopsy. Other concerns that might be considered when interpreting the PSA level are how quickly the PSA has risen (called PSA velocity), PSA isoform levels, the relationship between PSA and the size of the prostate, and the new urinary marker PCA3. Let's examine each of these important factors.

PSA VELOCITY

In the early 1990s, I had the unique opportunity to work with investigators at the Baltimore Longitudinal Study of Aging to understand what happened to PSA blood levels in aging men with and without prostate cancer. At that time, little was known about how to interpret PSA results.

We devised a study to measure the PSA levels over three decades in sixteen men without prostate disease, twenty men with benign prostatic enlargement, and eighteen prostate cancer patients. All of the participants had been enrolled in the aging study and had contributed frozen blood samples at about two-year intervals long before PSA was ever discovered.

Here is what we found: the most important factor affecting PSA levels as men grew older was the development of prostate disease. In men without prostate disease, average PSA levels remained around 1 ng/ml, with virtually no change over the decades. However, this was not the case for those who developed BPE or prostate cancer.

For those with age-related prostate enlargement, PSA levels started out in midlife around 1.0 ng/ml, on average, but increased to around 3.0 ng/ml over the course of the next one to two decades as the prostate grew in size. But the picture was very different for the men who developed prostate cancer. While their PSA started out in midlife at readings similar to those of men without prostate cancer, their levels rose much faster.

Five years before the cancer was diagnosed, the rate of rise in prostate-specific antigen could reliably distinguish men with and without prostate cancer. We coined the term PSA velocity (PSAV) to describe the rate of rise in PSA and, in an article published in the *Journal of the American Medical Association* in 1992, suggested that among men with PSA levels between 4.0 and 10.0 ng/ml, a PSA velocity greater than 0.75 ng/ml per year was predictive of prostate cancer.

Although some studies have suggested that PSAV is not useful for prostate cancer detection, many others have confirmed its value. Today no physician would ignore a rising PSA. He or she would either follow the PSA more frequently to gather information on the trend in PSA or recommend a prostate biopsy. This approach has led to earlier detection of prostate cancers.

Now fast-forward to 2006. The PSA test is now a routine part of clinical practice, and many investigators are concerned about the overdetection and overtreatment of cancers picked up through PSA testing—especially when prostate biopsies are performed at PSA levels below 4.0 ng/ml. But we now know that some men with low PSA levels have life-threatening or lethal cancers.

One unanswered question was whether or not PSAV could determine that if a man's PSA were below 3.0 to 4.0 ng/ml, would it be predictive of the development of a lethal prostate cancer decades later? If that were true, then PSAV could be used to stratify men into two groups: (1) those who should undergo a prostate biopsy despite low PSA levels, and (2) those who could wait longer to see what happens to their PSA level over time.

Through our collaboration with the BLSA, we determined PSA levels repeatedly among almost one thousand men for as long as four decades. In the 1992 PSAV study, we first selected men with and without prostate disease and then measured PSA levels to determine PSAV. This time we used a more powerful study design: we took the PSA measurements of 980 men and determined their PSAVs.

Of the 980 men, 856 never developed prostate cancer, 104 were diagnosed with prostate cancer but did not die of it, and 20 died of prostate cancer. The PSAV ten to fifteen years prior to the diagnosis of prostate cancer was closely associated with the risk of death from prostate cancer when most men had PSA levels below 4.0 ng/ml.

For example, for those men with a PSAV of 0.35 ng/ml per year or less, the probability of dying of prostate cancer twenty-five years later was 8 percent, whereas it was 46 percent for those men with a PSAV above 0.35 ng/ml per year. We concluded that PSAV was a useful indicator of the risk of dying from prostate cancer among men with PSA levels that ordinarily might not prompt a prostate biopsy, and that this could help identify patients who might otherwise be overlooked based on the PSA test alone. The National Comprehensive Cancer Network has recommended the use of PSAV as one indicator of prostate cancer risk among men with low PSA levels.

PSA DENSITY (PSAD)

To calculate PSA density, your physician divides the PSA value by the size or volume of the prostate, which is most commonly determined by a transrectal ultrasound or MRI scan. If your PSA is 5.0 ng/ml and your prostate is 45 cubic centimeters (cc), then your PSAD would be 0.11 ng/ml per cc.

Dr. Mitchell Benson, chairman of urology at Columbia University Medical Center in New York City, suggested in 1992 that adjusting PSA for prostate size (based on an ultrasound scan) could help distinguish between PSA elevations caused by BPE and those caused by prostate cancer. This certainly makes sense. If there is no prostate enlargement to explain the PSA elevation, then cancer is more likely present than if the prostate is enlarged. Without question, if two men have the same PSA, the one with the smaller prostate is more likely to have cancer discovered on a biopsy. While some believe that this is so because it is easier to detect cancer in smaller prostates, I don't.

When Dr. Jonathan Epstein of Johns Hopkins published his landmark 1994 paper in the *Journal of the American Medical Association* evaluating the predictors of indolent prostate cancer, PSA density was a strong predictor of larger, higher-grade malignancies. Numerous studies now confirm that men with higher PSADs are more likely to have more extensive cancers than those with lower PSADs.

Men with PSA levels that are less than 15 percent of the prostate volume (PSAD below 0.15) have a lower likelihood of cancer—and extensive cancer—when compared with men whose PSA levels are above 15 percent of the prostate volume (PSAD above 0.15).

Although PSA density is an imperfect predictor of cancer, it is an additional method of determining the risk that prostate cancer is present when someone's PSA level is below 10.0 ng/ml.

FREE PSA

The percentage of free PSA provides similar information to the PSAD. Prostate-specific antigen travels the bloodstream in two forms: free-floating PSA and complexed (attached) to proteins. The initial tests that were approved for early detection of prostate cancer measured both complexed and free PSA together. In the early 1990s, scientists discovered that men with prostate cancer have a greater percentage of blood PSA that is complexed—and a lower proportion of free PSA—than men without prostate cancer. Although the reasons for this are not entirely clear, the observation generated a lot of excitement, since scientists believed that this was the long-sought method to distinguish between PSA elevations due to prostate cancer and those due to prostate enlargement.

Dr. William Catalona demonstrated that the percentage of free PSA appears to be most useful in distinguishing between men with and without prostate cancer when total PSA levels fall in the range 4.0 to 10.0 ng/ml. In a large study combining data from multiple institutions, restricting biopsies to those with a free to total PSA below 25 percent would have detected 95 percent of cancers, while avoiding 20 percent of the unnecessary biopsies. The risk of cancer in this study ranged from 8 percent when the percentage of free PSA was more than 25 percent, to 56 percent when the percentage of free PSA was 0 percent to 10 percent.

In reality, however, most free PSA levels fall in the middle range, not the extremes above 25 percent and below 10 percent, where free PSA provides the most useful discrimination between prostate enlargement and cancer.

The percentage of free PSA is also associated with the presence of larger cancers that are more likely to cause harm. We used the frozen blood samples from the Baltimore Longitudinal Study of Aging to measure total and free PSA in men with locally advanced or high-grade aggressive disease, and in men without these features. In 1997 we reported that at ten years before a prostate cancer diagnosis, when PSA and free PSA alone did not distinguish between the two types of cancer, a free to total PSA ratio below 15 percent was associated strongly with the more aggressive type of cancer. Other investigators subsequently confirmed these findings.

The FDA approved the use of free-PSA testing for prostate cancer detection in 1998, and today there are specific assays for measuring free and complexed PSA. The percentage of free PSA and PSAD provide similar information, and are additional tools for risk stratification when deciding on the need for a prostate biopsy. Most urologists use free PSA to help determine the likelihood that a prostate cancer has been missed on a biopsy, or to help decide whether to biopsy a man with a borderline PSA indication. A new urinary marker called PCA3 also appears useful for this purpose.

PCA3 TEST

The prostate cancer gene 3 test, more commonly known as the PCA3 test, is a urine test that can be used when there is some doubt about whether or not a biopsy should be recommended. PCA3 is a nucleic acid—the information molecules in cells called messenger ribonucleic acid (mRNA)—that is found in higher amounts in prostate cancer tissue as compared with benign tissue. PCA3 was discovered at Johns Hopkins in the laboratory of Dr. William Isaacs. Subsequently, urinary assays were developed to measure PCA3 mRNA, and it was found that PCA3 urinary levels were associated with the likelihood of a positive initial or repeat prostate biopsy.

Although approved for use in Europe, PCA3 is still awaiting approval in this country by the Food and Drug Administration. Even so, many specialized diagnostic laboratories offer the test. Unlike the PSA test, PCA3 is specific for prostate cancer and not affected by benign prostatic enlargement and other noncancerous conditions that can elevate prostate-specific antigen.

When combined with other information such as the digital rectal exam and PSA, the PCA3 score can provide valuable information when you and your doctor are deciding between going forward with a biopsy or delaying it. The higher the PCA3 score, the more likely a biopsy will be positive for cancer. Scientists are currently investigating whether PCA3 is associated with prostate cancer aggressiveness, but to date the results are conflicting.

PSA ISOFORMS

Isoforms are different forms of the same protein. PSA isoforms have been shown to be present in different concentrations in the blood, depending on the type of prostate disease. One isoform is pro-PSA, or pPSA, which is a precursor form of PSA. Another isoform of PSA, BPSA, is found in benign tissue from the transition zone, the area of the prostate where benign prostatic enlargement begins. A larger proportion of pro-PSA has been found to be associated with prostate cancer.

Recent studies suggest that measuring these isoforms may improve our ability to predict the presence of prostate cancer over PSA alone, and work is ongoing. In the future, it is very likely that a panel of markers will aid your physician in determining the need for a prostate biopsy, and the likelihood that it will behave aggressively. For example, in a recent article published in 2011 in the journal *Science Translational Medicine*, a urine test that detected genetic alterations in two genes and also measured the activity of the gene PCA3, improved the prediction of cancer and the presence of high-grade cancer among men who gave a urine specimen before undergoing a prostate biopsy or a radical prostatectomy for cancer.

Early Prostate Cancer Screening: Navigating Results

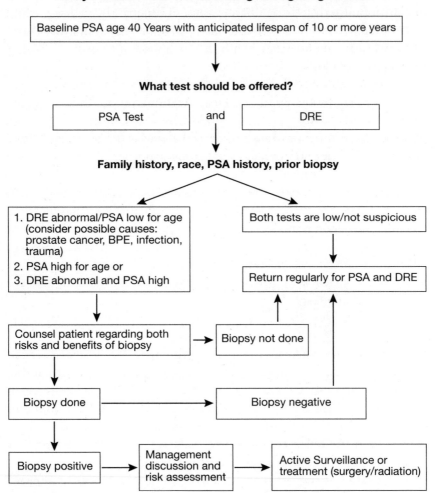

Baseline PSA age 40 Years with anticipated lifespan of 10 or more years

What test should be offered?

PSA Test　　and　　DRE

Family history, race, PSA history, prior biopsy

1. DRE abnormal/PSA low for age (consider possible causes: prostate cancer, BPE, infection, trauma)
2. PSA high for age or
3. DRE abnormal and PSA high

Both tests are low/not suspicious

Return regularly for PSA and DRE

Counsel patient regarding both risks and benefits of biopsy → Biopsy not done

Biopsy done → Biopsy negative

Biopsy positive → Management discussion and risk assessment → Active Surveillance or treatment (surgery/radiation)

Adapted from Greene, K. L., et al., "Prostate Specific Antigen Best Practice Statement: 2009 Update," *J. Urol.* 2009 Nov; 182(5): 2232–41.

THE BIOPSY: UNCOVERING IMPORTANT INFORMATION ABOUT YOUR PROSTATE

A PSA test and a digital rectal exam do not diagnose prostate cancer but only raise suspicion of its presence. A diagnosis of prostate cancer requires a prostate biopsy. If you are considered to be at risk of prostate cancer based on a PSA test or a DRE, a prostate biopsy may be recommended. Each year, more than a million men undergo prostate biopsy to determine if they have prostate cancer. In about 75 percent of the cases, the result is negative; there is no evidence of cancer.

Pathologists play a vital role in the process of analyzing the tissue removed from the body. They interpret the biopsy results, determine whether or not cancer is present, and if so, its degree of aggressiveness. Think of the pathologist as a detective and problem solver. He uses the tools of laboratory medicine to provide diagnostic and prognostic information to the treating physician, who guides management. A major challenge for urologic pathologists is to evaluate accurately the prostate tissue samples they view under their microscopes.

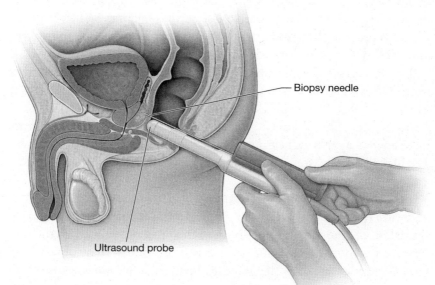

The prostate biopsy

Dr. Jonathan Epstein, the Rose-Lee and Keith Reinhard professor of urologic pathology at Johns Hopkins, is internationally recognized as the world's expert in prostate cancer pathology—the "chief justice," so to speak. To understand better what he and his fellow pathologists do, he recommends that you visualize the prostate as an oversized strawberry. Now imagine cancerous cells, if they are present, as tiny seeds just a few millimeters in size within the strawberry. When performing a biopsy with a spring-loaded biopsy gun, your urologist is on a delicate search mission to capture the tiny cancerous specks—typically found in the peripheral zone of the prostate, which extends along the sides of the gland. These prostate cells, among the hardest of all to analyze, are then sent to a pathologist for examination to determine if they are cancerous or not, and if so, what management is best.

Do you want to know what a prostate tissue specimen looks like under a pathologist's microscope? Imagine looking at a Jackson Pollock abstract painting, with countless shades and variations of color all swirled together. Within this mass are normal cells and in some cases cells that are not normal. By viewing this sample, the pathologist determines if cancer is present and, if so, how much.

What a pathologist is looking at are the patterns of the glands that make up the part of the prostate that produces seminal fluid and the proteins within. Prostate cancers arise in these glands. When prostate cancer is present, the glands are altered and can be divided into five recognizable patterns that are added together to form a score.

Dr. Donald F. Gleason, a pathologist, first described the five patterns in the 1960s when he served as chief of pathology at the Minneapolis VA Medical Center. He devised a scoring system that bears his name: the Gleason score. This system is still the most accurate predictor of a prostate cancer's aggressiveness and is used widely to guide management. The higher the Gleason score, the more virulent the tumor tends to be.

UNDERSTANDING THE GLEASON GRADING SYSTEM

There are five Gleason patterns or *grades*, from 1 through 5, that describe the extent of gland alteration. Think of the prostate glands like the furniture in a room, with some arranged more neatly than others. The Gleason grade describes the glandular patterns, or "orderliness of the furniture." The more orderly the furniture, the lower the grade.

Grades 1 through 3 describe glandular patterns that appear more normal and orderly, whereas grades 4 and 5 describe glands that no longer appear like glands—the furniture in the room is in complete disarray like the day after a raucous New Year's Eve party. Grades of 1, 2, and 3 are associated with a more benign clinical course, while grades 4 and 5 tend to behave aggressively and spread beyond the prostate.

The glands in a prostate cancer are often made up of an array of grades—not just one—some of which are fairly normal appearing and others quite disorderly. Dr. Gleason discovered that by adding the two most prevalent grades together to arrive at a *score*, the more precise the prediction of tumor aggressiveness.

For example, if the most prevalent, or primary, glandular grade seen is 3, and the second most prevalent, or secondary, grade is 4, the Gleason score would be 3 + 4 = 7, with 3 the primary and 4 the secondary grade. However, if the most prevalent grade is 4, and the second most prevalent grade is 3, then the Gleason score would also equal 7 (4 + 3), but with 4 the primary grade and 3 the secondary grade. The tumor scored 3 + 4 behaves less aggressively than the 4 + 3 tumor because the primary pattern is 3 rather than 4.

To complicate matters further, pathologists have decided to abbreviate the Gleason grading system, and only scores of 3, 4, and 5 are used to describe prostate biopsies for both primary and secondary grades, adding these to obtain scores from 6 through 10. Gleason score-6 cancers tend to behave less aggressively than Gleason score-7 cancers, which, in turn, behave less aggressively than cancers scored as 8, 9, and 10. Pathologists now often report primary, secondary, and tertiary patterns if a higher-grade component makes up a substantial amount of the cancer in addition to the primary and secondary grade.

Today 60 percent to 70 percent of cancers diagnosed on a prostate biopsy are graded as Gleason score 6; about 20 percent to 30 percent, Gleason score 7; and 5 percent to 10 percent, Gleason score 8 and higher. The vast majority of cancers picked up on a prostate biopsy are the least aggressive type. And because pathologists today tend to grade higher than in earlier years, many Gleason score-7 cancers would have been classified as score-6 tumors years ago. As you might expect, assigning higher grades contributes to the higher rates of prostate cancer treatment.

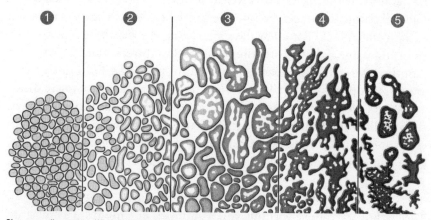

Gleason grading system: What the pathologist sees under a microscope
Low grades (1, 2, 3) behave less aggressively than high grades (4, 5)

THE BIOPSY PROCEDURE

The prostate biopsy is an outpatient procedure typically performed by a urologist and generally takes no longer than fifteen to twenty minutes. On the day before the procedure, an antibiotic—usually a fluoroquinolone (levofloxacin, or Levaquin; ciprofloxacin, or Cipro)—is started to prevent infection, which can occur if bacteria in the rectum seed the prostate or bloodstream. Since the ultrasound probe that's used only goes in the rectum on the day of the biopsy, you're to cleanse the rectum—a task that can usually be accomplished at home with a self-administered enema.

At the doctor's office, a mild sedative may be given to relax you, but usually the procedure is done using the analgesic lidocaine to block pain messages from the prostate, just like the dentist blocks a tooth before drilling a cavity. As you lie on your side with your knees drawn up toward your abdomen, an ultrasound probe is inserted into the rectum. The sound waves emitted by the probe are returned, processed, and produce images of the prostate on a video screen. These images help the physician to guide a needle through a hollow tube attached to the ultrasound probe so that different areas can be sampled systematically. The procedure is often referred to as transrectal ultrasound-guided prostate biopsy, or TRUS.

Usually ten to twelve samples or more are obtained. A spring-loaded device rapidly propels the needle through the rectum into the prostate, shearing off and capturing a small piece of prostate tissue each time it fires. Each needle collects a core of tissue 1/16th of an inch in diameter. Most men rate the discomfort level as minimal to none when lidocaine is injected through the rectum into the tissue beside the prostate and used as a prostate block. For a few days afterward, there may be blood in the stool and urine. Patients often report blood in the ejaculate for weeks to months afterward. Antibiotics are usually continued for a day or two after the biopsy.

Results are usually available within seventy-two hours after the procedure. Take the time to find out what the report means for you. I recommend that you review the pathology report with your urologist in person or by phone and also obtain a copy of the report for your records.

WHAT TO LOOK FOR IN YOUR PATHOLOGY REPORT

The pathology report will tell you a number of important things: do you have a precancerous condition called prostatic intraepithelial neoplasm (PIN), or atypical cells suggesting cancer, or cancer? If a malignant tumor is present, the pathology report will document its location and give an idea of how much of the tissue is involved with cancer. But most importantly, you will find the Gleason score of the cancer, which is the most important predictor of prognosis available. Here is what your biopsy can uncover and how it will be noted in your report:

Normal. When the report states, "Benign prostatic tissue," that means the prostatic glands are normal appearing. However, prostate biopsies can miss cancer, and the chance that it is present depends on a number of factors: your age, PSA level, percentage of free PSA, PSA density, PSA velocity, and whether or not previous biopsies were normal. In general, though, if cancer is found on a subsequent biopsy after having received a normal report, it is rarely a life-threatening type of cancer. A report of normal is good news if you had a carefully performed biopsy with at least twelve cores of tissue removed.

Repeat prostate biopsies after a report of normal are ordered if the PSA is persistently elevated, and especially if (1) the PSA density is high, (2) the PSA continues to rise, (3) you have a low percentage of free PSA, or (4) the digital rectal exam raises suspicion of cancer.

Atypical/suspicious. *Atypical* means that the tissue examined did not meet the diagnostic criteria for cancer but the diagnosis could not be excluded. Think of it as meaning "Maybe there is cancer." When a pathologist reports atypia on a prostate biopsy, a repeat prostate biopsy will turn up cancer about 40 percent to 50 percent of the time. If you get a report of atypia, it's a good idea to have the tissue sent to a pathologist who is an expert in prostate cancer to confirm the verdict. If the second opinion comes back as atypical, you need a repeat biopsy.

Dr. Epstein at Johns Hopkins found that men with atypia are more likely to have their "missed" cancer located in regions next to where the atypical glands were found, or in the same area where the atypia was found. Therefore, a repeat biopsy after the finding of atypia should focus on these areas, in addition to systematic sampling of the gland. Atypical findings on a biopsy occur about 5 percent to 10 percent of the time.

Prostatic intraepithelial neoplasia. PIN is considered to be a premalignant condition that is associated with prostate cancer but is *not* cancer. Under the microscope, the prostate glands appear normal, but the cells lining the glands are abnormal. The greater the extent of prostatic intraepithelial neoplasia in the prostate, the greater the likelihood that an associated prostate cancer was missed.

At this point, how to handle a finding of high-grade PIN is controversial. There is no such thing as low-grade PIN. Most experts believe that detecting only a small amount of prostatic intraepithelial neoplasia upon biopsy warrants no further biopsy without other reasons, such as a rising PSA. But if the PIN is widespread, then a repeat prostate biopsy might be recommended in a year or two.

Cancer. The finding of prostate cancer on a biopsy should prompt a discussion with your urologist about the stage of the cancer and the grade. Together with other factors, this will help determine whether or not treatment is necessary, and if it is, which therapy to pursue.

RED FLAG

Your PSA will rise immediately after a prostate biopsy, and it generally takes one to two months to return to baseline. The biopsy needles disrupt the prostate tissue, allowing PSA to leak into the blood.

SECOND OPINION: YOU REALLY SHOULD GET ONE

Making a diagnosis from prostate cells is one of the most difficult in all of pathology. The biggest mistake a pathologist can make is to call something cancer when it's benign. As part of a 1996 study published in the *American Journal of Surgical Pathology*, Dr. Epstein reviewed hundreds of prostate biopsies sent for a second opinion to Johns Hopkins over a one-year period. He found that 1.2 percent of the time a biopsy read as cancer was actually benign. While that may not seem like much, when you think that such a grave error can lead a man to undergo major surgery or radiation treatments unnecessarily, its rarity takes on more serious implications. Imagine for a moment that you were one of those men with the wrong diagnosis, and imagine if you'd never sent your biopsy specimen for a second opinion.

Furthermore, in 15 percent of the cases, Hopkins pathologists found major discrepancies in the Gleason scores. The most common prostate biopsy diagnosis that is changed when a second opinion is rendered is the finding of atypia suspicious for cancer. Upon reviewing the cases originally assigned this diagnosis, Dr. Epstein found that 60 percent of the time the atypical diagnosis was changed, most commonly to a benign diagnosis.

If you have a prostate biopsy, and the findings prompt your doctor to recommend either repeating the procedure or scheduling prostate cancer treatment, request a second opinion of the biopsy reading. To get a second opinion on your biopsy report at Johns Hopkins, your physician or hospital must send your slides and a summary of your case. The review process normally takes several days, after which a report of all findings will be sent to your physician.

The costs of a second opinion from Johns Hopkins may be covered by your insurance. Medicare will cover second opinion requested by a physician. If you have an HMO or PPO coverage, you will need an authorization to have a second opinion.

PROSTATE BIOPSY AND THE RISK OF INFECTION

To extract the necessary tissue samples in a routine fifteen-minute office biopsy procedure, a needle is inserted in the rectum and passed into the prostate. The test carries an infection risk because bacteria from the bowel can be transported by the needle into the prostate. Men are routinely given antibiotics beforehand to reduce this risk.

Unfortunately, despite the antibiotic, some men develop a serious life-threatening infection requiring hospitalization. This happens because the bacteria are resistant to the antibiotics. Most men recover after being treated with an alternative antibiotic to battle the drug-resistant bacteria, and the infection is rarely fatal.

Cognizant of the challenge of controlling these infections, my colleagues and I set out to determine just how safe—or unsafe—a prostate biopsy actually is. To answer that question, I, along with Drs. Edward Schaeffer and Stacey Loeb at Johns Hopkins, compared Medicare hospitalization rates for 17,472 men ages sixty-five and older who'd undergone prostate biopsies and for 134,977 men with similar characteristics during the same period who did not undergo a biopsy.

Surprisingly, the hospitalization rate was 7 percent within thirty days of a prostate biopsy, as compared with 3 percent for those who did not undergo the procedure. After accounting for a man's age, race, overall health, region of the country, and the year the biopsy was performed, we discovered that a prostate biopsy was associated with an almost three-fold increased risk of hospitalization within thirty days. When we looked at the reasons for the inpatient stays, we found that infections requiring hospitalization after a prostate biopsy were significantly greater in recent years, suggesting that the emergence of bacteria resistant to our currently used antibiotics has increased over time.

In the future, physicians will take a sample of the contents of the rectum using a cotton swab, culture the bacteria from the swab, and determine whether or not resistant bacteria are present. If so, an alternate antibiotic can be prescribed before the biopsy to prevent any infection from developing.

FINAL THOUGHTS ABOUT PROSTATE CANCER DIAGNOSIS

Surgery or radiation therapy can effectively prevent early stage prostate cancer from progressing to later stage disease. Although more than 240,000 men are diagnosed with prostate cancer each year, many of them do not need treatment of any sort, because of either advanced age, underlying health issues, or the low-risk nature of their cancer. Even so, overtreatment of prostate cancer—a common by-product of PSA screening in the United States—is common. And with overtreatment, often comes serious complications that can decrease quality of life.

My recommendation is to use the diagnosis of prostate cancer not as a knee-jerk response to immediately treat your prostate—something that 85 percent of men ages seventy and older do, many times owing to their underlying cancer fear—but rather as a vital piece of information that will help you decide what steps to take next. I will discuss these important decisions in greater detail in chapter 11.

THE TAKEAWAY

- Although the prostate-specific-antigen blood test is not cancer specific, it is the best test we have for predicting the likelihood of prostate cancer on biopsy, as well as the future risk that it will be diagnosed two to three decades after the test. PSA is predictive of both.

- PSA screening of men between the ages of fifty and sixty-nine can reduce the rate of death from prostate cancer by as much as

20 percent to 40 percent, even without treating all men diagnosed with the disease.

- Discuss the pros and cons of prostate cancer screening with your physician and then decide whether or not you want to undergo regular testing.

- Men younger than seventy who are in good health are most likely to benefit from prostate cancer screening, while older men or those in poor health are most likely to be harmed by screening.

- For men who decide to be screened, a baseline PSA level at age forty followed by infrequent testing could help identify those with an aggressive cancer early in life and those more likely to develop it later in life. African Americans and men with a first-degree relative who had prostate cancer are more likely to develop the disease early in life.

- There is no "normal" PSA level that excludes the presence of cancer. Rather, PSA levels should be used to stratify men into risk groups that need more or less monitoring, or a prostate biopsy.

- Additional tests—including PSA velocity, PSA density, percent-free PSA, and the PCA3 urine test—can help determine if a prostate biopsy is necessary.

- An eight- to twelve-core biopsy under transrectal ultrasound guidance is the standard approach to evaluate a man suspected of having prostate cancer based on a PSA test, digital rectal exam, or other tests.

- A pathologist's microscopic review of the biopsied tissue will provide information about the site, extent, and grade of the cancer. The Gleason score (the sum of cancer grades) is the best predictor of prognosis available today.

- Most men diagnosed with prostate cancer have Gleason scores of 6 or 7 that are considered low grade or intermediate grade and less likely to cause harm when compared with higher-grade cancers. Only 5 percent to 10 percent of men with prostate cancer have high-grade Gleason scores of 8 to 10.

CHAPTER ELEVEN

YOU'VE GOT (FAVORABLE RISK) PROSTATE CANCER

If Cure Is Necessary, Is It Possible?
And If Cure Is Possible, Is It Necessary?

—Willet F. Whitmore Jr., MD, chairman of urology,
Memorial Sloan-Kettering Cancer Center, 1951–82.
Dr. Whitmore died at the age of
seventy-eight from prostate cancer.

The voice on the phone was clear and direct.

"The biopsy was positive, Tom. You've got prostate cancer."

As Tom put down the phone that late Tuesday afternoon, the doctor's words were seared forever into his brain.

"Everything stopped for me with that phone call," he recalled. "I had no idea how I was going to deal with the cancer, how my life would change in the upcoming months and years, or whether my survival was now in serious question." One thing he knew for sure was that he was cancelling a long-planned wedding anniversary trip to Italy.

Tom was sixty-four and had hoped to retire from his commercial real estate job in a few years. He was living in a split-level home in a suburb of Baltimore with his wife, Barbara, fifty-nine, and their twenty-year-old son, Malcolm. Life was seemingly idyllic until last year, when he went in for his annual checkup. Tom's family doctor noted that his cholesterol was up, and so was his PSA. The doctor told him that screening the blood for prostate-specific antigen is the best test we have for detecting prostate cancer, but it has its problems.

Tom didn't think much about his cholesterol or PSA. He was working extra hours the past few months on a big shopping mall deal and had little time for personal concerns. He promised his physician that he would be more compliant in taking his daily statin, a cholesterol-lowering medication, and would return a few months later for a retest. When he did come back, his cholesterol had dropped significantly; such is the power of a statin drug. Unfortunately, his PSA had inched up to 4.8 nanograms per milliliter (ng/ml), and his doctor urged him to see a urologist, which he did. The urologist performed a digital rectal exam and a twelve-core biopsy to remove slivers of tissue from his prostate. Then Tom went home to await the results.

A week later, he received the devastating phone call.

"Why me?" he asked Barbara repeatedly. "Why me?" He had always tried to take good care of himself. And then he started weeping.

Tom was crying for his wife, who had survived a horrific car crash the year before and had come back to him after a week in the hospital, intact in mind and body; for their lost trip to Italy—he had only been out of the country once in his life; for his only child, who Tom wanted to see graduate from college; and for himself.

Tom's Gleason score was 6 out of 10, an indicator of a very treatable and curable prostate cancer. He was among the 40 percent to 50 percent of the 240,890 American men diagnosed with prostate cancer that year with favorable- or low-risk disease. The American Cancer Society estimated that more than 33,000 men would die from prostate cancer the year Tom was diagnosed. However, the more that he educated himself about prostate cancer, the more reason Tom had to be hopeful. Based on his Gleason score and PSA result, he soon felt that there was a good chance that he could be cured.

DESIGNING AN ACTION PLAN

Typically, the shock of a prostate cancer diagnosis has barely worn off before a man is asked to make a series of important decisions that can easily change the course of his life. These may include getting a second opinion, choosing the type of cancer treatment, and, for some men with low-risk cancers, opting for active surveillance, or close monitoring without any immediate treatment.

Each of these decisions is critical. In Tom's case, the good news was that low-risk prostate cancer—defined as low grade and low stage, with a PSA below 10.0 ng/ml—generally grows slowly, allowing time for careful thought and planning. And with this careful thought should come this all-important question: If I have favorable low-risk prostate cancer, do I really need to have it treated? In the majority of cases, though not all, the answer will be "Not now." Sometimes the best option for prostate cancer is no treatment.

The management of favorable-risk prostate cancer is highly controversial, although recent clinical trials may ease the debate in the future. But in the United States at present, the decision of what to do about prostate cancer treatment is driven primarily by patients' fears, doctors' professional experience, marketing initiatives from medical device manufacturers, and advertisements from hospitals, when it should be based on scientific evidence.

Therefore, it's up to each man to do his homework and get educated as best he can about his options.

Men with favorable-risk prostate cancer often undergo treatments that will not improve their overall health. This is the result of the misplaced enthusiasm for aggressively treating virtually all prostate cancers, regardless of the risk to patients. For example, two in three men between the ages of sixty-five and seventy-four with favorable-risk disease and a PSA below 4.0 ng/ml choose either surgery or radiation therapy. These are the very men for whom no treatment has been shown to be as effective as treatment for ten to fifteen years

WHAT I EXPLAIN TO PATIENTS

Two days a week, I counsel panic-stricken men with newly diagnosed prostate cancer, many of whom have fears of imminent death swirling around their heads. One day these men were seemingly healthy, and the next they were told they have prostate cancer and need treatment immediately. Plunged into crisis mode, most are frightened and hardly in any position to decide on what treatment—if any—they need.

My goal is to bring some sense of calm and order to a world that often becomes chaotic within seconds of receiving the diagnosis. First, I explain that the chances for cure are very high when the cancer is diagnosed and treated early. Then I walk them through the decision-making process step-by-step so that they fully understand their own particular situation. It's only then that they can develop a personalized treatment plan.

You may be in that same position and should be reassured that prostate cancer virtually never requires immediate action. There is no such thing as a favorable-risk prostate cancer emergency. If a man has been told that he has cancer, he should take the time to carefully review all options available with a knowledgeable physician who specializes in prostate cancer. A large medical center or a multidisciplinary cancer center is a good place to find these practitioners.

Time is not of the essence with favorable-risk prostate cancer. Let's put it in perspective: When a favorable-risk cancer is found in the prostate, it is microscopic and had probably been present for years. Granted, the emotional aspect of a prostate cancer diagnosis may make you feel that you want to get that cancer removed from your body immediately, but you have time to educate yourself, gather information, seek expert advice about available options, and develop your action plan that takes into account your age, cancer grade and stage, your overall health, and your personal preferences.

By personal preferences, I mean that not all men are alike. Some will take any steps necessary to avoid side effects of treatment, and may value their present quality of life more than the risk of possible harm from a lethal cancer fifteen to twenty years later. Others may simply not be able to live with the thought of having cancer and are more comfortable with immediate treatment. That's okay. You just need to figure out where you stand.

All treatments for prostate cancer have side effects, and impulsive decisions are rarely beneficial because some side effects can be permanent, such as urinary incontinence and erectile dysfunction. I recommend to my patients that they get different opinions and consult with their families and primary care physicians before making final decisions. You should too.

The words *prostate cancer* can be frightening, and many of my recently diagnosed patients will ask, "How can I take the time to do all of that asking around? If I have prostate cancer, don't I need immediate treatment?"

The short answer is no. With favorable-risk prostate cancer, it's not going to make any difference in cancer curability whether we act right away or commence therapy three to six months later. Take a deep breath, be thorough and methodical, and give yourself adequate time to learn about your options—all of them.

ASSESSING PROSTATE CANCER
AND DETERMINING YOUR RISK

When it comes to deciding who will likely benefit from prostate cancer treatment, newly diagnosed patients need to be categorized based on readily available information. This stratification of risk will help resolve whether or not a man's disease is likely to cause him harm.

To determine a patient's risk category, physicians take into account the stage and the grade of the cancer, the PSA level prior to the prostate biopsy, the amount of cancer detected on the prostate biopsy, and the PSA density. Let's start with stage.

CANCER STAGE: WHAT IT MEANS

Think of cancer stage as a means of assessing and classifying the extent or amount of cancer present in the body. In the oncology world, staging a cancer is an important component of determining a patient's prognosis and the most effective way to treat it. The staging system for prostate cancer, called the TNM system (see table 11.1 on page 310), assesses three key disease characteristics:

T = the local extent of the *tumor* in or around the site where the cancer arose (i.e., the prostate).

N = the presence or absence of lymph *node involvement*. Has the tumor spread there, or are the nodes clear? The pelvic lymph nodes are most commonly involved in prostate cancer, and they are located around the large blood vessels supplying the legs, just beside the bladder and prostate.

M = the presence or absence of *metastatic* spread to distant sites such as bones in the spine, hips, and ribs, the main destinations of metastatic prostate cancer.

A physician conducts a digital rectal exam to determine the extent of the cancer in and/or around the prostate (the T stage); orders a CT or

MRI scan, or a needle biopsy to determine if the cancer has infiltrated the lymph nodes or other areas; and a bone scan to ascertain if malignant cells have spread to the bones. Men with low-risk prostate cancer don't need an evaluation with scans because there is virtually no risk of disease spread beyond the prostate.

————————————————RED FLAG————————————————

A low-risk prostate cancer in a man older than sixty-five to seventy is unlikely to cause harm during life and sometimes the best option may be no treatment.

CANCER GRADE

Grading a cancer is another method of evaluating a patient's prognosis and determining the best management. The higher the grade, the more aggressive the cancer's behavior. In chapter 10, I reviewed the Gleason grading system that is used for prostate cancer. Let's recap quickly.

The Gleason system assigns a number from 6 to 10 to indicate the cancer's virulence. Gleason score-6 cancers tend to behave less aggressively than Gleason score-7 cancers, which, in turn, are not as aggressive as cancers scored 8, 9, or 10. Today 60 percent to 70 percent of cancers diagnosed by way of a prostate biopsy are graded as Gleason score 6; about 20 percent to 30 percent, Gleason score 7; and 5 percent to 10 percent are Gleason 8 and higher. Aggressive disease often requires more than one treatment to cure or halt it from progressing.

Prior to the 1990s, the grade and stage of the cancer were the only tools we had to determine prognosis and an optimal treatment plan. But then came PSA testing and the recognition that the level of prostate-specific antigen in the blood was associated with the extent of the malignancy. Although not perfectly correlated, the higher the PSA, the more likely it is that a cancer has extended beyond the prostate either locally or to lymph nodes and/or bone.

Johns Hopkins urologists Patrick Walsh, Jonathan Epstein, Alan Partin, and others began to wonder if combining grade, stage, and PSA would improve our accuracy in determining the cancer's extent as well as in rendering a prognosis. Dr. Partin, armed with data from the large volume of men who were coming to Johns Hopkins for prostate cancer surgery, wanted to see if he could predict more precisely the extent of the cancer, then physicians could better inform patients about the optimal management.

It turned out that the combination of PSA, grade, and stage did indeed help us to better predict the extent of the cancer. Out of this work grew the current concept of nomograms, or prediction tools, for prostate cancer. One of the earliest, the Partin tables, is named after Dr. Partin, the current chairman of the James Buchanan Brady Urological Institute at Johns Hopkins.

You are familiar with the nomogram concept if you have ever entered your personal information (age, family history of heart disease and cancer, race, marital status, income) into an online Internet tool that estimates your life expectancy. Just like nomograms for prostate cancer prediction, these life expectancy tools are estimates and not absolutes, with an accepted margin of error. Nevertheless, nomograms incorporating PSA, grade, and stage are useful aids to help patients and physicians understand the probability that a cancer has extended beyond the prostate.

Years later, Dr. Anthony D'Amico, the chief of radiation oncology at the Dana-Farber Cancer Institute in Boston, described what is now considered the standard risk classification system using PSA, grade, and stage. This scheme divides patients into low-risk, intermediate-risk, and high-risk categories that are closely associated with the probability that a prostate cancer will progress without treatment, or progress despite treatment. (More on this later.)

THE TNM STAGING SYSTEM

In medicine, the term *clinical* refers to aspects of a patient determined by observation or physical examination—in contrast to laboratory examination. Clinical staging relies on digital rectal exam and radiologic imaging to assess the extent of the prostate cancer, whereas pathologic staging is determined in the laboratory after the prostate has been removed surgically and evaluated, along with the seminal vesicles and pelvic lymph nodes if they too are resected. Obviously, the pathologic stage after removal of the prostate provides a more accurate prognosis when compared to tests such as a DRE or scans. Pathologic stage is denoted by the small letter p in front of other letters: for example, pT3a. (This stands for the examination of a radical prostatectomy specimen <p> with extraprostatic extension <T3a>.) The clinical stage is the first determination of the cancer's extent following a diagnosis and is not preceded by the letter p.

Table 11.1. Clinical* TNM Staging System

TNM	Description
T	**Tumor Assessment**
T1	• Tumor is not palpable on digital rectal exam.
T1a	• Tumor discovered when tissue is examined following a TURP. • Tumor is in less than 5 percent of the tissue sample. • Grade is Gleason score 6 or less.
T1b	• Tumor discovered when tissue is examined following a TURP. • Tumor is in more than 5 percent of the tissue sample. • Gleason score 7 or higher.
T1c	• Tumor discovered during prostate biopsy triggered by elevated PSA.
T2	• Tumor is palpable during digital rectal exam but is suspected to be confined to the prostate.
T2a	• Tumor involves no more than one lobe of the prostate.
T2b	• Tumor involves more than one lobe of the prostate.
T3	• Tumor extends beyond the prostate.
T3a	• Tumor extends beyond the prostate but only on one side.
T3b	• Tumor extends beyond the prostate on both sides.
T3c	• Tumor invades the seminal vesicle(s).
T4	• Tumor is fixed or invades adjacent structures (not seminal vesicles).
T4a	• Tumor invades bladder neck, external sphincter, and/or rectum.
T4b	• Tumor invades levator muscle and/or is fixed to pelvic wall.
N	**Lymph Node Assessment**
N0	• No lymph node metastases.
NX	• Regional lymph nodes cannot be assessed.
N(+)	• Involvement of regional lymph nodes
N1	• Metastases in single regional lymph node, 2 centimeters or less in dimension.
N2	• Metastases in (a) single lymph node (larger than 2 centimeters, but 5 centimeters or less) or (b) in multiple lymph nodes, with none larger than 5 centimeters.
N3	• Metastases in regional lymph node, larger than 5 centimeters.
M	**Metastases Assessment**
M0	• No evidence of distant metastases.
M(+)	• Distant metastatic spread.
MX	• Distant metastases cannot be assessed.
M1	• Distant metastases present.
M1a	• Involvement of nonregional lymph nodes.
M1b	• Involvement of bones.
M1c	• Involvement of other distant sites.

*Note the absence of *p*.
Adapted from Carter, H. Ballentine, et al., "Diagnosis and Staging of Prostate Cancer," in *Campbell-Walsh Urology* (9th ed.), ed. Alan J. Wein, Louis R. Kavoussi, Alan W. Partin, and Craig A. Peters (Philadelphia: W. B. Saunders Co., 2007), 2927.

RISK ASSESSMENT

The renowned Danish physicist Niels Bohr once commented tongue-in-cheek, "Prediction is very difficult, especially about the future." The most commonly used method for characterizing a man's risk that a prostate cancer will progress without treatment, or progress despite treatment, is called the D'Amico risk stratification scheme. Based on the work of Dr. Anthony D'Amico, a urologist from Brigham and Women's Hospital in Boston, the categories of low, intermediate, and high risk described by Dr. D'Amico are associated with the probability that a prostate cancer will cause harm without treatment, and the probability that a prostate cancer will recur despite treatment.

Like life insurance tables that estimate life expectancy, this tool estimates risk of harm from prostate cancer. However, a given patient may have a very different experience from the estimated probability based on the D'Amico risk categories. Nevertheless, the National Comprehensive Cancer Network (NCCN) has made recommendations for prostate cancer management based, in part, on these risk categories. (See table 11.2 on page 314.)

In 1994 my Johns Hopkins colleague Dr. Jonathan Epstein published a landmark paper in the *Journal of the American Medical Association* demonstrating a method for predicting the presence of a cancer unlikely to cause harm. At the time, urologists knew that around 30 percent of patients were undergoing surgery for PSA-detected prostate cancers that were very small and low grade and unlikely to cause harm if they remained so. The search was on for a method to identify these men in advance and possibly to avoid surgery for some.

By carefully studying the tumor volume and grade of the PSA-detected cancers (stage T1c) being removed at Johns Hopkins, Dr. Epstein devised the most accurate prediction tool for assessing the presence of a small, low-grade cancer before surgery. This assessment is based on the stage of the cancer, prostate biopsy findings, and the PSA density. (PSA divided by ultrasound-determined prostate volume.) PSA density is one of the strongest predictors of whether a cancer is small and low grade.

The NCCN now recognizes the category of very low risk prostate cancer based on the Epstein criteria, as follows:

- clinical stage (T1c);

- prostate-specific-antigen below 10 ng/ml;

- prostate-specific-antigen density below 0.15 ng/ml; and

- prostate biopsy findings (Gleason score of 6 or below, two or fewer cores with cancer, and 50 percent or less of any tissue core involved with cancer)

These are the men at the lowest risk of being harmed without treatment.

We now classify a prostate cancer as favorable risk if it meets either the Epstein criteria for very low risk or the D'Amico criteria for low-risk prostate cancer. These are the men who, if older, are the best candidates for no immediate treatment or active surveillance. (See chapter 12.)

WHO NEEDS TREATMENT: WHAT THE STUDIES REPORT

Two important clinical trials should inform a man's decision about management after a diagnosis of a favorable-risk prostate cancer. The Scandinavian Prostate Cancer Group Study Number 4 (SPCG-4) compared radical prostatectomy to no treatment for men who were diagnosed with prostate cancer without the help of the PSA test. Remember that the PSA test leads to a prostate cancer diagnosis five to ten years earlier, on average, than without the test. The men in the SPCG-4 had more advanced disease than the men diagnosed today with a favorable-risk prostate cancer. While the average age of subjects (sixty-five) was similar to the average age at diagnosis today (sixty-seven), unlike most men diagnosed today, three in four had palpable cancers, one in three men had Gleason scores of 7 or higher, and PSA levels were 10.0 ng/ml or higher in almost 50 percent of the subjects. Most of these men did *not* have favorable-risk disease.

A recent update from this important trial was published in the *New England Journal of Medicine* in 2011. After fifteen years of following the men who'd opted for surgery or no treatment, the investigators demonstrated both the effectiveness of treating prostate cancer surgically and the futility of treating most older men.

For the group overall, there was a significant reduction in the risk of dying from prostate cancer and of developing metastatic disease for those who underwent surgery when compared to no treatment. But the story was different for those men sixty-five and older. When compared to the untreated men, patients sixty-five and older who had surgery had no reduction in the risk of dying of prostate cancer or of developing metastatic disease.

If you recall from chapter 10, NNT—the number needed to treat—estimates how many people need to receive a treatment before one person experiences a beneficial outcome. Using NNT, we can estimate from this trial that seventeen men would need to undergo surgery to prevent one prostate cancer death; but among men sixty-five and older, thirty-three would need to undergo surgery to prevent a prostate cancer death. This does not mean that some older men with favorable-risk prostate cancer will not benefit from treatment. However, the likelihood of benefit is low if you are older—especially if you have other health problems that could limit your life expectancy.

The SPCG-4 trial findings strongly suggest that we are dramatically overtreating prostate cancer in the United States. If you are sixty-five or older and receive a diagnosis of favorable-risk prostate cancer, you should not rush to treat, but first consider active surveillance and see if it fits with your personal preferences.

THE PIVOT STUDY

PIVOT stands for Prostate Cancer Intervention Versus Observation Trial. In contrast with the Scandinavian study (SPGS-4), this large US trial enrolled men whose cancer had been detected in the early PSA era with the prostate-specific-antigen test. PIVOT, which compared radical prostatectomy with observation, followed the participants for twelve years. According to the authors, men with low-risk disease as classified by Dr. D'Amico did not benefit from surgery; their rates of dying from prostate cancer and of developing metastatic disease were no lower than if they'd been managed with observation.

Together, the SPCG-4 and PIVOT studies should urge caution to physicians recommending immediate treatment to older men with a favorable-risk prostate cancer. It would make more sense to individualize treatment for the older man with favorable disease rather than treating all with radiation or surgery.

Our current practice in the United States is also contrary to clinical guidelines developed by the National Comprehensive Cancer Network (see table 11.2).

CLASSIFYING YOUR PROSTATE CANCER

The risk of harm can be estimated based on factors that are easily deter-mined and shown in the table below. Not all prostate cancers are alike, nor should they all be treated in the same way. Review the four catego-ries below and see which category best describes you. Knowing which group you are in can affect your decision about what management is right for you.

Table 11.2. Risk Categories for Prostate Cancer

Risk	Percentage of Newly Diagnosed Cases	National Comprehensive Cancer Network Recommendations
Very Low • Stage T1c • PSA less than 10.0 ng/ml • Gleason score 6 or less and not more than two cores (biopsy tissue samples) with cancer • Less than 50 percent of any core involved with cancer • PSA density less than 0.15	15 percent	• Active surveillance when life expectancy is less than twenty years • Consider surgery or radiation therapy if life expectancy is greater than twenty years
Low • Stage T1c or T2a, and • PSA less than 10.0 ng/ml, and • Gleason score less than 6.	35 percent	• Active surveillance if life expectancy is less than ten to fifteen years • Active surveillance, surgery, or radiation therapy if life expectancy is ten years or greater
Intermediate • Stage T2b or T2c, or • PSA 10.0 to 20.0 ng/ml, or • Gleason score 7	40 percent	• Active surveillance or external radiation with or without hormonal therapy, with or without brachytherapy, or surgery if life expectancy is less than ten years • Surgery or external radiation with or without hormonal therapy, with or without brachytherapy if life expectancy is ten years or greater
High • Stage T3a, or • PSA 20.0 ng/ml or higher, or • Gleason score 8 or higher	10 percent	• Surgery or radiation plus hormonal therapy.

Adapted from Carter, H. B., "Management of Low (Favourable)-Risk Prostate Cancer," *BJU Int.* 2011 Dec.; 108(11): 1684–95.

THE OVERTREATMENT OF PROSTATE
CANCER IN THE UNITED STATES

The slow and prolonged natural history of low-risk prostate cancer, and the ease of detecting a disease with high prevalence among older men who are at greater risk of dying of a nonprostate cause, have led to extremely high rates of overtreatment of prostate cancer in the United States.

Data from the Surveillance Epidemiology End Result (SEER) program of the National Cancer Institute that keeps track of cancer diagnoses and treatments, show that between 1990 and 2007 the rates of men choosing no treatment for their favorable cancer have declined to about 8 percent. Among men with low-risk disease between the ages of sixty-five and seventy-four—an age group that would ideally benefit from active surveillance—only 12 percent of men choose it. Among men seventy-five and older, an age range in which treatment is generally not recommended, especially for a man with low-risk disease, only 20 percent opt for surveillance. Eighty percent of older men with low-risk cancer who are being treated choose radiation therapy, not surgery.

Today patients with favorable-risk prostate cancer find themselves in what Dr. Michael Barry, chief of the General Internal Medicine Unit at Massachusetts General Hospital, has dubbed the "prostate cancer treatment bazaar." Because of the overwhelming choice of options, a lack of evidence to support one choice over another, and a lack of consensus among doctors as to what works best for which men, there is a marked variation in how men are treated for their cancer in different parts of the country.

Given the high rates of treatment in the United States for prostate cancers that are considered low risk, the NCCN and European guidelines for management of favorable-risk (very-low-risk to low-risk) prostate cancer recommend that curative intervention options as well as active surveillance be discussed with all newly diagnosed patients. The primary treatment options, including external beam radiotherapy, brachytherapy, radical prostatectomy, and active surveillance, are reviewed in upcoming chapters.

While high-intensity focused ultrasound (HIFU) and cryotherapy have been used by some doctors to treat low-risk prostate cancers, patients should be aware that long-term data to support their use in this setting are lacking.

Also, treating part of the prostate by freezing or radiating it—something called focal therapy—assumes that it is possible to know precisely where a tumor is. Unfortunately, no imaging tests available today have the accuracy to pinpoint prostate cancers or exclude their presence. Therefore, focal therapy at this point is investigational, even though it is being advertised by many hospitals and doctors as more precise than has been proven.

Androgen deprivation therapy (ADT) is discouraged as a management option for favorable-risk disease because of the side effects, and the lack of evidence for benefit. In fact, some studies show that men with low-risk disease treated with ADT have a lower survival when compared to those not treated with ADT.

It's the job of the doctor to help patients make the right choice that works best for them, whether it be no immediate treatment or a curative intervention. When dealing with a disease like favorable-risk prostate cancer for which multiple reasonable options exist, a man should be encouraged to consider his own personal preferences and play a large role in decision making. No single answer is right for everyone.

TO TREAT OR NOT TO TREAT?
CONSIDER THE VARIABLES

The first part of the decision making for a man diagnosed with a favorable-risk prostate cancer is a decision about the need for treatment. This requires some soul searching that you may not have done before. Your urologist is likely to have helped countless men before make this important decision, and if you have a primary care physician who knows you well, he or she may be able to help you identify your personal preferences.

When I counsel patients, I ask that they factor the following four variables into their final action plan. If they decide on surveillance, then they will enter a program of careful monitoring (see chapter 12). And if they decide that treatment best fits their situation, we discuss their options.

VARIABLE 1. WHICH RISK CATEGORY ARE YOU?
Men with favorable-risk prostate cancer can have very-low-risk or low-risk disease. (See table 11.2 on page 314.) In our 2011 report on the Johns

Hopkins Active Surveillance Program, published in the *Journal of Clinical Oncology*, men with very-low-risk disease had a reduced chance of needing future treatment compared with those who had low-risk disease. That does not mean that men with low-risk disease should not consider surveillance, but the probability of requiring future treatment will likely be higher among those with low-risk compared to very-low-risk disease. Men in either group are very likely to have a good outcome without immediate treatment if they are older than sixty-five, especially if other health problems exist.

VARIABLE 2. WHAT IS YOUR LIFE EXPECTANCY?

Your age and your overall health status must be considered when deciding on whether or not to have your cancer treated. The average age at which prostate cancer is diagnosed in the United States is between sixty-five and seventy, when the average life expectancy is seven to fourteen years depending on health status. Based on careful trials of men with low-risk prostate cancer, most who go untreated will live out their lives just fine.

It is common for older men with serious health issues like coronary artery disease, diabetes, and obesity to come for a consultation for low-risk prostate cancer, believing that without treatment they are certain to die of their cancer. These men require a great deal of education about their disease, the potential side effects of the treatments, and the studies that demonstrate that their best option may be no treatment.

Men are often surprised to find out that when considering their remaining years of life, prostate cancer treatment makes little sense. Dr. Willett Whitmore, the Memorial Sloan-Kettering urologist who is considered the father of urologic oncology, once said, "Growing older is invariably fatal; prostate cancer is only sometimes so." This was a sage observation from a very smart doctor who realized the importance of life expectancy in any prostate cancer management decision.

Once a man looks at his current age on a life table (see table 11.3 on page 319) and the average number of years of life that are remaining, the reality of a finite lifespan may help him reconsider the need to do anything about treating a low-risk prostate cancer.

IF YOU ARE SIXTY-FIVE OR OLDER

In general, if you are over age sixty-five and have a low-risk prostate cancer—especially if you have other health issues—then you should consider surveillance as an option for management. That's because the risk that you will live with a side effect of treatment is much greater than the risk of the cancer causing you harm during the remaining years of your life. The major factors that determine the harm–benefit ratio in a man with low-risk prostate cancer considering treatment or surveillance are his age and health status.

David Liu, a medical student and a master of public health candidate working with me and my colleagues in the Bloomberg School of Public Health at Johns Hopkins, created a computer simulation to model the outcomes of the benefits and disadvantages of surgery compared with surveillance for low-risk prostate cancer patients. Using the most optimistic scenarios in the published literature for side effects from surgery, he reported that for the sixty-five-year-old man in excellent health, when compared with surveillance, surgery added one additional year of side effects for each year of life gained. If the man's health was average, surgery resulted in five additional years of side effects per year of life gained.

In other words, a man at age sixty-five with low-risk prostate cancer will likely pay a high price in terms of a quality of life reduction, without the added benefit of extending life, if he chooses surgery compared to surveillance.

WHO GAINS FROM TREATING PROSTATE CANCER?

When looking at averages, to benefit from surgery, a man with a very-low-risk prostate cancer would likely need to live an additional twenty years; someone with a low-risk prostate cancer would need to live beyond fifteen years. The younger and healthier man with favorable-risk prostate cancer is more likely to gain a health benefit from treatment when compared with the older man or one who is in poor health.

For the best estimate of your personal longevity, you should consult a life expectancy table, such as the one on page 319. This life expectancy table provides estimated years of life remaining for an American male in average health at any given age. The number you see for your remaining years is not a guarantee, of course; you may live longer than the number of years printed there if you are in excellent health, or you may live less if in poor health. Also, consider that you can add 50 percent to the estimate if you are in the best of health—the top 25 percent of the population—and subtract 50 percent if you have poor health—the bottom 25 percent of the population.

Having no family history of any cardiovascular problems is certainly a plus. It may indicate that you, too, have genes that protect against heart disease, stroke, diabetes, and even Alzheimer's disease. On the other hand, if your grandfather or father suffered a heart attack before the age of fifty-five, the odds are that you may be predisposed to heart disease.

You have to personalize your life expectancy, whatever it may be. For example, you may be sixty-five, in average health, and have seventeen more years of life left according to the life tables. But if you have heart disease, hypertension, and diabetes, which put you in the "poor" health category, nine years may be a more realistic estimate of your life expectancy. You would be much better off spending time addressing your other health issues than treating your prostate cancer aggressively.

Table 11.3. Life Expectancy for Men Forty to One Hundred Years of Age

The numbers in this table refer to those in average health who are in the two middle quartiles of health and similar to 25 percent to 75 percent of the population. Men tend to overestimate both their health status and life expectancy. Your primary care physician may be the best person to help you to determine where you stand.

Age	White Men: Remaining Years	African American Men: Remaining Years
40	37.9	33.5
45	33.4	29.2
50	29.0	25.2
55	24.9	21.6
60	20.9	18.2
65	17.1	15.1
70	13.6	12.3
75	10.5	9.8
80	7.8	7.7
85	5.7	5.9
90	4.1	4.5
95	2.8	3.5
100+	2.0	2.6

United States Life Tables, 2006, National Center for Health Statistics; http://www.ssa.gov/oact/STATS/table4c6.html.

THE IMPACT OF UNDERLYING HEALTH ISSUES ON LONGEVITY

Bill did not look well. He had not been taking care of himself. Although he was sixty-eight, he appeared much older, thanks to forty years of smoking Camels, and eating too much of the wrong foods. He had hypertension and diabetes. Two weeks earlier, Bill had been diagnosed with prostate cancer. Based on the tissue biopsy, he was given a score of 6 on the Gleason grading system and his tumor was staged as T1c. His prostate-specific-antigen level, which had prompted the biopsy, was 6.3 ng/ml.

Based on Bill's age and significant health issues, his life expectancy was seven to eight years. I advised him not to treat this cancer but instead to focus his efforts on managing his obesity, hypertension, and diabetes. Those were the primary health concerns that threatened his life, not his prostate cancer.

Bill decided that having prostate surgery was in his best interest, and he went to another hospital to have his prostate removed. A year later, Bill returned to see me, suffering from serious urinary incontinence issues caused by the operation. It had reduced his quality of life considerably, and he expressed his regret for having chosen cancer surgery.

After examining him, I told Bill that I could perform a surgical procedure to improve his urinary control, but he said he didn't want to undergo any more surgeries. He lived with this side effect for the remainder of his life, eventually dying from the complications of a stroke six years after I first saw him.

VARIABLE 3: WHAT YOUR DOCTOR HAS TO SAY—
ESTABLISHING A DIALOGUE

Your doctor will be able to present the options for managing favorable-risk prostate cancer, which include active surveillance, radiation therapy, and surgery. You should hear about all the options available, along with their associated risks. Your physician will understand that it's not easy choosing the option that is right for you.

Finally, your doctor should let you know that whatever you decide, in most cases there is no right or wrong decision. Every man is uniquely different, and there isn't a one-size-fits-all therapy when it comes to prostate cancer. Your ultimate decision is one that should be jointly made by you and your doctor.

VARIABLE 4. YOUR PERSONAL PREFERENCES

There are many very smart men who, even after hearing that they are not likely to benefit from treatment, conclude that because they have a cancer in their prostate, it needs to be treated, whatever the risk to their quality of life. "Damn the statistics," they say. "I want this cancer out."

I respect each man's choice and recognize that personal preferences are critical in choosing the most suitable form of therapy. Understanding what careful studies show regarding the likelihood of benefit and harm are also important considerations in the management decision process. However, deciding what you want is what matters most.

Do you want treatment for your cancer because you won't rest until you know that you've been cured? If that's the case, then surveillance may not be right for you. You may be more comfortable with treatment, understanding that, in exchange for a cancer-free life, you could develop side effects that will affect your quality of life for additional months or years to come.

Perhaps you are more concerned with potential side effects from cancer therapy—the urinary, erection, or bowel problems that may occur—and avoiding these is a top priority. You may value your present quality of life more than you worry about any potential harm that a cancer might cause a decade or more from now. In that case, active surveillance may be the best choice.

When you add your personal preference into the decision process, you will be better equipped to make a thoughtful decision. Only you can decide if the risks of treatment are worth the possible benefits. The right choice for another man may not be what's best for you, so be honest with yourself, gather all the information that you can about your cancer, and take ample time to weigh the possible risks of forgoing therapy versus the effect on your quality of life if you decide on treatment.

TOM MAKES HIS DECISION

I could tell that Tom was nervous and concerned when my assistant ushered him and his wife into my office for their consultation. I was happy to see that Barbara had come along. Studies have shown that patients hear only about 30 percent of what a doctor tells them during an office visit, so it's good to have more people involved.

"I know that you've been told that you have prostate cancer, but don't hit the panic button," I told the anxious couple. "You have the type of cancer that is unlikely to cause harm during your life."

I explained to Tom that he did not have an urgent case, since his PSA was 4.8 ng/ml, and nothing out of the ordinary was felt on his digital rectal exam. He had stage T1c cancer. This, together with his Gleason score 6 prostate cancer, put him in the category of low-risk disease. "The long-term outcomes for these cancers are excellent, even without treatment," I explained.

The couple looked relieved. "I sure feel a heck of a lot better now than when I first was diagnosed," Tom admitted.

I talked to the couple for an hour, explaining Tom's odds of needing treatment eventually if he enrolled in a surveillance program, as well as the odds that it would be successful. We also spent considerable time reviewing the treatment options and their associated side effects. Tom admitted that he was not the type to be comfortable living with cancer.

He told me that cancer removal, incontinence, and the continued ability to get an erection were his major concerns, in that order, so I detailed the two main side effects of prostate surgery—urinary incontinence and erectile dysfunction—for them.

Any incontinence after surgery, I explained, would very likely disappear within months after the catheter was removed. As for his ability to have an erection after surgery, that would depend on how strong his erections were before the operation, the results of nerve preservation during surgery, and the enthusiasm that he and Barbara have for this part of life. Because return of erections can involve a lengthy rehabilitation process post surgery, success is not likely for the couple that did not have sexual activity as a high priority before surgery.

With good erections pre-op—this is determined by a five-question self-test that Tom had taken called the SHIM (Sexual Health Inventory for Men)—and the retaining of his erectogenic nerves during the surgery, I told the couple that Tom would likely eventually recover erections strong enough for intercourse in the months following the surgery, but that the road to this recovery can be frustrating and long.

I reviewed with them the results from surgical procedures that I performed that assessed urinary control and sexual function before and up to four years after surgery. They were relieved to learn that only 5 percent of men had any urinary leakage requiring protection, and that 70 percent to 80 percent of men returned to within 95 percent of their baseline sexual function in four years depending on their age, prior success achieving satisfactory erections, and their level of sexual activity before the cancer diagnosis.

Both Tom and his wife admitted that they had been leaning toward radical prostatectomy to treat his cancer and felt most comfortable with this approach. We scheduled surgery for three weeks later.

LIFE PICKS UP AGAIN AFTER
A PROSTATE CANCER PROCEDURE

Despite the indiscriminate and potentially lethal nature of prostate cancer, people do recover from treatment and live normal lives—albeit a little scarred and changed, but oftentimes made stronger in both psychological and physical measures by their experience.

Just recently, my daily mail had been sorted by my assistant and placed in a neat pile on my desk. Sitting atop the many medical journals and letters that had come that day was a bright and colorful oversized postcard of the Italian Riviera. It read, "Life is great! *Grazie di tutto*, Dr. Carter! Best wishes, Tom and Barbara."

THE TAKEAWAY

- Not all prostate cancers are the same, nor should they be managed the same way.

- Favorable-risk prostate cancer is categorized as very low risk to low risk based on the prostate-specific-antigen test, PSA density, cancer stage and grade, and the extent of the cancer upon needle biopsy.

- A diagnosis of favorable-risk prostate cancer is not an urgent situation. Use your time to decide if treatment is necessary and, if so, which treatment is right for you.

- Men with favorable-risk prostate cancer should consider their overall health and life expectancy as a critical factor in the decision to treat. Treatment is likely to benefit only those with a fifteen-year life expectancy or more.

- With a favorable-risk prostate cancer, other critical factors in the decision of whether or not to treat are personal preferences, such as fear of living with cancer, and the side effects of treatment.

CHAPTER TWELVE

ACTIVE SURVEILLANCE

Diseases desperate grown
By desperate appliance are relieved,
Or not at all.

—William Shakespeare

When Mick was sixty-four years old, his local New Jersey urologist looked at the results of his PSA blood test that had risen from 2.0 nanograms per milliliter (ng/ml) to 2.7 ng/ml, and told him that he needed a prostate biopsy. The tissue sample tested positive for cancer and earned a score of 6 out of a possible 10 on the Gleason grading system for expressing a malignancy's aggressiveness. Mick's score put him in a distinctly gray area, leaving him bewildered.

What was going to happen to him?

How would he figure out what to do?

How would his life change?

How would his family be affected?

Hoping to hear better news—or perhaps that a mistake had been made—he consulted two other urologists. Much to his despair, both doctors proceeded to give him detailed descriptions of surgery and radiation therapy options. One of the urologists, a woman, told him that if he were her husband, brother, or father, she would recommend surgery.

Active surveillance as a management option wasn't recommended or mentioned.

After talking this over at great length with his wife and weighing every aspect of the situation—his chances of survival, of their sex life possibly being lost forever, and of his being left incontinent—Mick decided to go ahead with the operation. He would travel to New York City and have his prostate removed at a renowned cancer center there.

Just four days before he was scheduled to check into the hospital, Mick told his neighbor, an internist, about his upcoming procedure. The concerned doctor recommended that Mick postpone the surgery and go to Johns Hopkins, just a few hours away, for yet another opinion. After giving it some thought, he decided he had nothing to lose and contacted the New York surgeon to tell him of the change in plans.

The specialist warned Mick, "You're making a serious mistake," and urged him to reconsider.

MEETING WITH MICK AND ANDREA

When Mick finally sat down in my office with his wife, Andrea, I had in front of me a typical example of the baby boomer generation: a worried, stressed-out, and overworked couple; a man concerned about a serious, life-altering cancer that was having a physical and emotional impact on his very being, and a woman who was there to be supportive.

Mick's medical records sat on my desk. I asked simply, "What are your major concerns and your goals for today?"

Mick was apprehensive and worried both about harm from cancer and potential side effects of treatment. He'd cancelled the surgery that he had hoped would save his life. "What do you think I should do?"

"Based on your age, PSA, Gleason score, and cancer stage, I think you should hear about all of the options you have," I told him.

Mick and Andrea looked surprised. "We know our options already. We've already been to three urologists," Mick said.

I explained that there are different degrees of cancer of the prostate, and what Mick had was considered to be very-low-risk disease localized to his prostate. Based on what the biopsy had uncovered, I told him that it was likely that he had a small tumor that would not harm him even without treatment. But then, the biopsy *could* have missed a larger, more serious cancer within the prostate. We just didn't know that for sure.

Mick's disease was likely indolent and probably wouldn't impact his life, though it could eventually harm him at some point over the next few decades. I explained that surgery, radiation therapy, and active surveillance for his cancer were all considered reasonable management for someone his age. With active surveillance, I stressed to him that he would need to be willing to take some risk of losing the window of opportunity for cure, although this risk was small. I added that surveillance would be a bad choice if he was too fearful to go on living knowing he had a cancer inside him.

I then told Mick about the ongoing Active Surveillance Program at Johns Hopkins that encourages older men with very-low-risk or low-risk disease to consider active surveillance if it fits with their personal preferences. For the rest of the couple's office visit, we discussed the program, the patients who'd enrolled so far, and their outcomes to date. We spoke candidly about the downsides of surveillance, which included missing an opportunity for cure, as well as the possibility of not detecting a more aggressive cancer on a biopsy or imaging with magnetic resonance. I also mentioned that the need for repeated biopsies could cause some degree of harm, such as bleeding and infection.

When I finished, a bewildered Mick asked again what I thought he should do. I recommended that he consider all options, think hard about his preferences and fears, and then we could discuss this some more. Additionally, I stressed that if he was considering surveillance, he should undergo another biopsy; if he was leaning toward treatment, then another biopsy was not necessary.

Mick had the biopsy performed a week later, and nothing alarming was found. In fact, his biopsy showed no cancer, which is not uncommon in men with small volume disease. His PSA had dropped to 1.4 ng/ml, while his percentage of free PSA was high, almost 26 percent, an indicator of a low likelihood of harboring an aggressive cancer. I recommended that Mick return in six months for a repeat PSA and a digital rectal exam if he wanted to pursue surveillance, and have another biopsy in a year. And that is what he decided to do.

On his way home from Baltimore after that first appointment, Mick felt a great weight lift from his shoulders. He had never wanted to undergo surgery, because of the fear of side effects and a reduced quality of life. That was seven years ago. Since then, annual prostate biopsies have never found the prostate cancer that Mick's pathologist discovered originally, and his prostate-specific-antigen blood levels have varied from 0.9 to 1.0 ng/ml, well within the normal range for someone his age.

Scientists now believe that some cancers can regress—they're taken care of by the body's immune system. I don't know for sure, but this is one explanation for Mick's negative biopsies. Then again, the cancer might be so small that it was repeatedly missed on the serial prostate biopsies. Because no cancer has been found, Mick's follow-up now calls for a biopsy once every eighteen months.

Andrea was confident that her husband's decision to enroll in an active surveillance program was the right thing to do. They talked it over thoroughly, evaluating the pros and cons, discussing their fears and anxieties, and they were realistic about what would have to be done if a biopsy showed a change in his cancer, such as a higher Gleason score.

Mick has told me on more than one occasion that he considers himself lucky to have entered the active surveillance program at Johns Hopkins. Naturally, he is concerned, and he wonders if future test results will show an increase in disease activity. However, for now he is content to continue with surveillance and maintain his current quality of life. Sure, cancer is very scary, but he readily admits that he doesn't dwell on this too much. For Mick, these past seven years have been a gift.

WHO DOESN'T NEED PROSTATE CANCER TREATMENT

There is an ongoing debate in medicine about whether or not to treat a prostate cancer that is very low risk to low risk. (See chapter 11.) The decision is fairly straightforward in men older than seventy-five, who are more likely to die of a cause other than prostate cancer. But some experts believe that most other men—even if they have low-risk disease—should be treated to eliminate any chance of future cancer progression and possible metastasis. However, now that large clinical trials have demonstrated the lack of benefit over more than a decade in treating older men with favorable-risk cancer, a growing number of doctors—myself included—believe that a man diagnosed with low-risk cancer over the age of sixty-five, or any man with serious health issues, should consider surveillance as one option.

Prostate cancer is a prevalent cancer. Doctors know that most men over age seventy harbor some cancerous cells in the prostate. Because the PSA test is not specific for prostate cancer, many of these malignancies are uncovered when a prostate biopsy is performed for a PSA elevation that is unrelated to cancer. I call this serendipity. We also know from countless studies and autopsy reports that most of these small cancers will not cause harm during the lifetime of the patient.

It has been shown that from 30 percent to 50 percent of prostate cancers detected today with PSA testing would not have been discovered during the patients' lifetime if a biopsy had not been performed. Treating these cancers cannot prolong life but only reduce its quality. If we treat every man that we find with prostate cancer, overtreatment rates will continue to be unacceptable.

An alternative approach is to recognize that carefully selected men can be monitored, and if their cancer changes, treatment can be undertaken at that time. That is the thinking behind active surveillance as it is practiced at Johns Hopkins and other leading urology centers around the world. This approach is gaining more interest in the medical community because of the realization that prostate cancer is being overtreated.

THE FEAR FACTOR

Prostate cancer has a long, protracted course in most men. Today, in the United States, with widespread PSA screening of men who are free of any noticeable symptoms, prostate cancer is being detected at an extremely early stage in the natural course of the disease. When compared to men detected the old-fashioned way without PSA screening, most of the cancers discovered today by PSA are of low to moderate risk and unlikely to result in death from prostate cancer if left untreated among men over the age of sixty-five, especially those with other health problems such as hypertension and cardiovascular disease.

Still, in the absence of definitive tests that can guarantee a man that his cancer will not progress, most men today—even those whose age gives them a life expectancy of less than fifteen years—want a solution to their cancer problem. So they head off to the hospital or radiation center to undergo treatment for their prostate cancer even though the risks of treatment far surpass the risks posed by the cancer. It's the fear factor at work. Everyone fears cancer, and no one wants to die from it, so most men will take a pass on active surveillance.

THE PROS AND CONS OF ACTIVE SURVEILLANCE

Benefits for Low-Risk Prostate Cancer

- The side effects of surgery or radiation therapy can be avoided.

- Small, indolent cancers do not receive needless treatment.

- Quality of life is retained.

Potential Disadvantages

- Increased anxiety due to living with untreated prostate cancer.

- The need for frequent testing, including digital rectal exam, PSA, and biopsy.

- The uncertain possibility that the cancer will continue to behave nonaggressively.

- The possibility that the cancer will progress or metastasize before treatment can begin and the window for cure will be lost.

- If treatment is eventually needed, the cancer might be more difficult to treat later on.

ACTIVE SURVEILLANCE: IT'S NOT FOR EVERYONE

Active surveillance is an acceptable alternative for carefully selected older men who want to monitor their cancer rather than undergo immediate surgery or radiation. Even though these men have curable disease, they understand that it does not have to be cured right now. Instead they take an alternate course of active surveillance and regular testing, deciding to live with an uncertain future while still maintaining a high quality of life, free from any side effects of cancer surgery or radiation.

There is disagreement among physicians about who are the ideal candidates for surveillance. However, to ensure maximum safety, at Johns Hopkins we recommend this approach mostly for men who have a very-low-risk cancer and are, in general, older than sixty-five. Johns Hopkins pathologist Dr. Jonathan Epstein originally classified very-low-risk prostate cancers as having the following features (see chapter 11): Stage T1c, PSA density is below 0.15, and the results of a prostate biopsy showing a Gleason score of 6 or less, no more than two cores with cancer, and no core with more than 50 percent cancer involvement.

Many experts are recommending an MRI of the prostate as an additional means of ensuring that no larger and more aggressive cancer was missed by a prostate biopsy prior to entering surveillance. The value of this is yet to be proven.

A low-risk prostate cancer is defined as stage T1c or T2a, a PSA less than 10.0 ng/ml, and a Gleason score of 6 or less. Together, very-low-risk and low-risk prostate cancer are referred to as favorable-risk prostate cancer. (See chapter 11.)

I believe that the safest candidates for active surveillance have very-low-risk disease unless life expectancy is limited by other health issues, in which case men with higher-risk disease may also do well with surveillance. But for a man over age sixty-five who wishes to avoid treatment, studies show that harm is not likely over fifteen years without treatment if favorable-risk prostate cancer is present.

In my practice, men with very-low-risk prostate cancer and a life expectancy less than twenty years are ideal candidates for surveillance. Those with low-risk prostate cancer who have a life expectancy over fifteen years can consider surveillance as *one option*, while men with a life expectancy below fifteen years should consider surveillance as a *leading option*. Likewise, surveillance should be the recommended strategy for any man in poor health with favorable-risk prostate cancer and a life expectancy of less than ten years. See table 11.3 in chapter 11 for life-expectancy estimates.

If you are considering active surveillance, you should first review all other options carefully and understand their benefits and drawbacks. Understand, too, that active surveillance entails close monitoring by a physician on a regular basis. In the Johns Hopkins program, we monitor men with regular PSA measurements and a digital rectal exam twice yearly, and an annual or eighteen-month prostate biopsy up until the age of seventy-five. It goes without saying that if you decide to be monitored, you must stick to the recommended surveillance schedule. Just as importantly, active surveillance also requires that a man be able to live with the idea that he has cancer and will require long-term testing.

WHEN TO STOP ACTIVE SURVEILLANCE
AND SEEK CANCER TREATMENT

Patients in our active surveillance program ask, "How will I know if treatment is ever necessary?" We refer to "triggers" for intervention to describe the factors suggesting that surveillance should be abandoned and treatment initiated.

Even though the cancer can remain quiescent during the years of active surveillance, a follow-up biopsy may show more cancer or a higher-grade cancer (a Gleason score of 7 or above). Most experts believe that if a higher-grade cancer is found in the first three years after diagnosis while on surveillance, it was probably missed on the original prostate biopsy and did not change from Gleason 6 to 7 over that period. For this reason, we recommend that any man who had a diagnosis of prostate cancer made on less than a twelve-core biopsy undergo a repeat fourteen-core biopsy before entering surveillance, to decrease the likelihood that a more serious cancer was missed.

In most active surveillance programs, including our own, a Gleason score of 7 or above would trigger cancer treatment unless there was less than a ten-year life expectancy remaining. At Johns Hopkins, if a patient with very-low-risk prostate cancer no longer meets the biopsy criteria for very-low-risk disease (see table 11.2), then treatment is generally recommended—especially if the cancer grade was 7 or above on a surveillance biopsy and the man is in good overall health.

Some surveillance programs—not ours—use a rising PSA to trigger treatment. Dr. Ashley Ross, a urologist at the James Buchanan Brady Urological Institute, worked with data from our surveillance program and reported that that no PSA change over time could distinguish accurately between those men with and without the finding of high-grade cancer on subsequent surveillance biopsies performed after the PSA. Based on his work, experts are now questioning whether a rising PSA should be used as a trigger for intervention.

Summarizing the findings from surveillance programs throughout North America, at this point we can say the following:

1. The most common triggers for intervention are a rising PSA and finding a higher-grade cancer on a surveillance biopsy.

2. Upward of 25 percent to 50 percent of men will be treated within five to ten years of being on surveillance. Of these:

   a. 25 percent initiate treatment without a specific trigger for intervention,

   b. 30 percent to 40 percent have a higher-grade cancer on a surveillance biopsy, and

    c. 30 percent to 40 percent have a PSA rise as the trigger for intervention.

3. Over 95 percent of men have not died of prostate cancer over ten years on surveillance.

THE JOHNS HOPKINS ACTIVE SURVEILLANCE PROGRAM

The Johns Hopkins Active Surveillance Program was established in 1995 to reduce the overtreatment of prostate cancer among older men that we were seeing with small, low-grade cancers. Since that time, almost one thousand men have enrolled in the program, and no one has died of prostate cancer.

So, what have we learned about selecting men for the program and when to treat them? And what can we tell a man about the potential health risks that he will incur if he should he choose surveillance as an option?

First and foremost, only those men who can live with a cancer without worry should consider this approach. If constant worry reduces quality of life, a man should move to treatment.

Second, the older and less healthy a man is, the lower the risk of harm with surveillance. The younger and healthier the man, the greater the risk. The criteria used for selecting men are not perfect, and there are no guarantees. But if participants are selected judiciously and then monitored vigilantly, the risk of harm is low. We know this from large, carefully designed and executed clinical trials from our own program as well as others.

The greatest risk with surveillance is that a man harbors a high-grade tumor that has been missed on a prostate biopsy. We have estimated this risk to be about 4 percent per year. Hopefully, the future will bring new blood markers or imaging techniques that could lower this risk. Nevertheless, at present, men who have a cancer grade above Gleason score 6 should consider treatment unless their life expectancy is limited.

Of course, the safety of a surveillance program depends on just that: surveillance. In the Johns Hopkins program, about 97 percent of the men are compliant with follow-up appointments and biopsies. In large part, this can be attributed to having a coordinated program with staff who ensures that patients are aware of their upcoming appointments.

Dr. Jeffrey Tosian, a physician at Johns Hopkins, recently updated the results of our surveillance program, which were published in the *Jour-*

nal of Clinical Oncology in 2011. Table 12.1 shows the percentage of men each year who have events that we track in our program. Ten percent of the participants undergo treatment every year, and 9 percent have biopsy results that would trigger intervention. The difference of 1 percent stems from those men who opted for treatment without a specific trigger for intervention. These men likely become fearful of continued monitoring and move on to treatment. The rate of finding a Gleason score of 7 or above that would mandate treatment in any otherwise healthy man is 4 percent per year. And less than 1 percent per year die of a cause unrelated to prostate cancer.

Table 12.1. Event rates in percentage per year in the Johns Hopkins Active Surveillance Program

Event	Percentage Per Year
Exit from the program not because of death.	13 percent
Undergo treatment for prostate cancer.	10 percent
Biopsy reveals either more cancer or one of higher grade above Gleason score 6.	9 percent
Biopsy reveals Gleason score 7 or above.	4 percent
Death unrelated to prostate cancer.	0.5 percent

Adapted from Tosoian, J. J., et al., "Active Surveillance Program for Prostate Cancer: An Update of the Johns Hopkins Experience," *J. Clin. Oncol.* 2011 Jun. 1; 29(16): 2185–90.

Ruth Etzioni, an epidemiologist at the Fred Hutchinson Cancer Center in Seattle, has estimated the risk of death from prostate cancer over the long term for a man entering our program, accounting for the probability of death from a cause other than prostate cancer. According to Dr. Etzioni, if a participant with very-low-risk prostate cancer should need treatment while being monitored because a biopsy has discovered a cancer with a grade higher than Gleason score 6, the risk of death from prostate cancer twenty years later would be 4 percent compared to a risk of 2 percent had he undergone surgery immediately rather than choosing surveillance. This translated to an increase in life expectancy of less than six months. And while these are estimates, they are consistent with the results of comparisons of treated and untreated men in other studies.

FINAL THOUGHTS

Active surveillance is currently underutilized in this country. However, I believe it to be a feasible and safe option for carefully selected men. The National Institutes of Health convened a State of the Science Conference in December 2011 and came to the same conclusion after reviewing all of the data currently available. Although radical prostatectomy and radiation therapy are the options chosen by most men, for the patient who wants to maintain a high quality of life, active surveillance is an acceptable management strategy that should not be overlooked.

THE TAKEAWAY

- Four in five cancers diagnosed today are in men over age sixty-five, and half of them are favorable-risk disease (either very low risk or low risk) that is unlikely to progress and cause harm in this age group, even without treatment.

- For the older man with favorable-risk prostate cancer, active surveillance is a reasonable alternative to immediate treatment, because it avoids the risk of an unnecessary treatment while preserving quality of life.

- Active surveillance entails regular monitoring of the prostate and initiating definitive therapy only when a more serious cancer is found on a surveillance biopsy.

- The ideal candidates for active surveillance are older men—generally over the age of sixty-five and/or those with other health problems limiting their life expectancy—who have favorable-risk prostate cancer and can live with untreated cancer.

- Active surveillance requires repeat biopsies of the prostate, a procedure that can be harmful in some men.

- Men with favorable-risk disease on active surveillance are unlikely to be harmed by their cancer in ten to fifteen years, but there is a small risk that beyond this time the cancer could cause harm.

CHAPTER THIRTEEN

SURGERY FOR PROSTATE CANCER

Surgeons must be very careful
When they take the knife!
Underneath their fine incisions
Stirs the Culprit—Life!

—Emily Dickinson

Dr. Hugh Hampton Young performed the first radical prostatectomy—the surgery to remove a cancerous prostate—at Johns Hopkins Hospital on April 7, 1904. It was fitting that Dr. William S. Halsted, the surgeon in chief, and one of the four founding doctors of the hospital, assisted him during the procedure. Dr. Halsted, who developed the radical mastectomy for breast cancer, believed that his young colleague had come up with a unique surgery that would save men's lives.

Although initially hailed as a success, the operation was ultimately very difficult to perform because doctors had to operate in a virtual sea of blood, which made it extremely hard to see what they were doing. In addition, the surgery came with two devastating side effects. One in four men experienced severe problems with urinary control, and every man lost the ability to have an erection.

The end result was that both doctor and patient felt that the side effects from the surgery were almost worse than having prostate cancer. In the ensuing decades, not many men opted for prostate surgery. When the linear accelerator finally became available in the 1960s with its novel technology that delivered high-energy x-rays to tumors while sparing surrounding healthy tissue, radiation therapy became a more appealing prostate cancer treatment, and radical prostatectomies were rarely performed. By 1980, less than 10 percent of men with localized prostate cancer underwent surgery. (See graph below.) But that was about to change.

Incidence Rates of Prostate Cancer Therapy

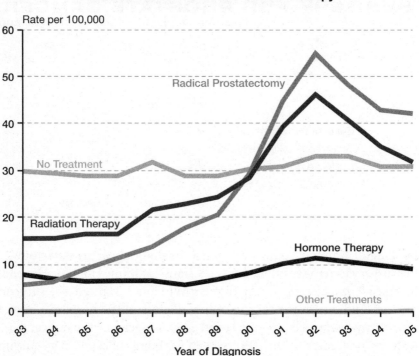

Incidence (on the vertical axis) refers to the rate of a given treatment shown in the graph per 100,000 men for each year (on the horizontal axis).
Adapted from Mettlin, C. J., et al., "Cancer: The National Cancer Data Base Report of Longitudinal Observations on Prostate Cancer," *Cancer* 1996 May 15; 77(10): 2162–66.

RADICAL PROSTATECTOMY 2.0

When Dr. Patrick C. Walsh came to Johns Hopkins in 1974 as director of the James Buchanan Brady Urological Institute, he decided that if the radical prostatectomy was the best way to cure prostate cancer, and if the major deterrent to performing the procedure was its significant side effects, then he was going to make it a top priority to minimize those side effects through a better understanding of the operation's shortcomings.

Dr. Walsh was appalled by the blood loss that occurred during surgery. Blood was routinely replaced during a prostatectomy by transfusions, putting patients at risk. What he found remarkable was that most doctors never mentioned this; blood loss was just an accepted part of the procedure that no one seemed to question.

The urologist went to the anatomy books in search of answers, and drawing on the work of others found the veins that were doing all the bleeding. It then became clear to him that the reason there was bleeding, the reason there was incontinence, and the reason there was erectile dysfunction was that the anatomy of the prostate and the surrounding regions was poorly understood.

In the past, anatomical studies of the prostate using cadavers had not been very helpful for surgeons. In the adult cadaver, chemicals used to preserve the body dissolved any fat, and as the abdominal organs settled in the postmortem state, they compressed the bladder and the prostate into a thin pancake of tissue that looked nothing like the prostate a surgeon would view in the OR when operating on a living person.

As he became even more familiar with the prostate, Dr. Walsh was able to study the anatomy of the veins draining blood from the gland. He soon determined that there was a common site overlying the urethra where the bleeding could be controlled, so he developed a surgical technique to stop it. And once he could control the bleeding, the radical prostatectomy became a more manageable procedure. He could then focus on improving other aspects of the operation in a bloodless field.

This was a big step forward, but there were still significant problems—particularly the erectile dysfunction that plagued men after the surgery. This is where chance and the prepared mind played a major role and offered Dr. Walsh his next important breakthrough. What follows is one of the great stories in modern medicine, with its themes of kindness, selflessness, inquisitiveness, persistence, and the lust for discovery that would improve patients' lives dramatically.

THE SEARCH FOR THE ERECTOGENIC NERVES

In February 1977 a recently married fifty-eight-year-old executive from Philadelphia arrived in Dr. Walsh's office for a consultation. After he left, the urologist noted in his file that he had advised the man that he probably had prostate cancer and that "this operation uniformly results in impotence; three months postoperatively a penile prosthesis could be used to restore sexual function."

The patient later discussed his options with his wife and decided to undergo a radical prostatectomy. Four weeks after the surgery, on March 11, 1977, he returned to Johns Hopkins for his first postoperative visit. He was voiding with a good stream and almost perfect control; he leaked only one or two drops of urine. A month later he saw Dr. Walsh a second time and announced happily that he wouldn't need a penile prosthesis, a surgically implanted device that allows a man to have an erection suitable for intercourse, because he was already having sex with strong erections several times a week.

Dr. Walsh was stunned. How could this man get an erection? Perhaps, he thought, he had somehow kept this patient's nerves intact during the surgery.

The key, then, was in finding the elusive nerves responsible for erections. If that were known, and they could be preserved while still eradicating the prostate cancer, then the radical prostatectomy would truly be a successful operation: controlling cancer while also preserving quality of life.

THE BREAKTHROUGH IN THE NETHERLANDS

While attending a urological conference in 1977, Dr. Walsh and his wife invited a doctor who was dining alone to join them at their table. Dr. Pieter Donker, a Dutch urologist and researcher, agreed happily, and the three chatted on through the night. Fast-forward to 1981. When Dr. Walsh traveled to the Netherlands for a surgical meeting at Leiden University, the man who was to be his guide during his visit turned out to be his dinner companion from four years earlier. Dr. Donker presumed that the American urologist would want to see the usual tourist sites, such as the windmills. But Dr. Walsh took a pass; he was more interested in the work Dr. Donker was doing in his laboratory.

Taking Dr. Walsh to his nearby lab, Dr. Donker showed him the cadaver of a stillborn male baby he was working on, along with a few pages of anatomical drawings he had created. He had been dissecting out the nerves to the bladder. The tiny cadaver was used because these nerves were not visible in an adult cadaver.

Peering closely, Dr. Walsh asked his host where the nerves were that controlled penile erections. Since Dr. Donker had never looked for them before, he and Dr. Walsh went to work for the next four hours, carefully dissecting the tiny prostate and looking for the nerves that he knew had to be there somewhere.

Finally, visible on either side of the prostate were the nerves they were looking for. Dr. Walsh hurriedly sketched them out on a piece of paper, along with his notes.

Eureka! On this special day, his forty-third birthday, Dr. Walsh now understood how it was possible to remove the prostate completely yet still preserve the nerves responsible for erections. The big question was whether he would be able to apply his new discovery in the operating room. The nerves in an infant are easier to see because they have less fatty fibrous tissue covering them than in an adult. Could he find these same microscopic structures in the deep recesses of an adult male's pelvis?

SUCCESS WITH PRESERVING ERECTION CAPABILITY

In March 1982 Dr. Walsh performed a radical cystectomy—removal of both the bladder and the prostate, to treat cancer of the bladder—on a sixty-seven-year-old man. Prior to the surgery, he told the patient that he had developed a new technique, and although he couldn't guarantee anything, it might be possible to maintain his sexual function. No surgeon had ever performed this type of radical surgery and preserved the patient's ability to achieve an erection.

The operation went well. Dr. Walsh located the blood vessels and nerves running together (bundles) on the sides of the prostate, dissected them gently from the gland, and then excised the prostate and bladder, leaving the nerve bundles intact. Ten days after the surgery, the patient awoke with an erection.

Dr. Walsh knew he was onto something important. A month later, on April 26, 1982, he performed the first purposeful nerve-sparing radical prostatectomy on a fifty-two-year-old professor of psychology from Cleveland. Within a year, the man regained his ability to have an erection, and is still cancer free—and free of all side effects—today. Every surgeon who performs radical prostatectomy and achieves favorable outcomes should attribute these results to Dr. Walsh's discoveries.

WHAT TO DO WITH A DISCOVERY

It's human nature to guard what is "yours." That is exactly what Patrick Walsh did *not* do. Instead he made it his lifetime goal to make sure that urologists learned the surgical technique that he'd perfected by extending an open invitation into his operating room for all to observe. And they came, as did patients from all over the world who wanted to be treated with this novel anatomic approach to radical prostatectomy that not only removed cancer but also preserved quality of life. From 1982 until June 29, 2011, when he performed his last surgery and stepped away from the surgical theater after performing what he described as his best surgery ever, Dr. Walsh trained visiting urologists and young trainees in urology. But the full impact of his discovery is often unappreciated.

Consider that deaths from prostate cancer began to fall long before the PSA test could have had a beneficial effect on mortality. Most experts now believe that the dramatic rise in radical prostatectomy rates (see graph on page 338) that began in 1983 as a result of Dr. Walsh's discoveries was in large part responsible for the earliest declines in prostate cancer mortality that began to occur a decade later, even before the prostate-antigen test had an impact.

DR. WALSH'S BREAKTHROUGH ACHIEVEMENTS

But there is more, because prostate tissue and blood samples from patients undergoing radical prostatectomy at Johns Hopkins were available for the first time, Dr. Walsh led a team of clinical and basic scientists who made the major discoveries in the prostate cancer field that continues today. From improvements in diagnosis with blood markers and charting the natural history of localized and advanced disease, to improving the assessment of prognosis before treatment and a better understanding of prostate cancer genetics, all of these advances and more stem from what appears on the surface to be a simple anatomic discovery in the Netherlands.

And then there is the realization by a surgeon—Dr. Walsh—that his discovery had the potential to lead to "too much" surgery among men not likely to benefit. Understanding this, he encouraged young urologists to consider active surveillance as a treatment option, which is now a standard approach to prostate cancer management today. (See chapter 12.)

WHO IS THE BEST CANDIDATE FOR SURGERY?

The ideal candidates for prostate surgery are men with a cancer that needs to be cured, and who can be cured. They have a prostate cancer that is likely confined to the prostate (stage T1 or T2), and they are young and healthy and can be expected to live long enough to reap the benefits of prostate cancer removal—with more than a ten- to fifteen-year life expectancy. They have low- to intermediate-risk prostate cancers, meaning that they also have a PSA below 20 nanograms per milliliter (ng/ml) and a Gleason score below 8. After all, these are exactly the men who, when randomized to a trial of surgery versus no treatment, had a 50 percent reduction in prostate cancer deaths and metastatic disease if under the age of sixty-five.

These men should have realistic expectations and not those based on unsubstantiated claims of "minimally invasive" surgery that does no harm as widely touted by physicians and medical centers alike. They need to understand the risks involved with an operation and the potential for side effects. This understanding cannot be overemphasized. In a study comparing satisfaction and regret after robotic radical prostatectomy and open surgical removal of the prostate (described in detail on pages 358 and 359, respectively), investigators found that those undergoing robotic surgery were three times more likely to be dissatisfied and have regret when compared to those undergoing open radical prostatectomy. The investigators believe that men who chose robotic surgery had unrealistic expectations about their recovery that were based on unsubstantiated claims made by physicians, medical centers, and hospitals, which heavily promoted the machine.

CHOOSING THE RIGHT SURGEON FOR YOU

Once a man chooses to undergo a radical prostatectomy, the most crucial decisions are who will perform the operation and where will it be done. Finding the surgeon and the hospital that are right for you requires some homework, but there is no need to rush such an important decision. It is best to take time to plan rather than hurry to treat a disease that progresses slowly.

Radical prostatectomy may be a common procedure, but it is still complex and challenging, and the surgeon's expertise has a significant influence on whether or not the cancer will recur, and whether or not urinary control and erectile function will return. Studies have shown that surgeons who have performed the operation many times have higher success rates with cancer control and quality of life outcomes when compared with surgeons who do not routinely perform radical prostatectomies. And surgeries performed in high-volume centers of excellence appear to be associated with better outcomes when compared with hospitals where radical prostatectomies are not performed as often.

A highly experienced surgeon is most likely to achieve clear margins, which means that the outer edge of the surgical specimen contains no cancerous cells—an indication that all the malignant tissue was removed. An experienced surgeon also is more likely to know how to avoid damaging the erectogenic nerves that are necessary for return of erections. The risks of other complications, such as urine leakage or incontinence, and urethral strictures—the narrowing of the urethra by scar tissue—are also reduced when an experienced surgeon performs surgery.

And then there is the matter of managing complications from surgery, because no matter how often a surgeon performs this operation, there are going to be unforeseen complications. An experienced surgeon knows how to manage the case that has a less-than-perfect outcome.

No one knows for sure how many radical prostatectomies a surgeon needs to do before becoming an "expert." In his book, *Outliers: The Story of Success*, journalist Malcolm Gladwell suggests that an expert is one who has devoted at least ten thousand hours to his craft. Assuming that an average major pelvic operation takes two to four hours, the surgeon who has performed more than two thousand pelvic operations is probably highly qualified to remove your prostate, although the learning curve may actually be far less than this.

Your quality of life and, ultimately, *your life*, will be in the hands of the doctor that treats your prostate cancer, so choose carefully. Ask questions about your prospective surgeon's personal results with cancer control, sexual function outcomes, and urinary control, as well as the number of procedures he or she has performed. That said, major medical centers, especially those in the annual *U.S. News & World Report*'s Best Hospitals rankings (see page 345), have attracted some of the best doctors around, and the nursing staff in these hospitals can't be beat. These facilities are also multidisciplinary, so that medical oncologists, urologists, and radiation oncologists are working together to improve patient outcomes.

One of my patients passed on to me a tip that you may want to try during your search; he used it himself before coming to me for surgery. Call the doctor's office and see who picks up. You want to get his office assistant, not a lengthy recording, only to end up with an answering machine. If you cannot talk to anyone in the doctor's office before surgery, don't think it will improve afterward when you might have a pressing question.

Finally, no matter what you hear, regardless of the surgeon or technique used, radical prostatectomy impacts the quality of life of virtually every patient. My experience has been that even with a less-than-perfect outcome in all areas, men adjust and tend to be happy with the overall results if they have realistic expectations based on discussions with their physician before the surgery, and if their doctor cares enough about them to provide the postoperative support that the man will need.

U.S. NEWS & WORLD REPORT'S AMERICA'S BEST HOSPITALS, UROLOGY (2011–12 RANKINGS)

The magazine's annual ranking of the best hospitals in each major specialty is one indicator—albeit imperfect—of excellent care. Obviously there are many more hospitals not listed that provide excellent urological care. The complete listing of the best urology departments can be found at the *U.S. News* website (http://health .usnews.com/best-hospitals/rankings/urology). Here are the top five in the magazine's 2011–12 national ranking for urology:

1. Johns Hopkins Hospital, Baltimore

2. Cleveland Clinic, Cleveland

3. Mayo Clinic, Rochester, Minnesota

4. Ronald Reagan UCLA Medical Center, Los Angeles

5. Memorial Sloan-Kettering Cancer Center, New York

ASK FOR PATIENT REFERRALS

If you are considering prostate surgery, I encourage you to ask your prospective surgeon for names of patients he or she has treated. There are many reasons for this, but helping reduce some of the fear of the unknown is probably one of the biggest.

Almost twenty years ago, I had a prostate cancer patient from Greece named Kostas who was scheduled to undergo radical prostatectomy. However, he was terrified at the prospect of surgery, and nothing I said to this forty-nine-year-old man could comfort him. He was actually in a panic and was having serious thoughts about cancelling the operation, even though he had a high PSA of 9.0 ng/ml and a Gleason score of 7.

It dawned on me that if Kostas could speak to someone who'd been through the surgery, perhaps his fears would be allayed. I contacted a patient I had recently operated on, and he agreed to speak to Kostas.

After his surgery, the once anxious Kostas readily admitted that nothing was more comforting to him than being able to speak with a patient before his surgery who had already undergone a radical prostatectomy. It was the only thing that was able to calm him down enough so that he could proceed. What I learned from this was that while I can convey confidence and realistic expectations for recovery, there are other fears at work that can best be reduced by talking to someone who has "been there." From then on, I made it a point to ask in my discharge instructions if my patients would be willing to speak to potential patients in the future. Thanks to the willingness of these men, my prospective surgical patients now receive a twenty-page list of telephone contacts that spans almost two decades. It's an unbiased list in that I don't know whether these men had perfect surgical outcomes or not. The only thing I am certain about is that they agreed to relate their experiences about undergoing and recovering from surgery, which, in turn, gives potential patients realistic expectations about surgery, the hospital stay, and the recovery period.

THE PROS AND CONS OF RADICAL PROSTATECTOMY SURGERY

Advantages

- The possibility to remove all cancer from the body.

- The ability to determine accurately the extent of the cancer after prostate removal.

- The ability to remove the pelvic lymph nodes and assess them for disease.

- The ability to use PSA after surgery to determine accurately the success of the operation. The PSA should be undetectable in men who had successful removal of all cancer.

Disadvantages

- The risk of surgical complications, including incontinence and erectile dysfunction.

- The need for a catheter for one to two weeks.

- An average hospitalization of one to two nights and an average of two to three weeks before returning to work.

- The possibility that not all cancer cells were removed and that further treatment will be needed.

GETTING THROUGH THE CANCER EXPERIENCE AS A COUPLE: IT'S ALL ABOUT COMMUNICATION

When a prostate cancer diagnosis is made, it doesn't only strike men but also their partners. I encourage all men to discuss openly all aspects of their diagnosis, and their fears, with their mates.

Having both partners involved from the very beginning is the best way to ensure open communication between couples and the beginning of a successful journey to deal with prostate cancer as a team.

FRANK AND CARMEN: WE HAVE PROSTATE CANCER

When Frank was fifty-eight, he was diagnosed with prostate cancer. His PSA had doubled in less than a year to 4.5 ng/ml, and his free PSA was very low. A biopsy came back positive. "I was told that I had an aggressive cancer," recalled Frank.

Up until the final biopsy test result came in, Carmen, Frank's wife, was in a form of denial, in that she hoped that her husband didn't have cancer. But once she knew for sure, she jumped into action.

"She is the one who did all the researching," praised Frank. "She bought all the books on the subject of prostate cancer and later came up with a written list of questions we needed answered by the doctor to help us in the tough decision-making process. We were extremely well prepared for our appointment."

Frank admits that he was numb when he received the cancer diagnosis and that he didn't know what he would have done without his wife's help. "It later became very clear to me that you need a spouse or a good friend to be there for you, to keep you on level ground and to give you hope," he said. "Otherwise, saddled with the cancer diagnosis, it becomes so easy to think of your cancer as some sort of a dark hole, with no way out for you.

"Carmen and I are very lucky to have each other. I don't think I've ever felt closer to her than I did after I was diagnosed. Your partner is your partner in the truest sense of the word. After my diagnosis, I found that I began thinking a lot of negative things. Talking about it with Carmen, however, made it less morbid. And then there was a tremendous amount of medical information to absorb. A lot of it was conflicting and confusing. But I knew if I missed something or didn't really understand it, Carmen was there to talk it over with me.

" 'How did you deal with your prostate cancer?' is what so many people have asked me. Well, I knew for sure as the owner of my own business with a dozen employees that I had to start practicing what I preached. This basically boiled down to the fact that if you have a bad day or week, and if you or your business is not doing particularly well, you need to find effective ways to deal with it. You must become proactive and get into the attack mode, doing everything you can to get answers.

"This approach is what I had to bring to my own cancer treatment. What scared me initially, in addition to my cancer, was that I didn't have the answers I needed. It certainly was a very difficult time emotionally. I was a mess. My blood pressure had skyrocketed, all from being scared about the cancer and what I had to do about it.

"Dr. Carter went over all my test results in detail for us and eventually said that, based on the aggressiveness of the cancer and my age, he'd recommend that I have a radical prostatectomy. Carmen and I listened as he described the intricacies of the surgery and what my postoperative experience would be like. Hearing his description is what helped to calm me down enormously.

"The ultimate decision about what to do was mine. Carmen and I sat together, and we discussed the pros and cons of the various treatment options. We finally decided that surgery, with its strong chance for cure, even with the possibility of side effects, was what we wanted to do.

"My surgery went without any complications. In addition to getting all the cancer out, both nerves beside the prostate that controlled sexual function were saved. Back home from the hospital, I had some postoperative problems with incontinence but they cleared up very quickly. One thing I really noticed after the surgery, however, was a distinct energy loss. I felt that the fatigue came from a combination of factors, including the physical trauma of the surgery and just the psychological fatigue that comes from knowing that I had cancer. Put them all together, and you get pretty tired.

"People often ask me if I made any changes in the foods that I eat after my cancer diagnosis. Since I have heart disease in my family, I have always been conscious about eating healthful, low-fat meals. But since Carmen and I had read about the possible effects of nutrition on prostate cancer, we consulted with nutritionists after my surgery to find ways of replacing all the cholesterol-laden foods still in our diet.

"Regular exercise was an important part of my recovery program. I'm a believer in the power of exercise, so I was religious about my walking routine that I followed daily. I have to admit, though, sometimes I worked out too rigorously in the early going and had to back off in order to recover."

Carmen has her own thoughts about her role in her husband's cancer battle. "Prostate cancer is a difficult experience to go through," she reflected. "Although prostate cancer was first and foremost about my husband's life, it would be the two of us who would have to fight this disease, both on our own and as a couple. One thing every spouse can and needs to do is become educated about prostate cancer. Get all the information you can so you are on the same page as your doctor and can ask intelligent questions.

"Communication is critically important, also. Even though he may never verbalize it to you, a man with a diagnosis of prostate cancer is going through an extremely emotional time, with a variety of thoughts racing through his mind throughout the waking hours. One of the best things you can do is to console him as best possible. But perhaps just as importantly, you need to communicate and tell him exactly how you feel emotionally because of his diagnosis. Tell him your own fears and your hopes for the future.

"The day that I finally sat down with Frank and opened up to him, telling him how lousy I felt because of his cancer diagnosis, this was the icebreaker that let us then talk freely about what he and I were going through and it allowed us to make plans on how we could best take care of our problems. Prostate cancer is a long journey, and we knew we were going to have to confront some intimate issues, including possible erectile dysfunction and incontinence.

"What also proved to be very important for us was an effective and extensive support system. I was lucky enough to have my sisters, parents, and a wonderful group of friends who were there for me when I needed to cry on someone's shoulder. Having support, whether it is from your loved ones, or from a prostate cancer support group, allows you to feel less alone in a dark time. Outside support allows you to vent your feelings, to zero in on what's really important, and offers you the necessary arena for solving problems."

THE RADICAL PROSTATECTOMY: SURGICAL DETAILS

Radical prostatectomy removes the entire prostate gland, along with the seminal vesicles and some surrounding tissue. For cancer confined to the prostate, it is the only treatment that has been proven to reduce deaths from the disease when compared with no treatment. The surgery offers the possibility of a cure only if the tumor has not spread to the seminal vesicles, lymph nodes in the pelvis, or other parts of the body. However, because PSA testing is widespread and leads to an early diagnosis, today it is uncommon to find cancer that has spread to the lymph nodes at the time of diagnosis.

Radical retropubic prostatectomy usually begins with a vertical midline incision in the abdomen—just above the pubic area and going up toward the navel. Radical perineal prostatectomy—an incision in the perineum, the area between the scrotum and rectum—is an uncommon approach for prostate removal and rarely used today.

The abdominal muscles that run vertically and are absent in the midline are then spread apart—but not cut—to provide access to the prostate and bladder. With a radical retropubic prostatectomy, the surgeon does not enter the intestinal cavity called the peritoneum but remains below it. In contrast, with a robotic approach, the surgery is performed through the peritoneal cavity where the intestines are located.

In cases in which the likelihood of pelvic lymph node spread is high based on cancer stage, grade, and prostate-specific antigen, pelvic lymph nodes are removed and submitted together with the prostate for evaluation by a pathologist. The extent to which the pelvic lymph nodes are removed and the decision to remove them varies, depending on the surgeon. For intermediate and high-risk disease, most surgeons perform a thorough pelvic lymph node dissection. For low-risk disease, the decision is more variable.

To minimize bleeding, which can obscure the surgeon's view and increase the risk of complications, the surgeon then cuts and ties off the group of veins that lie atop the prostate and the urethra. Next, he severs the urethra close to the prostate, taking care to avoid the urethral sphincter muscles in order to preserve urinary continence but also making sure not to cut into the apex of the prostate—the section closest to the urethra.

At this point, the nerve-sparing part of the surgery begins, if appropriate. The erectogenic nerves run together with blood vessels on either side of the prostate and are commonly referred to as "*the bundle.*" Each bundle is carefully dissected away from the prostate, and the prostate is dissected off of the rectum. However, if cancer is suspected to have spread beyond the prostate in the area of the bundles—a distance the size of the period ending this sentence—then one or both bundles will be either partially or completely removed. With one bundle, erections can be achieved perfectly in some cases. With no nerve bundles left, however, a spontaneous erection will not occur, and other options will be necessary to produce sufficient firmness for penetration.

The surgeon then dissects out the seminal vesicles beneath the bladder and amputates the prostate from the bladder neck: the junction between the bladder and the prostate. Together the prostate and seminal vesicles are removed in their entirety.

Finally, the bladder neck is narrowed with sutures and reconnected to the urethra. A catheter is inserted through the urethra to drain urine from the bladder. This flexible tube is left in place for a week or more to allow the rebuilt urinary tract to heal.

Rare complications of radical retropubic prostatectomy at the time of surgery include damage to the rectum or ureters, the tubes brining urine down from the kidneys, and the surgical and anesthetic risks that accompany any surgical procedure. Postoperatively, narrowing of the urethra by scar formation called a urethral stricture or bladder neck contracture, can reduce the force of the urinary stream and cause urinary retention. If this happens, it's most likely to occur one to three months after surgery. Urinary incontinence and erectile dysfunction are common immediately after any form of radical prostatectomy, but when performed by an experienced surgeon, these complications almost always resolve with time.

HOW LONG IT TAKES

An anatomic radical retropubic prostatectomy with nerve preservation takes between one to two hours, on average. Certain factors can affect the surgical time, such as patient anatomy and weight, with the obese patient presenting a more difficult undertaking.

Some people have naturally stiffer or "stickier" tissue than others, which makes the operation more difficult. Some have more veins overlying and surrounding the prostate, which may cause more bleeding, and this can also add time to the operation.

Pelvis size is also a consideration. A man's pelvis is not as wide as a woman's, and it is harder to operate in because it is a smaller space. A man with a small pelvis and a prostate that is tucked deep underneath the pubic bone can present obstacles even for the experienced surgeon, regardless of the technique chosen to remove the prostate.

HAPTIC FEEDBACK:
GETTING "TOUCHY-FEELY" WITH THE PROSTATE

In some experts' opinions, one advantage of operating by hand as opposed to working with the aid of a robotic device is the ability to feel the prostate and the surrounding tissue. Haptic feedback—that is, using the sense of touch—during prostate surgery enables the surgeon to sense the consistency of tissue with his fingers and to understand just how much tissue is adhering to surrounding structures.

Surgery entails being able to dissect one tissue from another, and they don't all separate easily in the same way. If there is cancer infiltrating a section of tissue, it can make two pieces of tissue adhere to each other. The surgeon must sense that, or else he might tear tissue or the prostate itself, which could lead to cancer being left behind and necessitate another cancer treatment sometime in the future.

Robotic surgeons tell me that they can easily see the tissue as they operate, due to the great magnification afforded by the robotic device, and that over time they eventually develop a special feel that alerts them to tissue adherence, indicated by how the robotic arm reacts when they move it. Perhaps very talented robotic surgeons can indeed do this, but I don't think it replaces touch.

RECOVERY IN THE HOSPITAL

After surgery has been completed, you will be wheeled to the recovery room, where you will be watched over by a team of special nurses as the general anesthesia wears off. Once you are deemed fit by a nurse, you will be taken to your hospital room. In my experience, most men rate their pain as 2 to 4 on a scale of 0 to 10, with 10 being the worst. The night of surgery or the following day, a nurse will assist you with getting up out of bed and walking in the hallway. You will also begin to eat solid food and take oral pain medications if needed to ease discomfort from the operation. Most patients are typically discharged from the hospital the day after surgery, although some will stay until postoperative day two.

POSTSURGICAL PATHOLOGY RESULTS

In the week after your surgery, you should hear from your doctor about your pathology report. The pathologist will have examined under the microscope all tissue that was removed and determined (1) the extent of the cancer, (2) the presence or absence of positive surgical margins, and (3) the cancer's Gleason score. The most important pathologic criteria that predict a man's prognosis following radical prostatectomy are the tumor grade and the presence or absence of extraprostatic disease, seminal vesicle invasion, or pelvic lymph node involvement. (See table 13.1.)

Four medical centers that perform a high volume of prostate surgery joined forces to evaluate the risk of dying from prostate cancer among 23,510 men treated with radical prostatectomy from 1987 to 2005. The results were published in 2011 in the *Journal of Urology*. At fifteen years following radical prostatectomy, the overall death rate was 7 percent. The three factors associated most closely with a man's probability of dying from prostate cancer were the cancer grade, seminal vesicle invasion, and the year of surgery. Men operated on in more recent years had a better prognosis than patients who'd preceded them to the OR. This is probably due to the combined impact of a shift toward smaller-volume cancers detected with PSA testing in later years, as well as improvements in therapy for prostate cancer. Furthermore, when a pathology report indicates advanced disease or positive surgical margins, men today are more likely to receive adjuvant radiation (radiation in conjunction with surgery). And if the prostate-specific-antigen level becomes detectable after surgery, men are more likely to undergo salvage radiation (radiation therapy given after surgery fails to cure the cancer) to the area where the prostate was removed.

Radiation therapy has been shown to improve disease-free outcomes after surgery in some men, especially if the PSA is rising fast or the pathology report from surgery suggests a high chance that the cancer was not completely removed.

Table 13.1 shows that the risk of death from prostate cancer increases directly with the Gleason score and with the extent of disease spread. Besides providing information to physicians and patients about their prognosis after surgery, this important study has two very important messages. First, it would appear that prostate removal can provide a long-term benefit, even among men with high-grade, advanced disease, which is rarely curable. If the death rate from prostate cancer ranges from 17 to 31 percent for these men (see table below), then those not dying of prostate cancer would range from 69 to 83 percent.

Second, men with a Gleason score of 6 rarely die of their disease even twenty years after surgery, possibly in part because of the indolent nature of these cancers and not the surgical intervention. Therefore, we are most likely overtreating men with low Gleason scores, and surgically undertreating those with high-grade advanced disease.

Table 13.1. Prostate Cancer Mortality After Radical Prostatectomy

Factor+	10-Year Mortality (percentage)	15-Year Mortality (percentage)	20-Year Mortality (percentage)
Gleason Score	Age Less Than Sixty		
6 or less	0.1 percent	0.6 percent	1.2 percent
3 + 4	2.2 percent	4.7 percent	16 percent
4 + 3	5.6 percent	9 percent	9 percent
8 to 10	15 percent	31 percent	31 percent
Confined to prostate	0.5 percent	0.8 percent	0.8 percent
Extraprostatic disease	1.7 percent	2.9 percent	7 percent
Seminal vesicle invasion	8.4 percent	27 percent	33 percent
Lymph node metastases	18 percent	30 percent	41 percent
Gleason Score	Age Sixty to Sixty-nine		
6 or less	0.1 percent	0.2 percent	0.2 percent
3 + 4	1.7 percent	4.2 percent	9 percent
4 + 3	4.4 percent	11 percent	23 percent
8 to 10	13 percent	26 percent	39 percent
Confined to prostate	0.5 percent	1 percent	1.4 percent

Factor+	10-Year Mortality (percentage)	15-Year Mortality (percentage)	20-Year Mortality (percentage)
Extraprostatic disease	1.9 percent	3.9 percent	6.6 percent
Seminal vesicle invasion	8.8 percent	22 percent	26 percent
Lymph node metastases	12 percent	22 percent	42 percent
Gleason Score	Age Seventy to Seventy-nine		
6 or less	0 percent	1.2 percent	1.2 percent
3 + 4	1.3 percent	6.5 percent	17 percent
4 + 3	6.6 percent	6.6 percent	18 percent
8 to 10	18 percent	37 percent	37 percent
Confined to prostate	1.4 percent	1.5 percent	1.5 percent
Extraprostatic disease	0.5 percent	10 percent	20 percent
Seminal vesicle invasion	13 percent	15 percent	15 percent
Lymph node metastases	23 percent	23 percent	23 percent

Adapted from S. E. Eggener, et al., "Predicting 15-Year Prostate Cancer Specific Mortality After Radical Prosta-tectomy," *Journal of Urology* 185, no. 3 (March 2011), 869–75. Since these are estimates based on a number of factors that vary among individuals, a man's experience could be different from the rates in the table.

THE PSA TEST AFTER SURGERY

PSA testing is routinely performed after prostatectomy to evaluate the success of the operation in removing the cancer. The first postsurgical PSA test is usually performed one to three months following the operation. An undetectable PSA level (usually considered to be less than 0.2 ng/ml) after radical prostatectomy indicates that all prostate tissue— both benign and malignant—has been removed successfully.

A common question from patients before and after surgery is, "If my prostate is removed, how can there be any PSA remaining?" Since only prostate cells make PSA, if all prostate cells have been removed, then PSA should be undetectable in the blood. But if prostate cells are left behind because the disease was advanced and could not be removed completely, those cells continue to secrete PSA that can eventually be detected in the blood. That is why PSA is the best available test to indicate the success of surgery in totally removing the cancer.

Most urologists will advise men to have their PSA checked every six months after surgery. If the post-surgery pathology report was favorable and indicated complete removal of the cancer, they'll extend the intervals between tests. In fact, in a recent report from Johns Hopkins, investigators suggested that men with Gleason scores of 6 or below could safely discontinue PSA testing once they'd had undetectable PSA levels for ten years after surgery.

DETECTABLE PSA AFTER SURGERY

A detectable PSA immediately after surgery—in other words, the level never becomes undetectable—indicates that the cancer has spread beyond the area of surgery. Men in this situation should first have a bone scan and a CT scan—if these weren't done prior to surgery—to investigate for the presence of metastatic disease. If not seen on these imaging studies, the options for managing residual cancer could include investigational treatments, radiation therapy with or without hormonal therapy, and observation, with tracking of the PSA. (See chapter 16 on cancer recurrence.) Of course, prior to any evaluation or treatment, it is important to ensure that the PSA test is not falsely positive by repeating it.

A subsequent rise in PSA levels in the months or years after surgery indicates that residual cancer that was not removed during the operation has grown to an extent that PSA production can be detected in the blood. It is not usually possible to know whether the cancer is in the area of the prostate or at another site because the microscopic residual disease causing the elevated PSA cannot be seen with conventional imaging techniques. However, it has been shown that salvage radiation to the prostate area improves survival when administered within two years of the PSA's becoming detectable, especially for men with a rapidly rising PSA.

THE EARLY POSTOPERATIVE PERIOD:
A TYPICAL REPORT FROM A PATIENT

Dear Dr. Carter:

I thought I would provide this progress report for you. I feel like I am doing well, even better than I had expected.

I had my surgery the 27th of last month, went home the morning of the 29th, got my pathology report four days after surgery (good news), and had the catheter and staples removed nine days after surgery. Initially I had some issues with leakage and wore pads. However, that situation improved, and I stopped wearing pads one month from surgery.

Hopefully, the incontinence issues are behind me. I do notice that late in the evenings (after 9:00 p.m.), it takes some concentration to avoid leaking (fatigue, I guess). Sexual potency has not returned, but I feel like I am making progress. I am taking Viagra, which seems to help.

A little more than a month after surgery, I had my first post-op PSA. It came in at 0.01, which my doctor said was a good reading. I will see him again in three months and will have a telephone call with you soon.

I have been walking a lot, started swimming thirteen days from surgery, and I started playing golf again one month from surgery. I returned to work part-time fifteen days from surgery and full-time twenty-eight days from surgery. I have not experienced any bouts of abdominal pain or restriction of urine flow. I have had some constipation (I can't really figure that one out), for which I have taken Colace and other nonprescription medications, which seem to work.

Starting at twenty days after surgery, I have been doing exercises for my back and strengthening exercises (full plank and push-ups), and my abdominal and upper body strength are coming back well. I will start workouts with a trainer this week. I leave for two weeks' vacation in Maine soon and expect to be able to participate in all activities (i.e., hiking, boating, golf, swimming, and tennis).

I would be happy to talk to other prostate cancer patients about my experience. I feel like you are truly a master in your field and that the care I received at Hopkins was world class. I feel blessed to be feeling so well and am grateful to all who have helped me get this far.

Best wishes,
Bill

ROBOTIC-ASSISTED LAPAROSCOPIC RADICAL PROSTATECTOMY (RALP)

The introduction of the da Vinci robot system more than a decade ago quickly caught the fancy of many men diagnosed with prostate cancer, as well as surgeons who remove prostates, and hospital officials who make the decisions to purchase medical equipment. Many doctors and patients have since come to believe that this high-tech and ultraexpensive medical tool will somehow improve on the prostate trifecta—cancer cure and restoration of presurgery continence and erection capabilities—and give men a better outcome than if the surgery were performed by a doctor with a scalpel costing less than $50.

Hospitals hoped that the buzz created by the robot would entice patients into choosing their facility for cancer surgery over a competing hospital without the robot. Hospitals' and physicians' fears of losing market share led to what was likely the most rapid acceptance of any expensive technology in medical history. And it's an even more amazing story, considering the lack of proof that robotic-assisted laparoscopic radical prostatectomy (RALP) improves upon standard radical retropubic prostatectomy.

While most prostate cancer surgeries today are performed with robotic assistance, there are still no studies to back up claims that these heavily promoted million-dollar "helping hands" yield better results. This is not to say that the robot does not belong in the operating room. But because of the machines' high cost, their expensive upkeep, expensive disposable instruments used for each surgery, and the number of men needed to be treated in order for a hospital to see a return on its hefty investment, there are many claims being made about RALP that are not supported by peer-reviewed studies because hospitals and doctors want your business.

The claims touting robotic-assisted laparoscopic radical prostatectomy are, for the most part, marketing claims. A study presented at the American Urological Association annual meeting in 2011 provided evidence that the manufacturer of the da Vinci robotic system inflated usage rates for treatment of prostate cancer by about 20 percent.

Fewer side effects are often given as a major reason to choose a robotic-assisted surgery, so researchers from Massachusetts General Hospital recently asked 406 Medicare-age men to fill out a survey that included self-ratings about how bothered they were by urinary and sexual side effects a year or more after their RALP. An additional 220 men who had the traditional open surgery also returned surveys.

Reporting on their study in the *Journal of Clinical Oncology* in 2012, Dr. Michael Barry, the lead author, noted that about 90 percent of the men had sexual complaints, with 30 percent complaining of urinary incontinence. When comparing the two surgical procedures, no significant decreases in side effects were seen by men in either group.

It should come as no surprise that there are billboards, newspaper advertisements, Web sites too numerous to mention, and commercials paid for by hospitals and surgeons announcing the fact that they too "have the robot." It's all part of the business of medicine in the twenty-first century. And this advertising has paid off for those seeking to profit.

Over a ten-year period from 2002 to 2012, the stock price for the manufacturer of the da Vinci robot has increased almost twenty-five fold.

A study in the *New England Journal of Medicine* in 2010 demonstrated that prior to introduction of RALP, radical prostatectomies were declining among men aged sixty-five to eighty-four—the group least likely to benefit from surgery. But after robotic surgery technology was introduced, there was a 50 percent increase in the number of radical prostatectomies in this older age group between 2005 and 2008. According to another analysis, reported in 2011, at hospitals that purchased the robot, the numbers of radical prostatectomies performed rose by about thirty per year; whereas those institutions that did not acquire the technology saw a decrease of about five surgeries per year.

Most medical economists now recognize that new technology can increase the cost of medical care not just because the technology is more expensive but also because there is increased utilization. RALP seems to succeed in both regards.

CHOOSE EXPERIENCE, NOT EQUIPMENT

The surgical "robot"—not really a robot at all—is an impressive piece of medical equipment. And there are many supertalented surgeons around the world using it to remove prostates safely and with excellent outcomes. There are thousands of American men who are very satisfied with the results of their robotic-assisted prostatectomies. However, if you have been diagnosed with prostate cancer and are investigating various treatment options, it is not technology that should be your focus but rather the experience of the physician treating you.

We don't have head-to-head studies yet that compare outcomes using different techniques for prostate removal. However, an ongoing multi-institutional trial is comparing robotic and open radical prostatectomy. At the present time, there is no evidence that short-term and long-term results differ between these procedures when performed by an experienced surgeon. The length of hospitalization, need for pain medication, time back to work, urinary control, and return of erectile function all appear to be similar in the hands of an experienced surgeon performing an open radical retropubic prostatectomy or RALP.

My final advice: don't make a decision based on hype. Instead look for that surgeon who can achieve the best results with whatever surgical approach he or she is most comfortable using.

PROSTATE REMOVAL WITH ROBOTIC ASSISTANCE

Here's the scene in an operating room with a robot: the room is well lit and large, with thick cables running along the floor, from the command center console where the surgeon will sit, and right up to the bulky yet graceful-looking robot fifteen feet away. Its four articulating arms are positioned next to the anesthetized patient on the operating table.

Before a robotic-assisted laparoscopic radical prostatectomy (RALP) can begin, members of the surgical team first prep the patient after he has been anesthetized and positioned on his back, with his legs apart. Next, a needle is placed in the intestinal cavity, or peritoneum, and the abdomen is inflated with carbon dioxide gas to expand the area and make it easier to manipulate the robotic arms within the body.

Ports, which are entrances into the abdominal wall, are filled with tubular structures to maintain the openings through which the surgeon will place a tiny video camera and the surgical instruments that will be driven by the robotic arms. The robot is then wheeled to the foot of the operating table, its arms are attached to the laparoscopic instruments entering the body, and an assistant is at the ready to pass instruments through one of the ports for suction, retracting tissue, or placing clips to control bleeding.

Seated behind the da Vinci console, the surgeon looks into special eyepieces that provide highly magnified 3-D views from inside the patient via the camera inside the abdomen. The images provide a view of delicate structures surrounding the prostate gland, including the nerve bundles. It's this excellent magnification that surgeons say allows for greater visualization and preservation of vital structures.

Once surgery begins, the da Vinci system turns the movement of the surgeon's fingers at the console into precise movements of the robotic arms and instruments. As with any surgical procedure, trained surgical nurses are also part of the team that prepares instruments and sutures needed by the surgeon.

In lieu of his own hands being placed within the abdomen, the surgeon uses the da Vinci system to translate movement of his fingers into movement of the robotic arms that control the laparoscopic instruments. This technology allows the surgical instruments to be rotated 360 degrees. Watching an experienced surgeon perform RALP is a truly remarkable demonstration of the application of twenty-first-century technology. And without question, the instrumentation will continue to improve, allowing future surgeons to "feel" tissue and use imaging technology in real time while operating.

From the standpoint of surgically resecting the prostate, RALP relies on the same principles developed by Dr. Patrick Walsh in the early 1980s. After the prostate is detached from all surrounding structures, the surgeon places it in a small plastic bag that is removed at the end of the operation by slightly extending the incision at the patient's navel. The surgeon finishes his work by manipulating the robotic arms to suture the bladder and urethra together to restore continuity of the urinary tract.

Just as in an open radical prostatectomy, a catheter is placed through the penis to drain the bladder and allow healing of the bladder-urethra connection called the anastomosis. A small drain is placed around the surgical site and exits the abdominal wall, and the patient is off to the recovery room. Up and walking the evening of surgery, or early the next day, patients are typically discharged the day following surgery with the retropubic approach.

Proponents of robotic-assisted laparoscopic radical prostatectomy firmly believe that this form of surgery is "minimally" invasive. But I would argue that from the patient's perspective, no form of radical prostatectomy is minimally invasive. In fact, removing a man's prostate is about as invasive a treatment as there is for prostate cancer. Nevertheless, it is a very effective method for curing or controlling prostate cancer in those who need it.

THE TAKEAWAY

- Radical prostatectomy is an effective method for treating localized prostate cancer that reduces both the development of metastatic disease and death from disease by as much as 50 percent over a fifteen-year period after treatment.

- The men most likely to benefit from radical prostatectomy are under age sixty-five, are in good health, and have localized disease. Older men with more aggressive forms of cancer may also benefit from surgery.

- The major long-term risks of radical prostatectomy are quality of life outcomes such as loss of urinary control and the ability to achieve and maintain an erection sufficient for intercourse; either or both can occur even when an experienced surgeon is performing the operation.

- Cancer control and quality of life outcomes appear to be better when surgery is performed by a high-volume surgeon in a high-volume center of excellence, as compared with surgery performed by a less experienced surgeon in centers where radical prostatectomy is less often performed.

- The important outcomes of radical prostatectomy (cancer control and quality of life) appear similar for open retropubic radical prostatectomy (RRP) and robotic-assisted laparoscopic radical prostatectomy (RALP), when performed by high-volume surgeons.

- There is no evidence that robotic-assisted laparoscopic radical prostatectomy is less invasive than a well-executed open retropubic radical prostatectomy.

CHAPTER FOURTEEN

TREATING PROSTATE CANCER WITH RADIATION THERAPY

The physician should look upon the patient as a
besieged city and try to rescue him with every
means that art and science place at his command.

—Alexander of Tralles,
Greek-born physician (ca 525–ca 605)

Radiation therapy is one of the recommended standard treatment options for prostate cancer. A man undergoes multiple treatment sessions in which radiation produced outside the body (external beam radiotherapy, or EBRT) is aimed at the prostate to eradicate the cancer cells within. Another type of radiation called brachytherapy, or BT, involves a single-session procedure to implant radiation "seeds" into the prostate. Most men can resume normal activities and return to work within a week.

Dr. Hugh Hampton Young of Johns Hopkins—the pioneer of prostate cancer surgery and the father of modern urology—began experimenting with placing radioactive radium pellets into the prostate as a treatment for prostate cancer in the early 1900s. But radiation injury to patients and physicians limited the application of these early attempts at brachytherapy. Fast-forward to the 1990s. With a much better understanding of radiation and improved technology that saw the advent of three-dimensional imaging using computed tomography (CT) scanners,

combined with linear accelerators that could produce a high-energy photon beam, it became possible to deliver high dosages of radiation more
precisely to the prostate deep within the pelvis. Computer programs
were developed to plan radiation dosages based on a three-dimensional
image of the prostate. Now referred to as three-dimensional conformal
radiotherapy, or 3D-CRT, this approach allowed the use of high dosages and at the same time reduced the injury to rectal and bladder tissue from radiation.

THE BEST CANDIDATES FOR RADIATION THERAPY

I tell patients with localized prostate cancer, "The good news is that there
are multiple ways to treat your prostate cancer. And the bad news is that
there are multiple ways to treat your prostate cancer."

There is no scientific evidence that any one treatment for localized
prostate cancer—whether radiation or surgery—will result in a better
cancer-free outcome than another. This means that a man and his family
will have to play a much larger role in decision making. The same men
who are candidates for surgical treatment of stage T1 and T2 cancers
are also eligible for radiation therapy. Historically, surgery has typically
been recommended for the younger prostate cancer patient, and radiation for the older man. And that trend continues today.

The conventional wisdom in the prostate world has been that if a
man has many more years to live, there is an intrinsic value in removing
a cancerous organ—the thought being that if radiation does not completely eradicate the cancer, it could return. However, there are no strong
data to support the contention that surgery is "best" for the younger
man; only a generalized instinct within the medical community. Even
so, some radiation oncologists are hesitant to recommend radiation as
first-line treatment for a young man with localized prostate cancer. And
then, given enough time, there is the greater risk of a secondary cancer
caused by the radiation.

Talk to radiation experts, and they'll agree that thanks to the great
cancer-killing potential of radiation, younger men with prostate cancer can benefit from either surgery or radiation therapy. Therapy with
today's high-tech machines has several other advantages, including no
hospital stay or lengthy at-home rehabilitation. External radiation treat-

ments are administered daily but are brief, and men can lead relatively normal lives around their treatment times. The side effects—fatigue, bladder irritation, and diarrhea—are generally mild and can be eased with medication and changes in diet.

While it may sound counterintuitive, daily exercise can lessen fatigue from external radiation treatments. Basic workouts can include brisk walking and other thirty-minute aerobic activities. Resistance training sessions a few times a week focusing on the muscles of the upper and lower body are also helpful.

HOW RADIATION KILLS CANCER CELLS

Normal cells in the body divide and replace themselves in an orderly process, keeping you healthy and repairing structures as needed. However, cancer develops when the cells lose the ability to control their own growth. The cancer cells are immortal and keep dividing, eventually forming clumps of tissue called tumors, or sometimes infiltrating throughout normal tissue and spreading beyond the organ where they originated—a process called metastasis.

DNA is the genetic information inside the cell necessary for life. Radiation therapy kills cells by damaging their DNA—either directly or by creating the charged particles called free radicals that can cause DNA damage. When the injured DNA cannot be repaired, cells die. But radiation kills normal cells as well as cancerous cells, and so treatment must be directed precisely at the tumor. Since the prostate is a dispensable organ, radiation can be given at doses that will destroy all prostate tissue, normal and cancerous.

However, radiation dosages are limited by the damage caused to surrounding structures. So the radiation oncologist must achieve a delicate balance between delivering enough radiation that it destroys all the cancer but without causing collateral damage to neighbors such as the bladder and rectum, which can bring about serious side effects—some of them permanent. These can include urinary and bowel frequency and urgency, pain with urination and bowel movements, and bleeding caused by damage to these tissues. And, just as with radical prostatectomy, there is the potential for the radiation to damage the erectogenic nerves, resulting in erectile dysfunction.

YOUR RADIATION ONCOLOGY TEAM

The American Board of Radiation Oncology certifies radiation oncologists, those doctors who have special training in using radiation to treat cancers. Radiation oncologists oversee a team that is involved in tailoring treatment to a particular cancer and the patient with the cancer. Members of the oncology team may include a radiation physicist, a dosimetrist, and a radiation therapist, all working together to ensure that the appropriate dose of radiation is delivered precisely at the most appropriate intervals.

It starts with simulation, which involves creating three-dimensional images of the prostate and surrounding structures for planning the radiation delivery, and using molds or casts of the body to ensure that the patient is in the same position every day.

Radiation dosages for treating cancer are measured in gray (Gy), which is defined as the amount of radiation energy absorbed per unit of tissue. The more Gys that can be delivered safely, the higher the cure rate. Going too high, however, can produce those serious side effects I just discussed.

Both external beam radiotherapy and internal radiation therapy (brachytherapy) can be effective for treating early stage prostate tumors (T1 and T2), while EBRT is often used to treat more extensive prostate cancers (T3 and T4) that have moved beyond the prostate. In addition, EBRT is used to reduce the pain and destruction caused by metastatic deposits in bones.

TYPES OF RADIATION FOR
PROSTATE CANCER TREATMENT

Radiation produced outside the body and focused onto a cancer is called external beam radiotherapy (EBRT). It is usually administered in daily doses for weeks. Brachytherapy, or seed therapy, delivers high doses of radiation from within the prostate, killing cells over the course of weeks while minimizing radiation to nearby healthy tissue.

THE PROS AND CONS OF RADIATION THERAPY

Advantages

- Avoiding surgery, as well as the recovery from a surgical procedure.

- Reduced risk of urinary incontinence and erectile dysfunction associated with surgery for some men.

Disadvantages

- Treatment with external beam therapy requires daily sessions over six to eight weeks.

- Treatment involves the addition of hormonal therapy for men with more aggressive cancers.

- Cancer within the prostate could be resistant to the effects of radiation, and the cancer may recur.

- Recurrences following radiation therapy are difficult to treat, especially surgically.

- Unlike with surgery, the tissue is destroyed, leaving behind no pathological information on the grade and extent of the cancer.

- Damage of adjacent tissues (bladder and bowel) can result in irritative urinary and bowel symptoms that are difficult to treat.

EXTERNAL BEAM RADIATION THERAPY

EBRT involves directing high-energy beams produced outside the body to the prostate. These beams are delivered by a linear accelerator that produces a photon beam (x-ray), or by a cyclotron, that produces protons to destroy cancer cells within the prostate. The length of the treatment depends on the total amount of radiation to be delivered, and that, in turn, depends on the aggressiveness of the tumor, and whether the radiotherapy is being used as primary treatment, in combination with another intervention, or for a cancer recurrence.

Advances in EBRT have been made by improvements in guiding the beam of radiation to the target, and shaping the beams so that the target receives more radiation and sensitive surrounding tissues less. These advances are referred to as conformal radiotherapy, intensity modulated radiotherapy, and image-guided radiotherapy.

THREE-DIMENSIONAL CONFORMAL
RADIATION THERAPY (3D-CRT)

With the advances in CT scanning and the ability to integrate information gained from the use of imaging, radiation oncologists can plan a course of radiation that is more precise when compared with the two-dimensional images of the past. The process of 3D-CRT calls for producing three-dimensional images of the prostate with the patient immobilized and in the same position that will be used for daily treatments. These 3D-images are used to define precisely the volume of the tissues to be radiated.

Earlier conventional external beam radiation could be likened to an off-the-rack suit. The high-energy x-ray beams were targeted to the location of the prostate but not tailored to the volume of the tissue to be treated. On the other hand, 3D-CRT can be thought of as the highly detailed, customized version of external beam radiation, with radiation beams expressly tailored to a given person.

Every man has a prostate of distinctive size and shape, a different extent of cancer, and the location of his nearby bladder and bowel varies as well. Whereas conventional EBRT would treat all prostates with identically designed beams of radiation, conformal radiation conforms those beams to fit each patient's unique anatomy.

HIGHER DOSES OF RADIATION ARE
MORE EFFECTIVE AT CURING CANCER

A randomized clinical trial comparing external beam radiation at a total dose of either 70.2 Gy (conventional dose) or 79.2 Gy (high dose) for men with localized prostate cancer was published in the *Journal of the American Medical Association*. Researchers from Massachusetts General Hospital reported that the proportions of men free from disease at five years were 79 percent for conventional-dose therapy and 91 percent for high-dose therapy. The risk of severe urinary or rectal side effects was only 1 percent for patients receiving conventional dose and 2 percent for those receiving high-dose EBRT.

INTENSITY-MODULATED RADIATION THERAPY (IMRT)

After the overall dosage to be delivered has been calculated, intensity-modulated radiation therapy, or IMRT, relies on computer software to determine the orientation, number, and intensity of the radiation beams. Think of IMRT as an even more precise 3D-CRT. Collimators, or beam-shaping devices, are used to deliver different dosages of radiation to areas within or around the cancer. This shutter-like attachment at the end of a linear accelerator filters the radioactive rays. The longer a collimator stays open, the stronger the dose of radiation that's delivered.

Using IMRT, specific portions of the prostate can now be treated with higher or lower dosages in an infinite number of patterns. The goal of intensity-modulated radiation therapy is to deliver the highest dosage necessary to eradicate all cancer while sparing surrounding tissue. In one study published in 2011 in the *International Journal of Radiation Oncology • Biology • Physics*, researchers compared the bowel, urinary, and erectile complications after 3D-CRT and IMRT to see if the latter technique reduced complications after prostate cancer treatment. They evaluated data collected by the National Cancer Institute and linked to Medicare claims for men over age sixty-five treated with EBRT—5,845 men with IMRT and 6,753 treated with 3D-CRT—between 2002 and 2004.

The investigators reported that IMRT was associated with a small reduction in bowel complications and bowel hemorrhage when compared with 3D-CRT, but no reduction in urinary and erectile complications. Publishing in the same journal in 2011, investigators at Fox Chase Cancer Center in Philadelphia reported that both early and late gastrointestinal toxicity was reduced significantly among men who were treated with IMRT when compared with 3D-CRT.

SINCE THE PROSTATE MOVES:
IMAGE-GUIDED RADIOTHERAPY (IGRT)

Understanding that the prostate does not stay in the exact spot on a daily basis due to the amount of air in the rectum, urine in the bladder, and patient weight change, researchers developed newer three-dimensional imaging technologies that could be used daily to make certain that the radiation would reach the prostate even if it had shifted slightly from where it was the day before.

Daily CT scans can be used to create three-dimensional images of the prostate and surrounding structures before each radiation treatment. This critical information is then transmitted to a computer and allows doctors to compare the current image taken from that of the previous day to see if the treatment area needs to be adjusted. This approach to IMRT is called image-guided radiation therapy, or IGRT.

Think of IGRT as a sort of GPS for your prostate. A CT scanner can be combined with a linear accelerator that rotates around the patient to capture images of the prostate before each daily treatment. Also, miniature electromagnetic sensors can be implanted in the prostate during treatment planning to monitor the prostate position and motion continuously, improving the targeting. If the prostate has moved, then the therapist can make necessary adjustments to redirect the radiation.

PROTON BEAM RADIATION THERAPY

Proton beam radiation therapy, which uses subatomic proton particles instead of the photons used in standard EBRT, has caught the attention of patients and hospitals, but for all the wrong reasons. Even though no studies demonstrate proton therapy's superiority compared with other forms of radiation therapy for prostate cancer, it is being heavily marketed to men nonetheless. That's because the few institutions in this country with proton beam therapy centers receive more than $50,000 in reimbursements from Medicare—almost twice the amount for other external radiation therapies for treating a prostate cancer patient.

For a medical center to offer proton beam radiotherapy, it must construct a facility the size of a football field to house the equipment—with its 222-ton cyclotron that can create the subatomic charged particles— at a cost of $150 million or more. Where is the value? Granted, proton beam therapy has been demonstrated to be safe and effective for a variety of pediatric cancers and some brain tumors. But when it comes to an adult malignancy such as prostate cancer, there are no data to warrant its extra expense for treating prostate cancer.

For a therapy that comes with such a high price tag, one would expect much more than equivalence when compared to IMRT in improved cancer control and reduced side effects. Although proton beam therapy may be considered state-of-the-art, it still has a long way to go in proving its ultimate medical value—if any—in the treatment of prostate cancer.

INTERNAL RADIATION THERAPY (BRACHYTHERAPY)

In the 1920s, Dr. Hugh Hampton Young of Johns Hopkins was on the right track with his early attempts at placing radioactive pellets near the prostate, but his tools for doing so were too primitive to be successful. He had no way of controlling the radiation so that patients—and their physicians—were not harmed by it, and no way to plant the radioactive material accurately. More than ninety years later, many men with prostate cancer choose a different form of internal radiation therapy:

brachytherapy. During a brachytherapy treatment session, radiation oncologists insert dozens of radioactive rice-size pellets, or seeds, into the prostate to kill cancerous cells.

There are two types of brachytherapy used in the treatment of prostate cancer. In low-dose-rate brachytherapy, permanent radioactive seeds deliver radiation slowly over a period of several months, after which they no longer emit radioactivity. Although the seeds are left in the patient's body permanently, they do not cause any untoward side effects.

In contrast, high-dose-rate brachytherapy utilizes seeds that are temporarily placed and deliver a much higher dosage per unit time. With this therapy, the radiation is administered through hollow needles that are placed in the prostate temporarily, with about twelve hours between treatments. During the treatment course, a man remains in the hospital.

There is no high level of evidence to demonstrate that high-dose brachytherapy improves cancer control when compared with other forms of radiation, so it's not possible to say with any certainty that this is as good as or better than other radiation therapies. The most commonly used internal radiation treatment for prostate cancer is low-dose brachytherapy.

A TYPICAL BRACHYTHERAPY TREATMENT

Weeks before the treatment is delivered, the radiation oncologist constructs a detailed three-dimensional map of the patient's prostate based on an MRI or CT scan. These images determine the number of seeds and their exact placement. Each radioactive seed releases radiation within a confined area, with all of the seeds contributing radiation to the overall implant. If the implant is not implanted precisely, there can be "cold spots," or areas of under-dosing, and "hot spots" (areas of overdosing). Underdosing could leave cancer cells inadequately treated, while overdosing could expose surrounding tissue to harmful radiation.

AT THE HOSPITAL

Brachytherapy is performed under anesthesia with a catheter in the bladder. With legs apart and raised in stirrups, needles loaded with the radioactive seeds are inserted through the skin of the perineal area between the scrotum and the rectum. Precise targeting is ensured with ultrasound or CT guidance. On average, between 70 and 120 seeds are used. The entire procedure takes approximately two hours or more.

Most men leave the hospital the same day without a urinary catheter in place. Sometimes, though, swelling from the implant causes urinary retention, in which case a week of catheterization becomes necessary. Patients experience some soreness in the perineum and burning upon urination that can last for several weeks afterward. Full activity, however, can usually be resumed in the first week after the implant.

Because of the radiation that the seeds emit, during the first two weeks after the procedure, children should not sit on the patient's lap for more than thirty to sixty minutes at a time. And for two days following brachytherapy, women who are pregnant—or who *could* be pregnant—must stay at least twelve inches away from the patient and avoid contact beyond six hours a day. At a distance of six feet, however, any visitor can be with the patient indefinitely.

BRACHYTHERAPY: IDEAL FOR SOME BUT NOT OTHERS

Brachytherapy is used most often to treat men who are thought to have a low-risk cancer that is confined to the prostate (stage T1c or T2a, a PSA level below 10.0 ng/ml, and a Gleason score of 6 or less). For more extensive cancers that are classified as intermediate risk (stage T2b or T2c; or a PSA of 10.0 to 20.0 ng/ml; or a Gleason score of 7), radiation oncologists don't recommend the use of permanent brachytherapy as a stand-alone treatment; instead they might recommend a combination of low-dose brachytherapy with external beam radiation therapy. The concept here is that higher dosages can be delivered to the prostate via the implant, while EBRT can treat any cancer that may have extended beyond the prostate and also keep side effects to a minimum. There is no strong evidence that men treated with a combination of brachytherapy and EBRT have improved cancer control when compared to EBRT alone.

As for treating high-risk cancers (stage T3 or higher, or a PSA above 20.0 ng/ml, or a Gleason score of 8 or above), brachytherapy is not recommended, either alone or in combination.

Certain situations also make brachytherapy less than optimal for treating prostate cancer. Patients with very small or very large prostates are more difficult to implant. In some cases, radiation oncologists use androgen deprivation therapy to shrink the prostate prior to implantation. Men who exhibit symptoms of bladder outlet obstruction (a high International Prostate Symptom Score above 15; see chapter 5), or who have undergone a transurethral procedure to remove prostate tissue (TURP; see chapter 6) could have an increased risk of side effects with brachytherapy. If the prostate extends into the bladder or if the prostate is positioned under the arch of the pubic bone, this could make an implant more difficult and produce increased side effects or result in areas of the prostate not being treated completely.

MAKING YOUR RADIATION THERAPY CHOICE

External beam radiation therapy has the broadest indications and selection criteria for patients with prostate cancer and is used to treat cancers that are low risk to very high risk. For brachytherapy, the eligibility and indications narrow somewhat. Men considering radiation may want to think about other options if they have severe lower urinary tract symptoms due to prostatic enlargement and obstruction, because radiation can exacerbate these symptoms if they are not addressed beforehand. Also, a person with chronic inflammatory bowel disease risks making that condition worse by undergoing any form of radiation.

Major considerations in selecting a treatment for prostate cancer are the extent and aggressiveness of the disease. (See the risk groups below.) This will give the radiation oncologist a sense of the pace of the disease and the likelihood that a given treatment will be successful.

A patient's overall health status must be considered as well. Diabetes and coronary artery disease put a man at higher risk for developing side effects from the combination of EBRT and androgen deprivation therapy. A man's personal preferences should play a large role in treatment decisions. Some patients consider the side effects of radiation and then choose surgery instead, while others want to avoid surgery altogether. Learning about the risks of each treatment will help in making the personal choice that is right for you.

RISK STRATIFICATION FOR RADIATION THERAPY

In order to get some sense of how aggressive your cancer is and what the possibilities are that radiation therapy will be successful, a radiation oncologist will stratify a newly diagnosed patient with prostate cancer into one of the following risk groups based on clinical stage, prostate-specific-antigen level, and Gleason score.

We have already reviewed the very-low-risk category (see chapter 12 on active surveillance). That is not included here because these men are ideal candidates for no immediate treatment, unless they have more than a twenty-year life expectancy. If they do have more than a twenty-year life expectancy, the options would be similar to those for low-risk disease shown below.

Keep in mind that for low-risk disease, no option has been shown to have a cancer control advantage over any other. Therefore, personal preferences with regard to the inconvenience of treatment and treatment-related side effects should play the largest role in decision making. Also, when more than one option is considered reasonable, that means that scientific studies have not proven a definite benefit for one option over another.

Low Risk

- Clinical stage T1c or T2a, and

- PSA less than 10.0 ng/ml, and

- Gleason score of 6 or lower

There is a major concern that these prostate cancers are being over-treated, especially in men in their seventies and eighties who have a reduced life expectancy due to their age and also have underlying health issues. Remember that according to carefully designed clinical trials, unless a man has more than a fifteen-year life expectancy, treatment for low-risk prostate cancer is not likely to provide a survival benefit when compared with no treatment at all. If this sounds like you, ask your physician if active surveillance might be just as reasonable a treatment, and if not, why not?

For those men whose life expectancy is more than fifteen years and who have a low-risk prostate cancer, reasonable options for treatment could include surgery, EBRT, or brachytherapy. Note that combining EBRT and brachytherapy would not be appropriate (nor would the addition of androgen deprivation to any form of radiotherapy), because the combination does not improve survival, and only increases the risk of complications.

Intermediate Risk

- Clinical stage T2b or T2c, or

- PSA between 10.0 and 20.0 ng/ml, or

- Gleason score of 7

Radiation alone may not be able to eliminate all of the prostate cancer in a man with intermediate-risk disease, so radiation oncologists may recommend adding a short course of hormone therapy referred to as androgen deprivation therapy. The rationale is that the combination of two cancer-killing approaches is better than one alone in fighting more aggressive prostate cancers. A study published in the *New England Journal of Medicine* in 2011 compared the survival of men with low- and intermediate-risk prostate cancer who underwent external beam radiation therapy alone with those who had EBRT in conjunction with a four-month course of ADT. Only 11 percent of the men in the study had high-risk disease.

The authors reported a significant reduction in prostate cancer deaths with the addition of ADT to the treatment regimen; 8 percent for the EBRT-alone group as compared with 4 percent for the combined-treatment group. But only the men with intermediate-risk disease benefited from adding androgen deprivation therapy. Therefore, ADT is not recommended for men being treated for low-risk prostate cancer. A caveat of the study was that the external beam radiation dosages were lower than what is delivered today with IMRT, IGRT, and brachytherapy. So a benefit of short-course ADT in combination with modern radiotherapy techniques is not proven for men with intermediate-risk disease, but it will be evaluated in a separate study later.

Androgen deprivation therapy in older men with cardiovascular disease carries some risk of increasing cardiovascular side effects such as heart attacks. Radiation oncologists take this into account and may choose to withhold ADT in patients meeting this profile.

For men with intermediate-risk prostate cancer who have less than a ten-year life expectancy, reasonable options for management could include (1) active surveillance, (2) EBRT with or without a short course of ADT for up to six months, or (3) a combination of EBRT and brachytherapy with ADT.

For those men with more than a ten-year life expectancy, active surveillance is not recommended for men with intermediate-risk disease. Reasonable management options could include (1) surgical treatment, (2) EBRT with or without a short course of ADT, or (3) a combination of EBRT and brachytherapy with or without ADT.

Some radiation oncologists recommend combining EBRT and brachytherapy for men with intermediate-risk disease, although I am not aware of any scientific evidence that this improves disease-free survival.

High Risk

- Clinical stage T3a, or

- PSA greater than 20.0 ng/ml, or

- Gleason score of 8 or higher

Very High Risk

- Clinical stage T3b or T4

Men who are diagnosed in a risk category above the intermediate classification need the most aggressive treatment or combination of treatments. Data from large trials demonstrate that men with high-risk, very-high-risk, or lymph node metastases that are going to be treated with external beam radiation therapy benefit from a combination of radiotherapy and extended androgen deprivation therapy for two to three years—maybe even longer. ADT is now standard of care for men in the high-risk category or above who are being treated with EBRT.

For those with high-risk and very-high risk disease, the addition of ADT in these cases is supported by high-level evidence. However, surgery is sometimes considered appropriate for men with high-risk prostate cancer if their tumor is thought to be surgically resectable, based on a physical examination and imaging studies that reveal no definite extension of disease to surrounding structures.

RADIATION FOR METASTATIC DISEASE

For men whose disease has metastasized to lymph nodes or bone, there is no proof that EBRT combined with ADT will provide a distinct survival advantage over androgen deprivation therapy alone. For men who have lymph node involvement but no distant metastases, either ADT or EBRT with two to three years of ADT would be options to consider. If ADT is used alone, then it can be used continuously for the remaining years of life. Alternatively, as a way to escape ADT side effects such as fatigue, hot flushes, loss of muscle mass, and decreased libido, it can be used intermittently for the rest of a man's life

Most oncologists believe that treating the primary cancer in the prostate benefits patients—if not in terms of a cure, then in reducing local and distant progression of disease with lymph node metastases. However, in the setting of distant metastatic disease to bone or other sites,

ADT alone is the recommended initial treatment, since at that point, it is not likely that irradiating the prostate would help to prolong life.

Keep in mind that androgen deprivation therapy alone is an acceptable form of management for a man thought to be too ill to undergo other forms of treatment; although bear in mind that a man with a limited life expectancy due to other medical conditions might fare better without any treatment at all.

ANDROGEN DEPRIVATION THERAPY (ADT) AND RADIATION

The recommendations for using androgen deprivation therapy in combination with radiation therapy are based on large trials of men who were not always similar in terms of risk. Clearly, there are some men who benefit from the addition of ADT with EBRT, and some who do not. It is not possible at present to identify with certainty those men who will and will not benefit.

Evidence supports the concept that ADT should not be used in men with low-risk disease, because the potential downsides of the hormonal treatment far outweigh its benefits. For most men with higher-risk disease, it can be stated definitively that the benefits more than compensate for the disadvantages, while with intermediate-risk disease, the evidence that the benefits outweigh the risks is less clear.

Your car mechanic does not put all the cars whose engines are "skipping" a beat in one corner and apply the same repair. Instead, he looks under the hood, finds the problem, and then repairs the problem for each individual car. I anticipate that in the future, an evaluation of the genetic makeup of a man's prostate cancer will reveal which men have cancers that will turn out to defy the effects of radiation and/or hormonal therapy. An understanding of what drives some prostate cancers to resist certain treatments and others to respond will lead to treatments that are more successful.

SIDE EFFECTS OF RADIATION THERAPY

The side effects of radiation therapy for prostate cancer have not been assessed very carefully. Many studies don't consider the delayed toxic effects of radiotherapy that are often most important to patients and occur six to twelve months after treatment and beyond. The major late side effect that limits the dosage of external beam radiation therapy is rectal toxicity or injury that causes bleeding and diarrhea that cannot be easily treated.

Another limitation in many studies is the lack of a baseline assessment against which to compare late-occurring side effects. Without a basis for comparison, it is not possible to know if patients had the complaint before starting the therapy. This is important because men undergoing radiation therapy are often older and in worse health overall than those undergoing surgery. Baseline urinary, bowel, and sexual dysfunction are often very different prior to treatment in those choosing radiation and surgery.

Then there is the problem of physicians reporting the outcomes versus patient reported outcomes using validated questionnaires. Doctors tend to downplay the side effects of a treatment they administered—it's human nature. Let's look at some studies that have been carried out carefully, albeit not perfectly.

PCOS STUDY

The Prostate Cancer Outcomes Study (PCOS) of the National Cancer Institute systematically evaluated quality of life issues for prostate cancer patients with diverse ethnic backgrounds. Four-fifths of the men had clinically localized disease, with 42 percent treated surgically, 24 percent treated with radiation, 13 percent with hormonal therapy, and 22 percent who went untreated. The PCOS investigators sent questionnaires to patients six, twelve, twenty-four, and sixty months after their cancer treatment in order to assess quality of life in the areas of urinary, sexual, and bowel dysfunction—the areas that are the most problematic in prostate cancer patients. Here is a summary of the most interesting findings:

- Surgically treated patients have more urinary control or incontinence problems than those treated with radiation five years after treatment.

- Surgically treated patients and radiation patients have similar overall sexual function at five years after treatment because with radiation therapy, sexual function continues to decline between two to five years after treatment.

- The majority of men treated for localized prostate cancer are satisfied with their treatment choice.

RESULTS FROM OTHER RADIATION STUDIES

- In one randomized trial comparing short-term side effects of low-dose brachytherapy and surgery at six months after treatment, low-dose brachytherapy patients experienced substantially less incontinence, while surgically treated patients experienced substantially less urinary irritation.

- A 2010 study published in the *International Journal of Radiation Oncology • Biology • Physics* evaluated the short-term and long-term effects of three modern high-dose radiation techniques and found striking differences. The investigators compared brachytherapy alone (BT), image-guided EBRT (EB-IGRT), and external beam with high-dose-rate brachytherapy (EBRT + HDR).

  Moderate to severe gastrointestinal and urinary toxicities occurred in 35 percent of the BT patients, 49 percent of the EB-IGRT patients, and 55 percent of those who underwent EBRT + HDR. Patients treated with EBRT + HDR were more likely to develop urinary obstruction, and those treated with BT were more likely to experience pain on urination.

  The greatest differences in side effects were found for rectal bleeding. After three years, less than 1 percent of BT patients, 20 percent of EB-IGRT patients, and 6 percent of the EBRT + HDR suffered this problem.

- A 2008 study reported in the *New England Journal of Medicine* explored the quality of life outcomes for men treated for localized prostate cancer with brachytherapy, external beam radiation therapy, or radical prostatectomy. The investigators evaluated the areas of sexual, urinary, and bowel function, as well as vitality. They specifically asked questions before and up to two years after treatment about irritative and obstructive urinary symptoms (blood, pain, frequency, weak stream), incontinence, bowel symptoms (frequency, urgency, blood, pain, incontinence), sexual function (quality of erections, in terms of both firmness and reliability, difficulty with orgasm), and vitality. They also questioned the patients' wives about distress caused by a spouse's symptoms.

  The baseline questionnaires uncovered substantial differences in symptoms before treatment, with 37 percent of the patients undergoing EBRT reporting preexisting erectile dysfunction, as compared to 14 percent in the surgery group. Nevertheless, the important findings from this study emphasized that each treatment was associated with a unique pattern of side effects that influenced a man's satisfaction with treatment. Here's a summary of the findings:

1. The addition of ADT—even short-term ADT—made the long-term side effects of radiation therapy worse, especially decreased sexual function and vitality.

2. Nerve-sparing surgical procedures reduced the side effect of sexual dysfunction.

3. Patients who were obese, African American, old, had a large prostate, and/or high PSA before treatment had worse side effects from treatment.

4. Obesity was associated with more side effects—especially vitality and sexual function—after EBRT and brachytherapy.

5. A large prostate size together with hormonal treatment worsened urinary irritation (frequency and pain) after brachytherapy or EBRT, but a large prostate was associated with improvement in urinary irritation after surgical treatment.

6. Quality of life changes that occurred in patients caused distress in their partners.

7. Sexual dysfunction was reported as a big problem one year after treatment in 26 percent of surgery patients, 16 percent of EBRT patients, and 16 percent of brachytherapy patients. By contrast, 44 percent of partners in the prostatectomy group, 22 percent of those in the radiotherapy group, and 13 percent of those in the brachytherapy group reported distress related to erectile dysfunction.

8. Urinary incontinence requiring any pad use two years after treatment was reported by 20 percent of surgical patients, 5 percent of EBRT patients, and 8 percent of brachytherapy patients.

9. A moderate to severe urinary problem at two years after treatment was reported by 7 percent of surgery patients, 11 percent of EBRT patients, and 16 percent of brachytherapy patients.

10. A moderate to severe bowel problem two years after treatment was reported by 1 percent of surgery patients, 11 percent of EBRT patients, and 8 percent of brachytherapy patients.

The bottom line: for the overwhelming majority of men with localized prostate cancer, control of the cancer will not be improved with one form of management over the other, including no treatment. Therefore, be very familiar with the side effects of treatment before making a choice. Understand the following:

- When compared to radiation without added ADT, surgery is more likely to cause erectile dysfunction and incontinence that is bothersome.

- When compared to surgery, radiation is more likely to cause irritative and obstructive urinary symptoms and overall urinary and bowel complaints.

- The addition of ADT to radiation increases the side effects of radiation, especially in the areas of sexual function and vitality.

CHOOSING A RADIATION THERAPY FACILITY

As with any prostate cancer treatment, pay less attention to marketing and more to the experience of the physician and the radiation center. Patients give too much weight to the particular machine or the technology rather than the expertise of the doctor, the treatment team, their years of experience, and the excellence of the hospital or cancer center.

Not all hospitals are alike, and the same goes for radiation therapy centers. Since it's very hard for a patient to assess what makes a good radiation team, one critical factor that applies across many disciplines in medicine, is patient volume. Find out how many prostate cancer patients the hospital or cancer center treats annually. A major center for prostate cancer care would see thousands of patients annually.

BE AN INFORMED CONSUMER

If your doctor has recommended radiation therapy for you, it pays—as it does in all areas of medical treatment—to be an informed consumer. Understand that in this highly competitive cancer treatment marketplace, some hospitals and cancer centers funnel patients to a particular treatment, perhaps because they have more expertise in that therapy, or because they are motivated by other factors, including profit. As a prospective patient, you should be given a balanced view of all prostate cancer treatment options in order to make an informed decision. When the options are presented to you, it's a very good sign if you hear about all management choices—including active surveillance—and why you would or would not be a good candidate for each. On the other hand, if you hear only about one option, it's probably time to look elsewhere.

HOW SUCCESS IS DETERMINED
WITH RADIATION THERAPY

Repeated PSA testing is the best measure for determining the success of any prostate cancer treatment, including radiation therapy. You might remember that the FDA first approved PSA for this purpose. After radiation therapy for prostate cancer, PSA tests are given every three to six months for the first several years, and then usually at intervals of six to twelve months afterward, depending on the cancer's aggressiveness. If the PSA level or rise in PSA indicates a recurrence, it is called a biochemical recurrence and is defined differently for radiation and surgery.

After EBRT, radiation oncologists want the PSA to go under 1.0 ng/ml and stay there. However, radiation does not completely destroy all prostate tissue, so after external beam radiation therapy, PSA values below 0.2 ng/ml are uncommon in contrast to surgery, where levels above 0.2 ng/ml would be considered biochemical recurrence.

After brachytherapy, the situation is more complicated because of what is called a "bounce," which is a temporary rise in PSA unrelated to cancer recurrence. It's important to understand that most patients without a biochemical recurrence have PSA levels of 0.1 to 0.4 ng/ml after brachytherapy. Although PSA should drop after radiation therapy—and this includes both external and internal radiation—a detectable PSA does not mean that the cancer is recurring.

One thing that is almost certain is that a consistently rising PSA after any treatment indicates treatment failure. This is the basis for the commonly used definition of biochemical failure after radiation treatment called the Phoenix definition—so named because it was decided by consensus at a meeting of the American Society of Therapeutic Radiation Oncology (ASTRO) in Phoenix in 2005.

According to the experts, treatment/biochemical failure is based on the rise in PSA after the PSA nadir is reached. The PSA nadir is the lowest PSA value ever obtained after radiotherapy is completed, and this can take anywhere from twelve to thirty-six months to achieve. The experts then add 2.0 ng/ml to that nadir. If a man reaches that number, it probably means that the radiation did not eliminate all cancer cells.

No definition is perfect, and the Phoenix definition is no exception. It was chosen because among men with a cancer recurrence, it correctly identified most men (high sensitivity); and among men without a cancer recurrence, it correctly identified most men (high specificity). The longer the PSA stays low and stable, the greater the probability that radiation treatment has been successful. But because the definitions of biochemical failure are different for surgically treated and irradiated patients, it is not possible, using PSA, to compare treatment success easily in the early years after therapy.

Here's an example of the Phoenix definition of cancer recurrence following radiotherapy: at diagnosis, George had a PSA of 7.4 ng/ml and a Gleason score of 7. Following two months of IMRT radiation treatment, his PSA eventually dropped to 0.5 ng/ml after sixteen months and stayed at that level for four more years. Therefore, his nadir was 0.5 ng/ml. George's PSA then started to rise. Using the Phoenix definition of biochemical failure, cancer recurrence would be defined once George's PSA level reached 2.5 ng/ml (0.5 ng/ml + 2.0 ng/ml).

BIOCHEMICAL RECURRENCES AND
CLINICAL RECURRENCES: NOT THE SAME THING

Keep in mind that a biochemical recurrence of cancer is not the same as a clinical recurrence. The latter term means that the disease has progressed to cause symptoms or is evident on imaging studies such as CT, MRI, and bone scans. On the other hand, a biochemical recurrence is based solely on the results of the PSA blood test in a patient without symptoms or evidence of disease spread. A biochemical recurrence predates a clinical recurrence by years in most cases, and when the only evidence of a recurrence is a rising PSA, it is not possible to determine whether the cancer cells are only present locally within the prostate or surrounding vicinity, or whether they have spread to a distant site.

Virtually all men with a clinical recurrence will have a biochemical recurrence, but a biochemical recurrence does not necessarily mean that a man will develop a clinical recurrence. In fact, most men with biochemical recurrences do not develop metastatic disease and do not die of prostate cancer.

PSA DOUBLING TIME AND DEATH FROM PROSTATE CANCER

The rate at which PSA is rising after both surgical treatment and radiation treatment for prostate cancer is a strong predictor of death from prostate cancer among men with a biochemical recurrence. Known as the PSA doubling time or PSADT, this measure is simply the time it takes in months for the PSA level to double after a PSA recurrence.

In one study after radiation, no men with a PSADT of greater than twelve months died of prostate cancer over five years after the biochemical recurrence; whereas 4 percent of those with a PSADT of six to twelve months, and 63 percent of those with a PSADT below six months, died of prostate cancer. As you might expect, there is a close correlation between PSADT after a biochemical recurrence and the risk category (low, intermediate, or high) based on clinical stage, cancer grade, and PSA before treatment—especially the cancer grade prior to treatment.

Writing in the *Journal of Clinical Oncology* in 2005, Dr. Anthony D'Amico, professor and chair of genitourinary radiation oncology at the Harvard School of Medicine, described the outcomes of men with biochemical recurrences after surgery and radiation therapy. For those treated surgically, the estimated rate of prostate cancer death five years after a PSA recurrence was 31 percent for men with a PSADT less than three months compared with 1 percent if the PSADT was three months or more.

In contrast, if the PSADT in men with a biochemical recurrence was less than three months after radiation therapy, the estimated rate of prostate cancer death five years after a PSA recurrence was 75 percent for men with a pretreatment Gleason score of 8 or more, compared with 35 percent if the Gleason score was 7 or less.

However, if the PSADT was three months or more, then the estimated rate of prostate cancer death five years after a biochemical recurrence was 15 percent for those with a Gleason score of 8 or more, compared with 4 percent for those with a biopsy Gleason score of 7 or less.

Oncologists helping patients make decisions about treatment for biochemical recurrences take into consideration not only how fast the PSA is doubling but also how aggressive the cancer was estimated to be prior to treatment.

TREATMENT FOR PROSTATE CANCER RECURRENCES AFTER RADIATION THERAPY

The first step in managing a biochemical recurrence after radiation therapy is to rule out the presence of metastatic disease with a CT scan or MRI scan and a bone scan. Some radiation oncologists might also order a ProstaScint scan, which uses radioactively tagged antibodies that seek out and attach themselves to prostate cancer cells. Since there are so many false-positive and false-negative results, however, the test is not used often.

In addition, some experts recommend a prostate biopsy before making a decision regarding management. A negative prostate biopsy implies the existence of distant metastatic disease causing the rising PSA.

If an evaluation for biochemical recurrence shows the presence of metastatic disease, then androgen deprivation therapy would be the most reasonable management option in a man without symptoms. In the absence of evidence of metastatic disease, the men most likely to benefit from further prostate treatment are those who had localized disease to begin with (stage T1 or T2), and at the time of biochemical recurrence have a life expectancy more than ten years, and a PSA below 10.0 ng/ml.

A clinical trial of an experimental drug is always an option for men with recurrent cancer after an initial treatment for prostate cancer. Cancer centers will post these on their Web sites, or else ask your oncologist if you are a candidate for a particular trial. An excellent place to start your search for available trials is ClinicalTrials.gov. This is a registry and results database of federally and privately supported clinical trials conducted in the United States and internationally. The site provides information about a trial's purpose, who may participate, locations, and phone numbers for more details.

SALVAGE THERAPY FOR RECURRENT CANCER

For those men with evidence of residual prostate cancer after radiotherapy, further treatment of the prostate gland is referred to as salvage therapy. The options include surgical removal (called salvage radical prostatectomy), salvage cryotherapy, and brachytherapy. These are complex decisions to make, and there are no hard and fast rules. Prior to considering salvage therapy, a number of factors should be considered. A prostate biopsy should be performed to confirm that residual disease is within the prostate gland. If the biopsy detects no cancer, that would suggest that the disease is elsewhere and that any salvage therapy directed at the prostate will not successfully eradicate the cancer.

The best candidates for salvage therapy have a disease that was localized to the prostate at the time of the original diagnosis, negative body scans, and a PSA that is not rapidly doubling. This suggests the possibility of localized rather than metastatic cancer. These men should also have a life expectancy of more than ten years.

Keep in mind that any salvage therapy is more likely to be associated with side effects when compared to an initial treatment. So observation or ADT is also a reasonable option for any man with recurrent disease wishing to avoid the side effects of a salvage treatment.

Table 14.1. Management Options for Men with a Biochemical Recurrence After Radiation Therapy

Evaluation Results (CT/MRI/Bone Scan)	Pretreatment Status	Current Situation	Management Options
Metastatic disease	Any stage or grade	No symptoms	Androgen deprivation therapy (ADT) or observation
No evidence of metastatic disease	Clinical stage T1 or T2	Life expectancy greater than ten years and PSA less than 10.0 ng/ml	If biopsy is positive, consider radical prostatectomy or cryosurgery or brachytherapy.* If biopsy is negative, consider observation or ADT.

*Salvage therapies for those considered to have disease still localized to the prostate gland

THE TAKEAWAY

- For most men with clinically localized prostate cancer that is not classified as intermediate risk or high risk, there is no evidence that any management option results in longer survival than any other, including no immediate treatment.

- Radiation therapy could be considered an appropriate management option for any man without metastatic disease.

- Radiation therapy can be delivered to the prostate to treat cancer either by producing a radiation beam outside the prostate and focusing it inward (external beam radiation therapy, or EBRT) or by implanting radioactive seeds inside the prostate (brachytherapy).

- Radiation oncologists have dramatically improved the delivery of radiation for prostate cancer treatment by targeting the prostate more accurately. This has resulted in the ability to use higher dosages with more cancer-killing power, while avoiding sensitive adjacent tissue and reducing the side effects of treatment.

- The ability to control the cancer with radiation therapy is closely related to the extent of the cancer and the cancer grade at diagnosis, similar to the situation with surgery.

- Radiation therapy can cause obstructive and irritative urinary symptoms, sexual dysfunction, and bowel symptoms.

- The side effects of radiation therapy depend in large part on the size of the prostate, the dosages necessary to treat the cancer, and whether or not androgen deprivation therapy (ADT) is added to the radiation treatment for men with more aggressive disease.

- After radiation treatment for prostate cancer, PSA levels rarely decline to an undetectable level in the absence of ADT, because radiation does not ablate all PSA-producing tissue.

- Biochemical recurrence—a PSA level that rises 2.0 ng/ml above the lowest point (nadir level) that is reached after radiation—is an indication that not all cancer cells were eradicated.

- Most men with a biochemical recurrence do not develop metastatic disease or die of prostate cancer.

- Options for managing a biochemical recurrence depend on many factors that include whether or not the residual disease is thought to be confined to the prostate, how fast the PSA is rising, the grade of the cancer before treatment, and the age and health of the patient.

CHAPTER FIFTEEN

MANAGING ERECTILE DYSFUNCTION AND INCONTINENCE AFTER PROSTATE CANCER THERAPY

Sex is one of the nine reasons for incarnation.
The other eight are unimportant.

—George Burns

There is no such thing as "minimally invasive therapy" for prostate cancer unless you are not the one being invaded. All treatments for prostate cancer can cause side effects, and physicians tend to minimize their rates of occurrence. There is now a greater emphasis on measuring patients' quality of life before and after prostate cancer treatments, and a greater emphasis on managing the treatment side effects that reduce a patient's quality of life.

In previous chapters, I reviewed the side effects of erectile dysfunction, incontinence, and irritation of the bowel and bladder, all of which could be caused by surgery and/or radiation. Radiation can cause long-term bothersome irritative side effects due to injury to the bladder and bowel, in addition to erectile dysfunction (ED). (See chapter 14.) In this chapter, I will discuss the long-term side effects of prostate cancer treatment that can be persistent if not treated.

The treatment for bladder and bowel irritation consists of attempts to reduce the symptoms of urinary and bowel urgency, frequency, and pain. Commonly used approaches are those drugs described in chapter 7 for treating the overactive bladder, and steroid suppositories, dietary changes, and antispasmodics to reduce bowel symptoms. Like treating the common cold, the goal is to reduce symptoms, recognizing that it is not possible to cure the problem if there has been injury to the bowel or bladder.

But herein lies a major difference in radiation and surgical treatment for prostate cancer. With surgery, it is possible to treat severe incontinence and ED successfully, whereas with radiation, severe irritative side effects are difficult if not impossible to erase completely. This being the case, I will focus here on management of ED that can result from both radiation and surgery, and incontinence caused by surgical treatment of prostate cancer.

WHAT IS ED?

Erectile dysfunction, or ED, is the consistent (defined as at least three months' duration) inability to attain or maintain an erection sufficient for sexual activity. Most men consider the ability to obtain an erection to be an essential part of their life, psychologically wrapped into the sense of being a male. Loss of erections or a decline in sexual function can have a large impact on a man's quality of life, reducing his overall mental and physical health. This occurs even in men who are not that sexually active and for whom sexual activity is not so important anymore. In fact, a recent study demonstrated that even among men who recover erections after surgery, the decrease in sexual function causes bother that can result in feelings of shame and embarrassment, and a reduction in a man's general happiness. The impact of ED on quality of life can be even greater than that of incontinence or urinary leakage, another side effect of surgery.

The good news is that since the 1980s, the area of sexual medicine has grown rapidly, with an increase in basic and clinical research that has led to an improved understanding of all aspects of sexual health in men and women—information that can be used to improve sexual function after prostate cancer treatments. Let's first review how erections occur.

FROM NOODLE TO STEEL: HOW AN ERECTION OCCURS

Sexual stimulation causes the release of chemicals from the nerves that innervate the penis, primarily nitric oxide (NO). This gas, won Molecule of the Year in 1992 from the American Association for the Advancement of Science as the first gas shown to be a chemical "messenger." NO carries information from nerves to cells necessary for normal functioning of organs and blood vessels in the body.

Nitric oxide plays a major role in erections. The shaft of the penis holds two individual chambers called the corpora cavernosa. A spongy tissue that is expandable fills the chambers, which extend from the base to the tip of the organ. This tissue also contains blood vessels and smooth muscles. In the normal, flaccid state, the smooth muscle keeps the blood vessels constricted, keeping blood out and the penis soft.

An erection begins when the brain senses something arousing. Impulses are then sent from the brain down the spinal column to the pelvic nerves, and finally, to the penis. Nerve stimulation induced by nitric oxide causes the smooth muscles of the corporal bodies to relax. This allows increased quantities of blood to flow in through the right and left cavernosal arteries, filling the space within the cavernosa. Like a sponge, the corporal tissues quickly expand with blood, compressing the veins that are the escape routes for blood, thereby engorging and enlarging the penis.

Erection drugs, which include Viagra, Cialis, and Levitra, block an enzyme that causes the smooth muscles to contract. This enzyme, called phosphodiesterase type 5 (PDE-5), causes contraction of smooth muscle in the penis and inhibits penile engorgement.

As nature arranged it, the enzyme happens to be in large supply in the penis to maintain a flaccid state that exists most of our waking hours. What a PDE-5 inhibitor drug like Viagra does is to increase blood flow and the trapping of blood in the penis by enhancing and prolonging the smooth muscle relaxing effects of nitric oxide.

The male erection involves a cascade of events, starting with sexual stimulation and requiring healthy nerves and blood vessels "feeding" the penile and vascular tissues, including smooth muscle cells within the penis. During a radical prostatectomy or radiation therapy to treat a cancerous prostate, the nerves and blood vessels supplying the penis can be injured.

THE CAVERNOUS NERVES INNERVATE THE PENIS
AND MAINTAIN HEALTHY PENILE TISSUE

The pathway of the cavernous nerves, discovered by Dr. Patrick Walsh at Johns Hopkins (see chapter 13), can be damaged during prostate surgery. In some cases, these nerves are removed purposely during surgery in order to remove all cancer. Either way, an injury to these erectogenic nerves that run alongside the prostate and on top of the rectum can cause permanent damage to the vascular tissue inside the penis, even when the nerves are intact. In other words, cavernous nerve injury causes penile tissue to change, reducing its ability to relax and fill with blood. This is much like the atrophy that occurs in muscles throughout the body when there is a nerve injury or the muscle is not used.

It was thought that by preserving the cavernous nerves during surgical removal of the prostate, men would recover erectile function. However, it is well known that even with nerve preservation, stretching of these nerves during surgery, or radiation injury to these nerves, can seriously injure penile tissue, resulting in ED. In the case of surgery, recovery can take years; and in the case of radiation, the damage to nerves and blood vessels continues to occur for years, resulting in declining erectile function over time.

PENILE REHABILITATION AFTER PROSTATE CANCER SURGERY

If injury to the nerves and blood vessels supplying the penis ultimately damages the penile spongy tissue, is it possible to prevent this tissue damage after a prostate cancer treatment?

The demonstration in animal models that cavernosal nerve injury causes cell death within the erectile tissues of the penis prompted physicians to attempt to prevent cell death after radical prostatectomy—a concept known as penile rehabilitation. The theory is that the promotion of blood flow to the penis, even in the absence of an erection, can protect the tissues from injury.

As I tell patients, after a stroke impairs someone's arm or leg, lying in bed will not improve function. In fact, just the opposite. The approach is rehabilitation through the use of that limb to promote recovery of function. Therefore, after prostate surgery or radiation, men should seek advice about methods for promoting penile blood flow that can prevent loss of function.

The idea of penile rehabilitation was first suggested by a group of investigators from Italy. To understand the concept, you need to know that injecting drugs such as alprostadil or phentolamine directly into the corporal bodies of the penis will relax smooth muscle and can produce an erection. This approach, called "penile injection therapy," was described in the 1980s, long before the understanding of the innermost workings of the erection process and the development of Viagra, the first of the PDE-5 inhibitors.

Penile injection of vasoactive drugs bypasses the normal cascade of events that take place during sexual activity: sexual stimulation, followed by the release of NO from the cavernosal nerves, and then relaxation of smooth muscle in the penis. Rather, injection of a vasoactive drug—prostaglandin, for example—directly into the penis leads to the direct relaxation of smooth muscle and production of a rigid erection, even in the complete absence of the erectogenic nerves.

The Italian investigators reported that the early use of penile injection therapy after radical prostatectomy promoted the recovery of spontaneous erections, suggesting a protective effect of the therapy. Prior to this, surgeons figured that if erections did not return after surgery, then the nerves must not have been spared. But this Italian study opened the door to the concept that even with nerve preservation, nerve injury can result in tissue damage within the penis that could potentially be prevented.

Although still not completely understood, it is believed that promoting smooth muscle relaxation within the corporal bodies of the penis soon after cavernous nerve injury can prevent the damage to the spongy tissues of the corporal bodies that is known to occur when the cavernous nerves are injured.

If injection therapy can prevent damage to corporal tissue in the penis after nerve injury, could the use of PDE-5 inhibitors or other methods for producing an erection prevent tissue damage?

A number of studies, while imperfect, support the early use of techniques to return blood to the penis after surgical treatment of prostate cancer. The options to enhance erectile function after prostate cancer treatment are:

- PDE-5 inhibitor drugs (Viagra, Levitra, Cialis).

- Vacuum erection devices or pumps.

- Vasoactive drugs that can be placed in the urethra or injected directly into the penis. The most commonly used vasoactive drug is prostaglandin, which can be administered by any of these two routes.

Remember this: sexual function may never be the same after surgery, despite claims suggesting otherwise. Listed here are some of the reasons why patients and their partners often have unrealistic expectations about the return of sexual function; recognizing these can help prevent disappointment with your surgical outcome:

- Failure to recognize that recovery of erections is often a long process that can take years, and the effort required to achieve and maintain an erection may be much greater than prior to surgery.

- Failure to recognize that at the time of orgasm, no seminal fluid will be released because the prostate and seminal vesicles—the organs that produce seminal fluid—have been removed.

- Surgeon-quoted results for the return of erections borrowed from the medical literature rather than from their own personal experience performing the operation.

- The patient believes, based on Web site advertisements, that "new" technology such as robotic surgery offers much better return of sexual function when compared with standard open surgery.

- The patient is not aware that older age and preexisting erectile dysfunction before surgery are risk factors for erectile dysfunction after surgery.

- The patient is unaware that preserving the erectogenic nerves does not ensure return of erections sufficient for intercourse.

- The patient is not aware that drugs for depression and hypertension, obesity, diabetes, and cardiovascular disease predict a greater likelihood of erectile dysfunction after surgery.

- There is a misunderstanding of how an erection occurs, and the many factors that can impact negatively on the ability to achieve an erection, including (1) a patient's overall mental and physical health, (2) strength of the relationship, (3) drugs, (4) the patient's age, (5) sexual function prior to surgery, and (6) surgical expertise.

THE IMPORTANCE OF AN INTIMATE RELATIONSHIP

When it comes to sexual function, I define the "successful" outcome after surgery as the ability of a man—even in the absence of the perfect erection—to adapt to his particular circumstances by continuing to have an intimate relationship with his partner. An intimate relationship can be present without a perfect erection. In my experience, the best predictor of this outcome is a well-informed patient and partner who both understand what is involved in recovery of sexual function after surgery.

This requires preoperative counseling regarding the options for rehabilitation, perhaps speaking to other patients who have been through surgery, and postoperative support for penile rehabilitation. The first step in the process is to find out where you are in terms of sexual function.

IT'S HARD TO KNOW WHERE YOU'RE GOING
IF YOU DON'T KNOW WHERE YOU ARE COMING FROM:
THE PREOPERATIVE ERECTILE FUNCTION ASSESSMENT

An assessment of sexual function prior to prostate cancer treatment is important for many reasons. First, it may uncover factors that are hindering sexual function that can be altered to improve the outcome after surgery. For example, medications that can be changed, better control of blood sugar, weight loss, and exercise programs can be initiated. Second, it will allow the starting point for an honest discussion regarding the expectations for recovery of sexual function.

I have seen many men with poor erections who believed that with nerve-preservation surgery, their erections would somehow miraculously improve. This misconception needs to be corrected before a trip to the operating room to prevent disappointment and regret. Documentation of sexual function prior to surgery will allow an accurate postoperative assessment for determining whether a man is back to his baseline score.

There are two questionnaires that are accepted for assessing a man's sexual function. The International Index of Erectile Function (IIEF) and the Sexual Health Inventory for Men (SHIM) are both validated methods for evaluating male sexual function. The cutoffs for normal are 26 on the IIEF and 21 on the SHIM.

I use the SHIM as my initial assessment of sexual function in men who have been diagnosed with prostate cancer. (See the SHIM questionnaire that follows.) If a man's SHIM score is greater than 21, it suggests that he has normal sexual function and indicates to me that he should have a very high probability for return of erections after a nerve-preserving radical prostatectomy. But with SHIM scores lower than 21, the odds for a return of erections decline, although with PDE-5 inhibitors such as Viagra, men with SHIM scores below 21 can return to baseline sexual function. But no man should mistakenly believe that his SHIM score will be better after surgery than before.

And it is important to recognize the limitations of SHIM. Notice that for all questions except one, it is possible to score a 0 if a man was not sexually active in the past six months. If the diagnosis of prostate cancer, loss of a loved one, losing a job, or any other psychological stress caused a man to be sexually inactive, he might score very low on the SHIM. But this may not be indicative of his true sexual function in the absence of psychological stress. Therefore, it is important to have an honest discussion about the score and the possible causes for a low score.

THE SEXUAL HEALTH INVENTORY FOR MEN (SHIM) QUESTIONNAIRE

Instructions

Each question has five possible responses. Circle the number that best describes your own situation. Select only one answer for each question.

Over the Past Six Months:

1. How do you rate your confidence that you could get and keep an erection?

    1   Very low

    2   Low

    3   Moderate

    4   High

    5   Very high

2. When you had erections with sexual stimulation, how often were your erections hard enough for penetration (entering your partner)?

    0   No sexual activity

    1   Almost never or never

    2   A few times (much less than half the time)

    3   Sometimes (about half the time)

> 4   Most times (much more than half the time)
>
> 5   Almost always or always

3. During sexual intercourse, how often were you able to maintain your erection after you had penetrated (entered) your partner?

> 0   Did not attempt intercourse
>
> 1   Almost never or never
>
> 2   A few times (much less than half the time)
>
> 3   Sometimes (about half the time)
>
> 4   Most times (much more than half the time)
>
> 5   Almost always or always

4. During sexual intercourse, how difficult was it to maintain your erection to the completion of intercourse?

> 0   Did not attempt intercourse
>
> 1   Extremely difficult
>
> 2   Very difficult
>
> 3   Difficult
>
> 4   Slightly difficult
>
> 5   Not difficult

5. When you attempted sexual intercourse, how often was it satisfactory for you?

> 0   Did not attempt intercourse
>
> 1   Almost never or never
>
> 2   A few times (much less than half the time)
>
> 3   Sometimes (about half the time)
>
> 4   Most times (much more than half the time)
>
> 5   Almost always or always

Please add up your totals for your score: Total _____

SHIM Score Results

> 1 to 7:   severe erectile dysfunction
>
> 8 to 11:   moderate erectile dysfunction
>
> 12 to 16:   mild to moderate erectile dysfunction
>
> 17 to 21:   mild erectile dysfunction

INTERPRETING SURGICAL RESULTS: SEXUAL FUNCTION

Every surgeon wants excellent results. However, there are many ways for a surgeon to report his or her results to prospective patients—and some may be misleading. I mentioned that a surgeon could report the "average" results for other surgeons who have published data, suggesting that he or she would obtain similar results. That may or may not be true.

In the early days of radical prostatectomy, questionnaires such as SHIM did not exist. Before surgery, doctors simply asked the patient if he could have intercourse. If the patient answered yes, it meant that he had a strong erection, while a no meant that he had erectile dysfunction.

But if a man said yes, was he trying to please the surgeon? And if he could have intercourse, to what extent was it now compared to a year earlier? And do both partners consider sexual function to be satisfactory? With the acceptance of validated instruments for assessing sexual health, patients can now have a much better understanding of their prospects for return of function.

I believe that an honest method for reporting a surgeon's personal experience regarding return to sexual function is to utilize a validated questionnaire, and to report the proportion of men who have return to baseline sexual function. That gives a patient an idea of his probability that at any given time after surgery, sexual function would likely return. For example, if you have a "normal" score on the SHIM for your age group and with nerve preservation, what is the likelihood that you will return to your baseline function?

I collected SHIM scores prior to and four years after surgery for more than seven hundred men undergoing radical prostatectomy. At one year after nerve-sparing surgery, 65 percent of men who were fifty-seven years old and younger and had no preexisting sexual dysfunction returned to within 95 percent of their baseline sexual function. Approximately 80 percent had a return to their baseline sexual function four years after their surgery.

OPTIONS FOR MANAGING SEXUAL DYSFUNCTION AFTER SURGERY

In the early 1990s, researchers working at the Sandwich, England, laboratories of Pfizer, the American-based pharmaceutical company, were looking to see if they could find a way to increase blood flow in the body to treat heart disease. Although their experimental drug did not turn out to improve blood flow in the heart, it certainly did in the penis. Men in the trial noticed that their erections improved. And so was born the drug sildenafil (Viagra), the first PDE-5 inhibitor approved by the FDA, in 1998. Clinical studies had reported that three in four men with erectile dysfunction caused by a variety of conditions were able to complete intercourse as compared to about one in five men taking a placebo.

Now there are two other PDE-5 inhibitors on the market: vardenafil (Levitra) and tadalafil (Cialis). As mentioned before, the drugs work by inhibiting an enzyme, phosphodiesterase 5, or PDE-5, that leads to smooth muscle contraction in the spongy (corporal) tissue of the penis.

PDE-5 inhibitors are first-line treatment for virtually every man with ED and are used routinely for penile rehabilitation after radical prostatectomy. But since the drugs work through the nitric oxide pathway by enhancing the effects of NO gas, PDE-5 inhibitors will not affect erectile function if there are no erectogenic nerves present. Also, the drugs do not increase sexual desire but rather enhance performance after sexual stimulation. And they don't magically produce an erection without sexual stimulation, although the TV advertisements would lead you to believe that satisfactory sexual activity can occur when partners are located in two different bathtubs!

WHO IS A CANDIDATE FOR DRUG THERAPY?

Not everyone is a candidate for using PDE-5 inhibitors. Anyone taking nitrate-containing medicines on a regular or as-needed basis for heart pain (angina) prevention cannot use the medications. Blood pressure could suddenly drop to an unsafe level, resulting in dizziness. In some cases, a heart attack or stroke could also be triggered. The more common nitrate-based medications include nitroglycerin (sprays, ointments, skin patches, or tablets), isosorbide mononitrate, and isosorbide dinitrate. Also, nitrates are found in recreational drugs, including amyl nitrate or nitrite, also known as poppers.

Alpha-blockers taken by men for lower urinary tract symptoms, when combined with PDE-5 inhibitors, could also cause a drop in blood pressure. Be sure to discuss this possibility with your physician prior to taking the two types of drugs together.

PENILE INJECTION THERAPY WITH VASOACTIVE DRUGS

As with so many discoveries in medicine, serendipity played a part in the development of the first drugs that could safely and reliably trigger an erection. In 1982 the French physician Ronald Virag reported that the pressure inside the penis increased after injection of papaverine, a nitrogen-containing substance derived from the opium poppy. Papaverine relaxes smooth muscle tissue inside the penis and causes the corporal bodies to fill with blood, thus creating an erection. This discovery set in motion serious research into the use of injectable medication for relief of ED.

In 1984 a New York urologist named Dr. Adrian Zorgniotti presented his first case studies of self-injection using a dual combination of papaverine and phentolamine, both agents that induce smooth muscle relaxation. Two years later, Japanese researchers presented evidence that injections of prostaglandin E-1 (alprostadil) produced powerful erections. Finally, modern medicine had injectable drugs that, used either alone or in combination, were able to give a man an erection whenever he wanted one.

Slowly, news of the favorable results with the injectable medication began to spread within the small international community of urologists who were treating erectile dysfunction. Most began utilizing all three—papaverine, phentolamine, and prostaglandin E-1—in what was referred to as "tri-mix."

HOW THE INJECTABLE DRUGS WORK

The specific formulation of an injectable drug or drugs to be administered is based on the type of erection achieved with test dosages. The urologist determines this during an office visit in which a patient is taught how to inject a sample formulation into the penis. The patient's comfort, the degree of erection obtained, and the time it takes for detumescence (return to flaccid state) are observed carefully.

Once the optimum dosage is determined, the medication is prescribed, and the patient can then self-administer the injection at home. Understandably, this takes some getting used to, since the medication is delivered directly into the base of the penis with a small hypodermic syringe. While this may sound painful, some men describe it as a mild pinching sensation, not unlike injecting insulin for diabetes.

Usually an erection occurs within five to ten minutes after injection. Erections can last between thirty and ninety minutes, becoming more rigid with sexual stimulation. However, the erection does not always disappear immediately after orgasm or ejaculation, and is prolonged in some men.

A prolonged erection, one that lasts for four to six hours, occurs in about 5 percent of patients using injection therapy. Priapism, an erection lasting for more than six hours, occurs in about 1 percent of patients. Prolonged erections can damage the penile tissue and it is treated as a medical emergency that requires irrigation of blood from the penis and injection of a drug that causes smooth muscle contraction and detumescence. If priapism occurs when using injectables, the patient should go to a hospital emergency department for immediate treatment.

The penile injections have a high success rate: more than 70 percent. The success rate with injectable drugs may be linked to the detailed instruction from the doctor or trained medical personnel to the patient in mastering the injection technique so that the patient feels competent and comfortable in self-administering the drugs.

The major cause of failure is generally due to the drugs' inability to override a man's poor blood flow to the penis or damaged spongy tissue within the penis. In some cases, men are not comfortable injecting a drug into the penis, and for them, other options are available.

INTRAURETHRAL SUPPOSITORY

If you are not comfortable with the idea of drug injections, another option to consider is MUSE, which employs a small, specially designed plastic plunger that is placed at the tip of the penis. Once the plunger is pressed in, a rice-size pellet of alprostadil—the same drug used for penile injection therapy—is pushed into the urethra. There, moisture causes the pellet to dissolve, triggering an erection minutes later. Of course, if a patient has incontinence after surgery, the pellet may be "washed" out before the drug gets absorbed. As with the injectable tri-mix, your doctor needs to titrate the correct dosage of MUSE for you.

Although not as successful as penile injection therapy, MUSE has the advantage of not requiring an injection. In one review, 40 percent of patients after surgery had successful intercourse at least once after surgery using MUSE. In a trial comparing MUSE to Viagra for penile rehabilitation in men without ED before their nerve-preserving surgery, there was a trend for better outcomes with MUSE. But dropout rates were only 19 percent for Viagra as compared to 30 percent for MUSE. The most common side effect with MUSE is penile pain from the drug.

VACUUM ERECTION DEVICE (VED)

Geddings Osbon developed vacuum erection therapy in the 1960s when he invented a plastic external vacuum that was capable of inducing an erection when placed over the penis. A reversible, noninvasive form of dealing with erectile dysfunction, the vacuum device was used successfully by Osbon for more than twenty years. In 1983 he was awarded a patent for his ErecAid device, and it continues to be a top seller.

The VED works in a very simple way. When a man wants to have an erection, he places a clear plastic cylinder over his penis, and either a manual pump or a special electrical pump is used to create negative pressure in the cylinder. Regardless of the source of the erection problem, this pressure causes vessels in the penis to fill with blood. But the blood is not oxygenated to the extent of blood that fills the penis with a spontaneous erection, or one that is produced by a PDE-5 inhibitor or injection therapy. However, there is evidence from small trials that men using a VED after surgery for penile rehabilitation are more likely to recover spontaneous erections and maintain penile length when compared with those not involved in penile rehabilitation.

Once an erection is achieved—it may take two minutes or so—a flexible tension ring is slipped off the bottom of the cylinder around the base of the penis to keep blood from flowing back out, thereby allowing the penis to stay hard when the cylinder is removed. The resulting erection may be safely sustained for at least thirty minutes. Allowing the erection to last longer than that could produce damage to delicate erectile tissue. The pump costs $200 to $500 and is available only with a physician's prescription. Most insurance plans will reimburse the full cost.

THE PENILE PROSTHESIS: ON-DEMAND ERECTIONS

Implant surgery is another option for men whose erections are damaged by prostate therapies. Prior to considering this option, men should have tried other simpler approaches such as oral medications, penile injection therapy, intraurethral suppository, and a VED, and concluded that they are not satisfactory solutions to their ED problem.

There are two types of penile prostheses; a semirigid rod that is folded into an erect state at the time of sexual activity, and an inflatable prosthesis that is flaccid when not inflated and erect when inflated. Most penile prostheses implanted today are of the inflatable type, because of their more natural appearance and greater rigidity.

Surgery to implant a prosthesis is straightforward and involves placing a pair of rods or cylinders in the penis. Extremely compact, the cylinders, which come in a variety of widths and lengths, are implanted inside the corpora cavernosa of the penis and therefore replace the spongy tissue permanently. A small container that holds fluid for the cylinders is implanted in the lower part of the abdomen and a pump is inserted into the scrotum. Whenever an erection is desired, the man squeezes the pump several times, which transfers the fluid from the receptacle to the inflatable cylinders, which then expand, widening and lengthening the penis. To deflate the implant after use, a valve at the top of the pump is squeezed, and the fluid returns to the abdominal reservoir, causing the penis to go flaccid.

Important considerations prior to undergoing an implant are that if removed later, the inside of the corporal bodies will scar, and the tissue will be unresponsive to other treatments for ED. An implant should be thought of as a measure of last resort when other options are not successful. Additionally, men should realize that some penile length will be lost, and that only restoration of penetration will be gained; not necessarily any improvement in sexual sensation or desire.

Possible complications from penile implantation surgery are infection requiring the removal of the prosthesis, pain, and mechanical failure of the device. Most patients and their partners are satisfied overall with penile implants as management for erectile dysfunction.

PENILE REHABILITATION PROGRAM FOLLOWING SURGERY

There are no definitive rules for a penile rehabilitation program. A physician may have his or her own approach based on patient experience. The idea behind penile rehabilitation and the use of PDE-5 inhibitors and/or other methods for enhancing or producing an erection early after surgery is based on animal and human data. These data suggest a protective effect on penile tissue for PDE-5 inhibitors and penile injection therapy when there is cavernosal nerve injury.

One approach described by investigators at Memorial Sloan-Kettering Cancer Center is the use of a low-dose PDE-5 inhibitor (25 milligrams of Viagra, for example) for two weeks each night prior to surgery and while the catheter is in place after surgery. Upon resuming sexual activity as soon as possible after the catheter is removed, a man would then take the low-dose drug six nights a week and the maximum dose (100 milligrams of Viagra, for example) one night a week at the time of sexual activity. After three to four weeks, if a man were achieving penetration after taking the high-dose PDE-5, he would use the low-dose pill five nights a week and a high-dose drug two nights a week while attempting penetration.

If successful intercourse were not possible with the PDE-5 inhibitor, then a recommendation for penile injection therapy twice weekly would be made. On noninjection nights, a low-dose PDE-5 inhibitor would be taken—but not Cialis because of its long half-life. Half-life is the amount of time it takes for the drug to reach half of its original concentration in your blood. Gradually, a patient on injection therapy would begin to experiment with a high-dose PDE-5 inhibitor to see if oral therapy could be substituted for injection therapy. Realistically, patients should understand that this rehabilitation process could take up to two years after surgery.

ERECTILE DYSFUNCTION AFTER RADIATION THERAPY

Erectile dysfunction can result from radiation damage to arteries and nerves that are responsible for normal erections. (See chapter 14.) Patients often assume that radiation causes ED less often than surgery does, but understand that the damage to arteries and nerves after radiation is cumulative over time and does not appear immediately in most cases. We know that when surgical and radiation patients are followed long term, the rates of ED appear similar. And when androgen deprivation therapy is added to external beam radiation therapy, erectile dysfunction is more likely to occur long term, even after androgen deprivation is discontinued.

It has been estimated that when followed for many years, 35 percent to 60 percent of men develop erectile dysfunction after EBRT, as do 25 percent to 50 percent of men after brachytherapy. And recall from chapter 14 that in a quality study published in the *New England Journal of Medicine*, sexual dysfunction was reported as a big problem one year after treatment in 16 percent of EBRT patients and 16 percent of brachytherapy patients; whereas distress related to erectile dysfunction was reported by 22 percent of those who underwent EBRT and 13 percent of those who underwent brachytherapy.

In a 2011 study published in the *Journal of Sexual Medicine*, men treated with Viagra after EBRT plus ADT had higher sexual function scores when compared with those taking a placebo, but only about one in five patients responded to treatment. And another study published in the same journal reported that both an "on-demand" dose of Cialis and a daily dose of Cialis produced significant improvement in erectile function scores after radiation therapy for prostate cancer.

The approach to managing ED after radiation is not different from that after surgery. While there is no strong evidence to support the success of penile rehabilitation programs after radiation, animal data would suggest that it might be possible to protect penile tissues by encouraging production of erections with oral drugs and other approaches similar to the recommendations after surgery.

MANAGING INCONTINENCE AFTER PROSTATE CANCER SURGERY

It's many weeks after your radical prostatectomy, but you're frustrated and embarrassed because you can't completely control the urine flow from your bladder. After coughing, sneezing, lifting a bag of groceries, getting up from a chair, or swinging a golf club, you suddenly leak urine. Incontinence, the inability to contain urine, has now affected your life.

Although the incontinence isn't life threatening, it's a significant quality of life issue. The stigma attached to the wet clothing and the offensive odor can inflict profound psychological consequences, including humiliation, helplessness, fear, and social withdrawal. And so you begin to cut back on social engagements. You stop exercising. Laughing is something you now try to stifle. Your sex life falls apart due to the fear of leaking, and is replaced by stress and anxiety.

On average, more than sixty thousand men undergo a radical prostatectomy each year for their cancer. When performed by a skilled surgeon, permanent incontinence—the inability to control urine—following a surgical procedure is extremely low. Unfortunately, not everyone has access to a talented surgeon who performs hundreds of radical prostatectomies annually. Then again, even the most experienced surgeons have patients who fail to recover urinary control.

The reported prevalence of urinary incontinence after radical prostatectomy varies from 5 percent to as high as 50 percent, and 5 percent to 10 percent of men will undergo another procedure for incontinence after radical prostatectomy. In the hands of an experienced surgeon, any incontinence requiring the use of an absorbent pad would be expected to occur in approximately 5 percent of patients, depending on age, and incontinence severe enough to require surgical intervention would be expected in 1 percent to 2 percent of patients.

Some men regain control within a few weeks of their surgery, while for others progress is slower and recovery takes months to a year. The time frame varies, depending on the extent of surgery, your age, and the surgeon's experience in performing a careful operation.

Most men experience some incontinence after their catheter is removed postsurgery. While incontinence is inconvenient and embarrassing, thankfully, it's manageable in all cases and curable in most. Permanent incontinence following prostate cancer surgery is rare because treatments for incontinence after surgery are quite effective. For most men, the problem will improve dramatically over time, and their lives will return to normal.

OTHER CAUSES OF INCONTINENCE

Although incontinence usually subsides spontaneously within a few months after surgery, even at this early stage, it is important that your doctor exclude two treatable conditions that may be causing or exacerbating the problem: urinary tract infection and urinary retention. A careful history can usually detect these problems.

A urinary tract infection is generally associated with pain at the time of urination and can be confirmed by urinalysis and a urine culture, and it's treated with a course of antibiotics.

Urine retention is usually associated with a slow urinary stream, pushing or straining to urinate, and a feeling of incomplete bladder emptying. Urinary retention can be confirmed with an ultrasound estimate of bladder volume after urination. This is called a postvoid residual. Retention might require placement of an indwelling catheter, depending on when it occurs in the postoperative period.

Patients with incontinence due to a weakened urinary sphincter (sphincter deficiency) usually describe leakage when standing or moving but less so while sitting or lying down. This is called gravitational incontinence. Also, patients with sphincter deficiency often have leakage at times of increased stress on the sphincter caused by coughing or laughing. Total incontinence without storage of any urine in the bladder is rare after radical prostatectomy, but it can occur when there is severe sphincter deficiency.

THE FIRST STEPS TOWARD RECOVERY

The first steps to improve retention of urine after radical prostatectomy are simple and require only lifestyle modifications. They involve optimizing the ability of the bladder to store urine and the bladder outlet to retain urine. While recovery is taking place, absorbent pads are used for protecting garments. Try out a number of different brands until you find the best ones to meet your particular needs. Some men are able to get by with just a thin minipad, which is similar to a feminine menstrual pad, while others with moderate to severe loss may require adult diapers or briefs to contain the urine. All products are available at your local pharmacy, supermarket, or surgical supply store.

You can also try the following measures to help improve your restoration of urinary continence:

- **Lose excess weight.** Now that you have less force being generated by the sphincter, you don't want excess weight adding to the stress on your remaining sphincter. If you are overweight, get to an ideal body weight with programs described in chapter 3.

- **Don't drink caffeinated beverages or alcohol.** Fluids that result in the bladder's filling rapidly by increasing urine output may worsen your incontinence. Space out fluid consumption over the day and drink when thirsty.

- **Pelvic floor muscle training (PFMT).** Often referred to as Kegel exercises, this program involving repeated pelvic floor muscle contractions should be taught by a health care professional. For some men, in-office sessions to learn how to contract the pelvic floor muscles could be beneficial.

   Pelvic floor muscle contractions to improve the function of the muscles are an accepted part of recovery to help reduce leakage after prostate surgery. Studies suggest that they hasten recovery of urinary control but may not necessarily affect the long-term outcomes. In other words, men who were destined to recover urinary control may recover whether or not they engage in PFMT.

   It may be best to do these contractions lying down so that little stress is placed on the muscles, although they can be done in any position. Here's how pelvic floor contractions are performed:

  - Contract your anal sphincter as if you were preventing yourself from urinating or beginning a bowel movement. Don't tighten your abdominal, quadriceps, or buttock muscles when performing the exercise.

- Perform three sets of eight to twelve maximal contractions that are held for five to ten seconds. Rest for five to ten seconds between contractions.

- At the end of each set, perform five to ten rapid contractions.

- Perform PFMT exercises five times per day.

ORAL MEDICATIONS FOR POSTPROSTATECTOMY INCONTINENCE

For more than two in three men who have incontinence after a radical prostatectomy, the cause is solely a weakness of the sphincter. This is called intrinsic sphincter deficiency. However, in fewer than 10 percent, the primary cause of incontinence is due to the bladder's inability to store urine properly. And in some men, there can be a combination of bladder and sphincter problems.

In my experience, if a man reporting incontinence after a radical prostatectomy has leakage primarily upon standing (gravitational) or with stress (stress incontinence), then medications are not likely to be beneficial. Also, those who have no awareness of leakage but rather drip like a leaky faucet are not likely to improve with oral medications. On the other hand, men who report urgency followed by an episode of incontinence may well benefit from oral medications.

For men who have bladder dysfunction contributing to the incontinence, oral medications that relax the bladder can be beneficial, as can medications that both relax the bladder and lead to a tightening of the outlet. Some of these drugs—often referred to as antimuscarinics—were discussed in chapter 7 on the overactive bladder. They work primarily by allowing more efficient storage of urine within the bladder and reducing unwanted bladder contractions that can contribute to incontinence.

Another class of medications called tricyclic antidepressants is often used in men who are thought to have bladder dysfunction contributing to incontinence. A commonly used drug is imipramine (Tofranil), because it can "relax" the bladder and increase outlet resistance.

No well-regarded clinical trials have been carried out to prove the beneficial effects of oral medications on postprostatectomy incontinence. Still, it is likely that some men will see improvement and others will not. However, it seems reasonable to try oral medications in men suspected of having bladder dysfunction as a component of postprostatectomy incontinence prior to proceeding to more invasive approaches.

PENILE CLAMP

A penile clamp fits on the penis and constricts the urethra between foam pads to prevent urinary leakage. A mechanical urethral compression device for incontinence was first described in a surgical textbook in 1750. Mechanical devices are not recommended in the immediate postoperative period, as they can delay or hinder the return of urinary control.

A number of penile compression devices are now available, including the Cunningham clamp, the C3 penile clamp, and the U-Tex device. They should never be worn for more than four hours straight without removal because continuous compression can cause a pressure injury to the penis.

Penile clamps are only for men who have sphincter deficiency, not those with bladder dysfunction. For the man with minimal leakage except during physical activity such as golf or tennis, and who does not want to pursue surgical treatments, placement of a penile clamp during exercise may be a reasonable solution.

While effective for reducing urinary leakage and pad use, clamps are not used often today because of the availability of minimally invasive approaches to treating postprostatectomy incontinence.

If your incontinence continues despite the noninvasive approaches that I've described, most physicians will recommend other options after a year from surgery, when it is evident that return of spontaneous control is not likely. Injectable agents, implantation of a sling, and an artificial urinary sphincter are considerations for the man who wishes to reduce pad dependency and who is bothered by the incontinence.

INJECTION THERAPY FOR POSTPROSTATECTOMY INCONTINENCE

Injectable agents are the least invasive solution when lifestyle measures and pelvic floor muscle exercises don't solve the leakage problem. They are placed around the urethra at the bladder neck and are meant to compress it and thereby reduce leakage. These materials are referred to as bulking agents, and they work by increasing the resistance at the bladder outlet.

Most physicians place bulking agents around the urethra by injecting the material through a cystoscope that allows visualization of the bladder neck and urethra. A needle is used to penetrate the lining of the urethra, and the substance is injected just beneath the lining, bulking up this tissue. The most commonly used bulking agents are collagen and silicone.

The downside to all bulking agents is that cure rates are low, and multiple injections are required to achieve improvement. In addition, the effect wears off over time, making retreatment necessary. Improvement rates or success with treatment are in the range of 33 percent to 67 percent of men, but fewer than 20 percent will actually become dry after injection.

Bulking agents do not work for men who developed scar tissue at the bladder neck (bladder neck contractures) and for those who've also been through radiation. The best candidates are men with mild incontinence, a well-healed urethra-bladder connection without scar tissue, and a generous length of urethra between the sphincter and the bladder neck in which to place the bulking agent.

The patient most likely to benefit from a bulking agent is one who might wear a few small liners a day for stress incontinence that occurs when coughing or laughing, or only when exercising. For severe cases of incontinence, especially if scar tissue developed after surgery, a sling procedure or artificial sphincter would be a better option.

If you have minimal stress leakage, your urologist can best determine if you are a candidate for injection therapy by taking a look at the area with a cystoscope. For men with moderate to severe incontinence not likely to improve with injection therapy, further evaluation is necessary prior to a surgical procedure to correct incontinence. Your urologist will want to directly visualize the urethra-bladder connection, and measure the pressures inside the bladder to make sure there is no obstruction or bladder overactivity that could doom a surgical procedure to failure.

When there is moderate to severe incontinence after radical prostatectomy, a more invasive approach to treatment is necessary, with either a sling or an artificial urinary sphincter.

MALE URETHRAL SLING

The AdVance Male Sling System is the latest procedure for mild urinary incontinence triggered by sneezing, coughing, and physical activity. This is a thin-strip synthetic mesh device that is implanted through a small incision in the perineum during an outpatient procedure that takes less than an hour. A catheter is usually left overnight.

The AdVance sling works by repositioning the urethra. While compression of the urethra may play some role in improving incontinence, it is believed that the major effect from this sling is support and repositioning of the urethra to a position that more effectively prevents urine leakage when abdominal pressure increases after standing up, laughing, exercising, or having sex.

The beauty of the sling is that it works immediately. Most patients go home without pain medication, not only surprised that they have little or no pain but also even more surprised that they no longer leak urine. Normal activities can be resumed in about a week, but the man should not spread his legs, participate in any sports, or do any heavy lifting for six weeks, to allow adequate time for the sling insertion points to heal. Sexual activity is discouraged for the first six weeks.

For carefully selected patients without severe urinary incontinence, the results with AdVance appear favorable. A recent study of over one hundred patients undergoing the AdVance for incontinence after radical prostatectomy defined a "cure" as no pad use or one dry prophylactic pad, and "improved" as one to two pads or a 50 percent or more reduction in pad use.

Patients were followed for more than two years. The overall success rate with the sling was about 75 percent, with 52 percent cured and 24 percent improved. Also, quality of life scores improved substantially after sling implantation. These improvements did not deteriorate over time, as would be expected with bulking agents used for treating postprostatectomy incontinence.

The ideal candidates for a sling procedure are those without severe incontinence, scar tissue, and prior radiation, and who leak fewer than 150 grams of urine in a twenty-four-hour period. It's easy to measure urine leakage by weighing your pads using a postage scale prior to putting them on, and then after they are removed. The difference in weight is the amount of urine that leaked into the pad.

By obtaining an average pad weight, and knowing the number used per day, you can easily determine and record for your urologist the average amount of urine leakage in a day. There are 28 grams per ounce and 30 milliliters per ounce, so the AdVance would more likely be successful for a man leaking less than about 5 ounces, or 150 milliliters per day.

When urine leakage after prostate surgery is more extensive, or there is scar tissue or prior radiation, the gold standard treatment is an artificial urinary sphincter (AUS).

ARTIFICIAL URINARY SPHINCTER (AUS)

The AUS is the most durable and effective means of treating moderate to severe incontinence due to sphincter deficiency. The device is implanted by making a small incision in the perineum between the scrotum and rectum—as for the sling procedure—and a separate small incision in the abdomen.

The sphincter prosthesis, made of a plastic-like material, consists of three parts that are interconnected: the sphincter cuff, a pump, and reservoir. The cuff is implanted around the urethra through the perineal incision and substitutes for the damaged sphincter. When the cuff is inflated, it compresses the urethra so that urine may not escape involuntarily. The pressure in the cuff is maintained by a liquid-filled balloon that transfers pressure from the balloon to the cuff. This is placed in the abdominal cavity during the implantation surgery. A pump placed in the scrotum makes up the third piece of the device and, when squeezed, transfers liquid from the cuff to the balloon, thereby opening the cuff to allow urine passage.

The scrotal pump is placed through the abdominal incision so that a separate incision is not required. There are no external parts for the AUS. For a man who is also considering a penile implant to correct erectile dysfunction, rest assured that there is adequate room for both devices in the body.

The operation to insert the artificial sphincter takes one to two hours for an experienced surgeon and can be done with general or regional anesthesia. The hospital stay is generally one night, with a catheter left overnight. When the catheter is removed prior to discharge, there will be no difference in urinary leakage because the device is not activated for about four to six weeks in order to allow healing. In this deactivated position, the cuff remains open. However, once activated by pressing the scrotal pump, the cuff fills and prevents urinary leakage until the patient presses the pump again, which allows the bladder to empty. Of course, only men who have the manual dexterity to operate the device are candidates for this procedure.

The major complications of the AUS are infection, with 1 percent to 3 percent of patients requiring removal of the device. Erosion of the urethra, where the cuff compresses it, occurs in less than 5 percent of patients, and this too requires removal of the device. Mechanical failure of the device can also occur in some instances, which necessitates revision or replacement. A patient can expect the device to last seven to ten years in the absence of the abovementioned problems.

Most patients with severe incontinence are very satisfied with the results of the artificial urinary sphincter. On average, three in four patients will report that they are dry, requiring one pad per day, or none at all. Another 13 percent will show improvement, for an approximately 90 percent overall success rate at two to four years after implantation.

SPEAK TO YOUR DOCTOR ABOUT INCONTINENCE

While urinary incontinence is still a socially taboo topic, you don't have to suffer in silence any longer. Remember that some urinary leakage is expected following a radical prostatectomy but that the vast majority of men will eventually regain urinary control. The good news is that it's a fixable problem.

THE TAKEAWAY

- Prostate cancer therapy can affect both urinary continence and sexual function.

- Erectile dysfunction (ED) is the consistent inability to attain or maintain an erection sufficient for sexual activity for at least three months.

- Most men regain sexual function after surgery and radiation if there was a high degree of sexual function before treatment.

- Should erections falter or vanish after a cancer procedure, there are a variety of options to consider, ranging from oral medications, vasoactive drugs delivered by a urethral suppository or penile injection therapy, to vacuum erection therapy or a penile prosthesis.

- The bladder neck sphincter is removed during prostate cancer surgery, leaving the distal or external sphincter to prevent urinary leakage. If this sphincter is weakened by surgery, minor to severe incontinence can occur.

- Incontinence following surgery is usually temporary and managed with absorbent pads and lifestyle changes. Recovery of urinary control may be hastened with pelvic floor muscle exercises.

- In men who do not recover urinary control after a year, options depend on a number of factors but primarily on the degree of urinary leakage.

- When urinary leakage is minor, injection of a bulking agent around the urethra is a simple outpatient option performed endoscopically.

- When urinary leakage is minor to moderate, placement of a urethral sling through the perineum is an option; whereas for severe incontinence, the artificial urinary sphincter (AUS) is the most effective therapy.

CHAPTER SIXTEEN

IF CANCER COMES BACK

When you come to the end of your rope,
tie a knot and hang on.

—Franklin D. Roosevelt

How can this happen again?

Shock, sadness, anger, surprise. These are just some of the reactions that men have when they're told that their prostate cancer has come back after treatment. For some, the news is more troubling than their original diagnosis because there is a chance that this cancer can take their life.

Most of these men were treated for presumed localized disease, but some time after treatment the PSA began to increase. For the majority, prostate cancer will not be the cause of death. For those men with a recurrence of prostate cancer after surgery whose disease takes their life, the time from recurrence to death is—on average—thirteen years.

The PSA test is the best indicator we have of whether or not a prostate cancer was successfully treated, and it was for this use that the FDA originally approved the test. A rising PSA after treatment signals that the initial attempt with surgery or radiation to eradicate the cancer was not successful. Thus begins the dilemma that plagues both patients and physicians: What to do next?

A PROBLEM WITH AN IMPERFECT SOLUTION

When PSA levels are rising after prostate cancer treatments, patients and physicians often refer to this as "recurrent" cancer or a "biochemical PSA recurrence." Actually, recurrence is not quite accurate because it's a residual disease that was initially treated inadequately. This can occur because of the unrecognized spread of cancer beyond the prostate at diagnosis, inadequate surgery, or resistance to radiation and/or androgen deprivation therapy.

In some cases a curable disease is treated inadequately with dosages of radiation that are too low or else do not hit all of the target, or the surgical technique is too "skimpy" or does not remove all of a cancer. For most men, however, the disease was too far advanced and already "out of the barn" at the time of diagnosis. Regardless, the residual prostate cancer cells continue to make prostate-specific antigen and eventually with enough cells producing PSA, it can be detected in the blood. This signals treatment failure.

But when a rising PSA indicates residual disease, is the cancer confined to one spot or multiple places throughout the body? Can it be treated successfully? Who should be treated? When is the best time to initiate treatment? These are some of the questions that, in large part, remain unanswered, mainly because there is no current imaging technology that can identify the microscopic disease that's producing the PSA in the body. Nor can anyone be sure, for example, if the cells are confined to the pelvis where the prostate used to be or if they are still within the prostate after radiation therapy. Or have cells left the prostate altogether and relocated at a distant site?

And then there is this conundrum: Most men with a rising PSA after treatment don't die of prostate cancer, so many don't need any treatment at all. They don't have symptoms from prostate cancer, such as bone pain or fatigue, and an additional treatment triggered only by a rising PSA might cause more harm than benefit. So, what's to be done? And when? It's currently estimated that this dilemma of the rising PSA after treatment for localized prostate cancer affects about seventy thousand men annually.

As you recall from chapters 13 and 14, it is easier to determine when failure occurs with surgery than with radiation. After surgery, the PSA should be undetectable at levels below 0.2 ng/ml if all cancer has been eradicated. But after radiation—whether external beam radiotherapy or brachytherapy—benign tissue remains that can produce PSA, clouding the picture as to whether the PSA is indicative of a failure to eradicate the cancer. And then there is the issue of androgen deprivation therapy (ADT) that is sometimes used in conjunction with radiation therapy. ADT lowers testosterone and PSA levels and may "falsely" indicate eradication of cancer when cancer is still present.

In this chapter, I will outline the options for management of a rising PSA after undergoing curative treatment with surgery or radiation for what was presumed to be localized prostate cancer. But remember, there is no one best answer for such men and a great deal of controversy regarding who should be treated, when, and how.

RISING PSA AFTER RADICAL PROSTATECTOMY

Most experts agree that a PSA level above 0.2 ng/ml on two separate occasions indicates a high probability that surgery did not completely eradicate all of the cancer. But if a detectable PSA does occur, what does it really mean for that individual? When the PSA first becomes detectable or is rising, no imaging studies such as bone, CT, PET, MRI, or Prosta-Scint scans can reliably pinpoint where the cancer cells are located. They could be residing solely in the pelvis where the prostate used to be, or they may be found at a distant site in lymph nodes or bone, or perhaps in both places.

What is known is that even without any treatment most men who face this dilemma don't die of prostate cancer. How could that be known when most American men with a rising PSA get treated? The realization comes from a unique study done at Johns Hopkins that followed men with a rising PSA after surgery who did not receive any treatment until they developed signs of metastatic disease and were then treated and monitored.

Johns Hopkins researchers reported in 1999 on a large group of men that underwent a radical prostatectomy, had a detectable PSA (PSA relapse) at some point after surgery, and were then carefully monitored without any treatment until they were found to have metastatic disease on a bone or CT scan. Of the group:

- Thirty-four percent of those who developed a PSA relapse developed metastatic disease that occurred in half of the men by eight years.

- Once metastatic disease developed, half of the men died of prostate cancer by five years.

- On average, death from prostate cancer occurred thirteen years after the development of a detectable PSA.

Three primary factors in the Hopkins study that were associated with the development of metastatic disease were (1) a shorter time from surgery to development of a detectable PSA, (2) a higher Gleason score at the time of surgery, and (3) a faster doubling of the PSA known as PSA doubling time or PSADT.

Following up on this group of men who developed a detectable PSA after surgery, researchers from Johns Hopkins reported in 2011 that the PSADT and the Gleason score could be used to stratify men into risk groups for the development of metastatic disease. The table below shows how this works.

Table 16.1. Proportion of Men with PSA Relapse After Radical Prostatectomy Free of Metastatic Prostate Cancer After Surgery

Observation	Gleason Score of Cancer at Surgery			PSA Doubling Time in Months*			
	6 or less	7	8–10	15 or more	9–15	3–9	Below 3†
Percentage of men free of metastatic disease at ten years after detectable PSA	94	52	19	72	51	7	—

*Time it takes in months for the PSA level to double; †Not enough men in this group to make an accurate estimate
Adapted from Antonarakis ES et al., BJU Int 2011.

WHO SHOULD BE TREATED AFTER SURGERY AND HOW

The options for management of a rising PSA after radical prostatectomy include observation without immediate treatment, radiation to the prostate bed (called "salvage" radiation), and androgen deprivation therapy. Choice should depend on a man's overall health and life expectancy, preferences regarding living with cancer, desire to avoid side effects, and the risk that the cancer will progress to metastatic disease and death from prostate cancer.

For men with a low risk of progression, no immediate treatment may be the best choice of all. In general, the men most likely to do well without treatment are those with:

- PSA levels below 10 ng/ml before radical prostatectomy
- Gleason grade 6 or below
- T1 or T2 disease stage
- a longer time from surgery to PSA relapse and long PSA doubling times

For those with a short PSA doubling time and high Gleason score, radiation and/or androgen deprivation may be a better choice. There are no rules and much controversy in this area. However, several studies strongly suggest that for some individuals, especially those that receive salvage radiation therapy within two years of a detectable PSA and before the PSA rises above 0.5 ng/ml, survival is improved with treatment.

Androgen deprivation, on the other hand, is most likely to benefit those men with rapid PSA doubling times of less than six to twelve months who also had Gleason scores of 8 to 10 at surgery. About half of the men in this country who undergo treatment following a PSA recurrence opt for salvage radiation therapy, with about half also treated with androgen deprivation therapy.

Today, most oncologists recommend that intermittent androgen deprivation therapy be given after a detectable PSA following surgery. This involves alternating cycles of therapy with a period away from the drugs. First, anti-androgen treatment drugs are given for at least six months until testosterone and PSA levels are at their lowest level (nadir) and remain there. The drugs are then stopped until PSA levels rise again to a predetermined level, at which point the hormone treatment resumes. This cyclic therapy approach appears to delay tumor progression and provides a drug-free period in which the patient experiences renewed vigor, increased sexual function, and a greater overall sense of well-being.

RISING PSA AFTER RADIATION THERAPY

Remember from chapter 14 that a biochemical failure or recurrence after radiation therapy is now defined as a PSA rise of 2 ng/ml above the lowest PSA achieved after treatment. Once a recurrence is documented, as with a rising PSA after surgery, oncologists will perform imaging studies to make sure there is no evidence of metastatic disease. But as with the rising PSA after surgery, these studies are not likely to reveal the microscopic cancer.

The major difference between a surgical PSA recurrence and recurrence after radiation therapy is that the prostate is still in place following radiation therapy. The possibility that the cancer is present only within the prostate means that another prostate-directed treatment could potentially lead to a cure. Successful salvage treatment directed at the prostate at this time is more likely among men who (1) had PSA levels below 10 ng/ml before radiation therapy, and (2) had Gleason scores below 8, and (3) still have PSA levels below 10 ng/ml after radiation.

Most oncologists would first recommend a prostate biopsy to prove the presence of cancer within the prostate before proceeding with a salvage therapy such as radical prostatectomy, cryosurgery of the prostate, or brachytherapy. Of course, just as with a rising PSA after surgery, no immediate treatment is the best choice for some men.

In general, a salvage radical prostatectomy is only offered to those men with a life expectancy of more than ten years who had suspected prostate-confined cancer before radiation and a Gleason score of 7 or less. Following radiation, they should have PSA levels less than 10 ng/ml if surgery is to be considered. The risk of incontinence and rectal injuries associated with this salvage prostatectomy procedure discourage most men from undertaking this approach. In addition, more than 60 percent of patients would be expected to have a biochemical relapse within ten years.

Other approaches, such as cryosurgery, are thought to have a lower risk of side effects when compared to salvage surgery. About 50 percent of patients have PSA levels suggesting treatment success five years after cryotherapy. Unfortunately, should the PSA begin to rise rapidly, there are no long-term studies proving that any salvage treatment prolongs survival when compared to less invasive approaches like observation with androgen deprivation therapy.

WHEN ANDROGEN DEPRIVATION
THERAPY (ADT) IS APPROPRIATE

Withdrawal of androgens, which is called androgen deprivation therapy or ADT, was initially performed with surgical castration (orchiectomy) to remove testosterone produced by the testes. This was the standard of care for men with metastatic prostate cancer from the 1940s through the 1980s, because androgens, particularly testosterone, are required for maintenance of prostatic tissue and their withdrawal results in regression of prostate tissue, including cancer.

In lieu of surgical castration, the standard treatment for metastatic prostate cancer since the 1980s has been *medical* castration with drugs that block the brain signals for testosterone production by the testicles. These drugs are called luteinizing hormone-releasing hormone agonists or antagonists, or LHRH agonists/antagonists for short.

Although androgen deprivation therapy can result in long-term remissions of metastatic prostate cancer, it is not a curative treatment. The reasons for this are not entirely clear yet, but this area is one that has recently generated a great deal of research interest.

It was accepted by many scientists that when ADT no longer held the cancer at bay that it was androgens from sources other than the testes that must be fueling the cancer. In addition to the testes, surgeons in the early days tried removing the adrenal glands, another source of androgens, in an attempt to remove all testosterone from the body. Pharmaceutical companies soon developed drugs to block not only production of androgens, but also the receptors to which androgens attach, thinking this would result in improved outcomes when compared to halting testosterone production only. This attempt at total androgen blockade was to no avail, however, as metastatic prostate cancers progressed despite all attempts at ADT, no matter how complete. When this occurs, we call it castration-resistant prostate cancer.

Scientists now believe that prostate cancer cells continue to grow despite androgen deprivation therapy by manufacturing their own androgens, and they are searching for alternate methods to block cell growth. Regardless, it is not likely that any approach to ADT, no matter how complete, will be successful at arresting prostate cancer progression.

Because ADT can result in erectile dysfunction, breast swelling and pain, loss of muscle and bone mass, fatigue, depression, anemia, and metabolic syndrome, physicians try to avoid or delay ADT unless it is evident that a man will benefit from the treatment.

There is no controversy about the use of ADT in men with evidence of metastatic disease on imaging studies such as bone and CT scans, especially if metastatic disease is producing symptoms. And there is some evidence that men who have lymph node metastases will benefit from ADT initiated soon after surgery. In addition, there is no controversy that ADT should be used in combination with radiation therapy in more aggressive cases. ADT improves survival for men with more aggressive disease, as discussed in chapter 14. But prior to the development of metastatic disease, physicians still debate whether starting ADT is associated with more benefit than harm.

In the absence of radiographic evidence of metastatic prostate cancer, the men most likely to benefit from ADT are those with Gleason scores of 8 to 10 or a rapidly rising PSA. Like many other choices in medicine, when the evidence of benefit is not clear cut, a man's personal preferences should play a large role in decision making.

WHEN ADT STOPS WORKING:
MANAGEMENT OF CASTRATION-RESISTANT DISEASE

The FDA has approved several promising new drugs for the treatment of metastatic prostate cancer. Exciting progress has been made, not so much because survival is improved to a great extent, but rather because these new medications prove that alternate approaches to treatment can be successful in halting the progress of this disease.

The standard approach to improve the survival for men with castration-resistant prostate cancer since 2004 has been to use the chemotherapy agent Taxotere (docetaxel)—an approach that lengthened life about three months when ADT stopped working. Now, two new nonchemotherapy agents have been approved for men with castration-resistant prostate cancer. Provenge (sipuleucel-T) received FDA approval in 2010, with Zytiga (abiraterone) getting approved the following year.

Provenge is a vaccine that uses a man's own immunity to kill cancer cells. The vaccine is created in a multistep process that takes immune cells from the patient's blood and exposes them to a protein on the surface of prostate cancer cells. This exposure activates the immune cells that are then injected back into the man to treat the cancer. For men with castration-resistant prostate cancer who participated in the Provenge clinical trial, survival was improved by four months compared to men not receiving it, prompting FDA approval.

Because Provenge doesn't really have a direct tumor-killing effect, it doesn't usually produce PSA declines and visible tumor shrinkages. Although patients are living longer after taking Provenge, oncologists don't really know why. Some researchers think the vaccine might work by preventing the formation of new tumors, and others say that it may stimulate the immune system to attack the cancer.

Zytiga is a more potent method of reducing androgens that can lead to cancer progression. FDA approval for this drug was based on about a four-month increase in survival for men who had failed both androgen deprivation therapy and chemotherapy with Taxotere.

The exciting prospect for these alternatives is that if they can increase survival in those men who have metastatic disease with extensive tumor burden, they may be even more effective for men who are at high risk of cancer recurrence after surgery and radiation but have not yet manifested the recurrence.

The goal in the future will be to better predict those men who will develop metastatic disease after radiation or surgery and then use these new therapeutic approaches before metastatic disease becomes evident. In so doing, it might be possible to turn aggressive prostate cancer into a chronic disease that a man lives with and does not die from.

THE TAKEAWAY

- Biochemical or PSA recurrence is the progression of prostate cancer after surgery or radiation therapy for prostate cancer.

- For men with a rising PSA after surgery, no immediate treatment, androgen deprivation therapy (ADT), or salvage radiation therapy are viable options.

- After radiation therapy, management options for a rising PSA most often include no immediate treatment, androgen deprivation therapy, or treatment of the prostate with surgery or cryoablation (freezing).

- ADT is the standard first-line treatment for men with metastatic prostate cancer, but the timing of therapy is controversial and this approach is not curative.

- When ADT no longer works to control the cancer, chemotherapy, immunotherapy, and more potent androgen withdrawal drugs are now available to prolong life.

A

abiraterone (Zytiga). This FDA-approved oral medication blocks the synthesis of male androgens and is prescribed for men with hormone-refractory prostate cancer.

active surveillance. A strategy for managing prostate cancer for men with low-risk disease thought to be small volume and low grade in which the patient is closely monitored, with curative treatment initiated if the cancer progresses.

acute urinary retention. A complete inability to urinate despite having the urge to do so; requires immediate medical attention.

adenocarcinoma. A cancer that develops from glandular tissue like the prostate and breast.

adjuvant therapy. Any additional treatment given before, during, or after a definitive cancer therapy, to increase overall effectiveness and the possibility of a cure. This can include radiation therapy, chemotherapy, hormone therapy, and biological therapy.

age-specific PSA. An adjustment of the PSA value that accounts for the natural, gradual increase in PSA that occurs with age as the prostate enlarges.

alpha-1-adrenergic blockers. A class of drugs that treats lower urinary symptoms that are often caused by benign prostatic enlargement (BPE; also called benign prostatic hyperplasia, or BPH) by relaxing smooth muscle in the prostate. Also called alpha-blockers.

androgens. Sex hormones, such as testosterone, that produce and promote male characteristics. These hormones are responsible for normal male development in utero and maintain the function of androgen sensitive tissues in the body, including prostate cells.

androgen deprivation therapy. A strategy designed to decrease circulating levels of testosterone, the male androgen, either by removing the testicles (orchiectomy) or by giving medication to block the production or action of testosterone. (See hormone therapy.)

antiandrogens. Drugs (bicalutamide, flutamide, and nilutamide) that block the action of testosterone and dihydrotestosterone at the cellular level by interfering with androgen receptors in cells.

antibiotics. Medications that kill bacteria.

angiogenesis. The formation of new blood vessels; a necessity for cancer progression.

angiogenesis inhibitors. Drugs that block angiogenesis.

antibody. A protein made by the immune system of the body to eliminate substances recognized as foreign (e.g., bacteria, cancer cells).

antigen. A molecule that promotes the production of an antibody.

anus. The opening at the end of the digestive tract where unabsorbed bowel contents leave the body.

apoptosis. Programmed cell death triggered by cellular stress. An imbalance between cell death and proliferation—a reduction in cell death—results in tumor formation.

artificial sphincter. A surgically implanted device to treat severe incontinence.

B

benign. The absence of cancer; the opposite of *malignant.*

benign prostatic enlargement (BPE). Noncancerous enlargement of the prostate gland resulting from a decrease in cell death that often increases with age and can result in a rise in PSA and a variety of urinary symptoms.

benign prostatic hyperplasia (BPH). The increase in noncancerous prostate tissue that can result in benign prostatic enlargement (BPE) and urinary symptoms.

biopsy. A procedure in which tissue samples are removed from the body for examination under a microscope often done to determine the absence or presence of cancer.

bladder. The hollow, muscular pelvic organ that collects and stores urine made by the kidneys.

bladder neck. The junction between the bladder and the prostate in a male.

body mass index (BMI). A measure of body fat that is determined by a person's weight and height.

bone scan. A nuclear medicine imaging study involving an injectable radioactive compound to identify areas of increased bone cell activity in the skeleton; typically used to screen for bone metastases (e.g., prostate cancer).

brachytherapy. A prostate cancer radiation treatment that entails implanting multiple tiny radioactive seeds into the prostate. Also called seed therapy or interstitial radiation therapy.

C

cabazitaxel (Jevtana). A second-line chemotherapy medicine approved for the treatment of castration-resistant prostate cancer no longer responding to docetaxel.

cancer. A general term for a group of diseases characterized by uncontrolled cell growth. Unlike benign cells, cancer cells exhibit properties of invasion and metastasis and can spread through the blood and lymph systems to other parts of the body.

castrate. Removal of the gonads. In the context of prostate cancer, refers to lowering the levels of testosterone by removal of testicles (orchiectomy) or blocking the production or action of testosterone by medications to treat prostate cancer; sometimes called hormonal therapy.

castrate-resistant, castration-resistant. A prostate cancer that continues to progress despite androgen withdrawal (castration).

catheter. A tube that is inserted through the urethra to drain urine from the bladder.

cell. The fundamental structural and functional unit of all living organisms.

clinical trial. A study designed to determine the safety and/or effectiveness of a medical intervention.

chemotherapy. Treatment of a cancer with a drug designed to eradicate cancer cells.

combined androgen blockade. The use of an antiandrogen to block the action of testosterone at the cellular level, together with an intervention (drug or castration) to block the production of testosterone.

computed tomography (CT scan). More detailed than traditional x-rays, this is a radiologic imaging study in which cross-sectional images (called slices) of the body are obtained from x-rays and computer technology. Commonly used in treatment planning for prostate cancer radiotherapy.

core. A piece of tissue obtained from a prostate needle biopsy.

corticosteroid. A drug used to relieve swelling and inflammation.

CP/CPPS. A painful condition involving the male genitourinary system that is not associated with a bacterial infection.

cryotherapy. The use of cold temperatures to eliminate prostate cancer cells. Sometimes used to treat localized prostate cancer.

cystoscopy. An examination in which a tube (rigid or flexible) called a cystoscope is inserted through the urethra to directly view the inside of the bladder.

D

diethylstilbestrol (DES). A synthetic estrogen (female hormone) that was used to treat prostate cancer by suppressing testosterone production.

digital rectal exam (DRE). An examination in which a doctor inserts a gloved and lubricated finger into the rectum to feel for abnormalities of the prostate and rectum.

dihydrotestosterone (DHT). A testosterone derivative that has a higher biologic activity within the prostate than testosterone. DHT can be blocked by 5-alpha reductase inhibitors, medications such as finasteride (Proscar) and dutasteride (Avodart) used for treating urinary symptoms caused by benign prostatic enlargement.

docetaxel (Taxotere). The first FDA-approved chemotherapy for advanced prostate cancer.

E

ejaculate. Discharge of seminal fluid through the penis during orgasm. Together with sperm, the fluid contains secretions produced by the prostate gland and seminal vesicles.

elevated PSA. An outdated phrase that was used to indicate a PSA value considered above the "normal" range. Experts now advise using PSA as a risk-assessment tool rather than characterizing levels as normal and abnormal.

epithelium. Cells that line an organ and are capable of producing secretions. Epithelial cells in the prostate manufacture numerous substances including PSA.

erectile dysfunction (ED). The inability to achieve an erection suitable for sexual intercourse.

external beam radiation therapy (EBRT). The use of photons or protons for treating cancerous tissues, including the prostate gland.

extracapsular. The tissues surrounding the exterior boundary of the prostate gland.

extracapsular disease. Cancer that has spread to the tissue surrounding the prostate gland.

F

5-alpha reductase. An enzyme that converts testosterone to dihydrotestosterone (DHT), the most potent androgen within the prostate.

5-alpha-reductase inhibitors. A class of drugs that block the conversion of testosterone into dihydrotestosterone and can lead to a reduction in prostate size. These drugs are often used to treat urinary symptoms caused by prostate enlargement.

filling cystometry. A test that involves measuring the pressures inside the bladder with filling to determine the ability of the bladder to store urine normally.

flare. An increase in testosterone caused by drugs that initially stimulate testosterone production (LHRH agonist), but then lead to castrate testosterone levels for the treatment of advanced prostate cancer.

focal therapy. A treatment for prostate cancer with radiation, heating or freezing, that attempts to ablate an individual prostate tumor instead of the entire prostate gland in an effort to reduce side effects of treatment.

follicle-stimulating hormone (FSH). A pituitary hormone that stimulates sperm production by the testes.

G

glandular cells. Cells in the prostate that produce part of the fluid portion of semen.

Gleason grade and score. A numerical value given to prostate cancer that describes tumor aggressiveness. Grades are assigned to the most common cancer pattern and the second most common pattern, and range today from 3 to 5, from least to most aggressive appearing. The Gleason score is obtained by adding the two Gleason grades, yielding totals that range from 6 to 10.

GreenLight laser prostatectomy. A high-energy laser that is used to vaporize or ablate prostate tissue in men with lower urinary tract symptoms caused by benign prostate enlargement (BPE). Sometimes called photoselective vaporization.

gynecomastia. Male breast enlargement sometimes caused by androgen deprivation therapy (ADT) used for the treatment of prostate cancer.

H

hematuria. Blood in the urine; either seen by a patient and referred to as gross hematuria; or seen by a physician/technician when examining urine under a microscope and referred to as microscopic hematuria.

high-dose-rate brachytherapy. A focal radiation treatment involving temporary placement of a radioactive source in the prostate that is removed after each brief (five to twenty minutes) treatment.

high-intensity focused ultrasound (HIFU). A treatment for prostate cancer that uses the energy created by ultrasound waves to destroy prostate tissue.

histology. The study of cells and tissues under the microscope.

hormone. A chemical made by glands in the body that circulate in the bloodstream and control the actions of various organs and cells.

hormone therapy. Usually refers to the withdrawal of the male hormone (testosterone) from the body by blocking its production or action with drugs to treat prostate cancer.

hot flashes/flushes. A side effect of hormone therapy (androgen deprivation therapy) for prostate cancer that causes a hot or flushed feeling similar to the symptoms of female menopause.

hyperplasia. An abnormal increase in the number of cells in a tissue or an organ such as the prostate.

I

imaging studies. Tests such as ultrasound, computed tomography (CT), magnetic resonance imaging (MRI), and x-rays that produce images of the inner structures of the body.

immunotherapy. A type of treatment that harnesses the immune system to fight disease. Provenge (sipuleucel-T) is the first prostate cancer vaccine.

incontinence. A loss of bladder control that results in leakage of urine from the bladder.

intensity-modulated radiation therapy (IMRT). An advanced form of three-dimensional conformal radiotherapy (3D-CRT) that allows for the changing of radiation intensity for each radiation beam.

intermittent androgen suppression. An approach to androgen deprivation therapy for treatment of prostate cancer that involves the use of drugs to lower testosterone, with discontinuation of the drugs when PSA levels fall, and restarting the drugs when PSA levels rise. This on/off treatment allows drug holidays that can reduce the side effects of the treatment.

interstitial laser coagulation. A minimally invasive therapy to treat urinary symptoms due to benign prostate enlargement (BPE). The treatment involves placing a needle into the prostate to deliver laser energy to ablate prostate tissue.

K

Kegel exercises. Exercises to strengthen the pelvic floor muscles by tightening and then releasing the muscles.

L

laparoscopy. A surgical technique in which small holes are made in the abdominal wall through which specially designed instruments are passed for performing surgical procedures.

laser prostatectomy. A treatment for urinary symptoms caused by benign prostate enlargement (BPE) in which laser energy is used to ablate excess prostate tissue.

libido. The desire or drive for sexual activity that is affected by hormones such as testosterone.

LHRH agonists. Drugs used to treat advanced prostate cancer that work by reducing the secretion of luteinizing hormone-releasing hormone from the hypothalamus in the brain. LHRH agonists cause release of luteinizing hormone from the pituitary gland, which triggers testosterone production by the testicles.

linear accelerator (Linac). A machine used to deliver external beam radiation therapy for treatment of cancer .

lower urinary tract symptoms (LUTS). A nonspecific term that refers to any combination of urinary symptoms, or as a more specific term to refer to those symptoms primarily associated with storage and/or voiding disturbances common among older men.

luteinizing hormone-releasing hormone (LHRH). A hormone released by a portion of the brain (hypothalamus) that stimulates the pituitary gland in the brain to produce luteinizing hormone and follicle-stimulating hormone.

lymph nodes. Organs of the immune system located throughout the body that house the cells responsible for ridding the body of foreign invaders such as bacteria, viruses, and cancer. Lymph nodes can become enlarged when bacteria/viruses or cancer are lodged within the organ.

M

magnetic resonance imaging (MRI). A diagnostic procedure that uses a combination of large magnets, radiofrequencies, and computer software to produce detailed images of organs and structures within the body.

margin. The outermost portion of a tissue or organ. In prostate surgery, the outermost surface of the gland that is removed and examined under the microscope for the presence or absence of cancer. A margin is referred to as positive when cancer cells are present at the outermost surface.

medical castration. The use of medication to interfere with the production or actions of testosterone.

metabolic syndrome. A dangerous cluster of ailments that can include high blood pressure, abdominal obesity, abnormal blood lipids or fats, and high fasting blood glucose levels, that together increase the risk of developing heart disease, stroke, and diabetes.

metastasis. The spread of cancer from the organ of origin to another organ such as lymph nodes or bone, the most common sites of spread for prostate cancer.

metastatic prostate cancer. Secondary growth of prostate cancer that has spread to other organs.

moderately differentiated cancer. The appearance of a cancer that resembles its tissue or organ of origin to a moderate degree and in between well and poorly differentiated.

N

nadir. The lowest level.

neoadjuvant hormonal therapy. A treatment administered before a definitive therapy; for example, the use of androgen deprivation therapy before the start of radiation treatment for prostate cancer.

nerve-sparing radical prostatectomy. The technique during a radical prostatectomy in which one or both of the neurovascular bundles that contain the nerves responsible for male erections are preserved.

neurovascular bundles. The band-like structures running along the sides of the prostate gland that contain the nerves and blood vessels necessary for obtaining and maintaining a penile erection.

nocturia. Frequent nighttime urination that can be caused by an increased nighttime production of urine or inability to store urine efficiently.

O

oncologist. A doctor who specializes in treating cancer.

orchiectomy. Surgical removal of the testicles to eliminate testosterone production; used to treat advanced prostate cancer.

open prostatectomy. A surgical procedure in which prostate tissue is removed through an incision in the abdomen or laparoscopically through holes in the abdominal wall.

overflow incontinence. Urine leakage that occurs when the pressure from urine in the bladder exceeds the resistance at the outlet. Overflow incontinence can occur from obstruction by the prostate or the lack of sensation of bladder filling caused by diabetes.

P

palliative therapy. Treatment aimed at relieving pain and limiting disease complications rather than providing a cure.

palpable cancer. A cancer that can be felt by touch; in the case of prostate cancer by digital rectal examination.

pathologist. A physician who renders diagnostic and prognostic information using tissue samples removed from the body.

PDE-5 inhibitors. Drugs that block PDE-5, the enzyme that leads to smooth muscle contraction in penile tissue causing detumescence or loss of rigidity. These drugs, sildenafil, tadalafil, and vardenafil, help men achieve and maintain an erection.

pelvic lymph node dissection. Removal of lymph nodes in the pelvis near the prostate to examine for the presence of prostate cancer.

penile clamp. A device that compresses the penis to prevent urine from leaking.

penile rehabilitation. Post-prostatectomy therapy designed to increase penile blood flow and the chances that erections will return spontaneously.

percent free PSA. The proportion of PSA not attached to blood proteins. Men with prostate cancer have a lower percentage of free PSA than men with benign prostatic enlargement (BPE).

peripheral zone. The outermost area of the prostate gland, where most prostate cancers originate.

perineal prostatectomy. An approach to prostate removal for cancer in which the incision is made in the perineum, the area between the scrotum and the anus.

phytotherapy. The use of plant-derived substances to treat symptoms such as lower urinary tract symptoms from benign prostatic enlargement.

pituitary gland. A gland located at the base of the brain that produces a variety of hormones, including one (luteinizing hormone or LH) that stimulates the testes to produce testosterone.

postvoid residual. The amount of urine left in the bladder following urination.

pressure-flow urodynamic studies. Tests that measure bladder pressure and flow during urination to help determine the cause of lower urinary tract symptoms.

prostate gland. A gland in the male that surrounds the neck of the bladder and urethra. Secretions produced in the prostate contribute to the seminal fluid or ejaculate.

prostate-specific antigen (PSA). An enzyme produced by the epithelial cells of the prostate and secreted in the seminal fluid released during ejaculation. High blood levels of PSA may indicate the likelihood and extent of prostate cancer, as well as the size of the benign prostatic enlargement, or BPE.

prostatectomy. A surgical procedure for removal of the prostate; a radical prostatectomy involves complete prostate removal for cancer, while a simple prostatectomy involves removing only the inner obstructing tissue to treat urinary obstruction from benign prostatic enlargement or BPE.

prostatic intraepithelial neoplasia (PIN). A precancerous prostate lesion.

prostatic stent. A plastic or metal device placed in the urethra to treat blockage from prostatic enlargement in men who cannot tolerate a more invasive surgical procedure.

prostatitis. Inflammation of the prostate that may cause pain or discomfort in the perineum, testicles, and lower back; can be accompanied by urinary symptoms and fever.

proton beam radiation therapy. A highly focused form of radiation therapy for prostate cancer that uses protons instead of photon beams.

PSA density (PSAD). The PSA level divided by the size of the prostate gland as measured by ultrasound examination. PSAD, a method for adjusting the PSA for the prostate size, can help a physician interpret whether a given PSA level is due to benign prostate enlargement or prostate cancer.

PSA nadir. The lowest point to which a person's PSA drops following a prostate cancer treatment; most often used to describe the lowest PSA after radiation treatment for prostate cancer.

PSA velocity. A measurement of the changes in PSA values over time.

R

radiation oncologist. A physician who specializes in treating cancer using radiation therapy.

radiation therapist. A person trained to operate the linear accelerator and administer radiation treatments.

radiation therapy. Cancer treatment with high-energy x-rays (photons or protons) that cause cell death in cancerous tissues.

radical prostatectomy. A treatment for a localized prostate cancer that involves the surgical removal of the entire prostate gland and seminal vesicles.

radical retropubic prostatectomy. Surgical removal of the prostate gland for cancer that is performed through an incision in the lower abdomen.

radiologist. A doctor that uses imaging technology to diagnose and/or treat disease.

rectum. The last six to eight inches of the intestine leading to the outside of the body.

refractory. Unresponsive. In the case of cancer treatment, refractory describes a state in which a cancer treatment is no longer effective.

remission. Cancer that is under control and responding to a cancer therapy.

residual disease. Cancer that was not completely eliminated by a treatment.

residual urine. Urine retained in the bladder after voiding. It can become infected or lead to the formation of bladder stones.

retrograde ejaculation. Ejaculation of semen into the bladder rather than out through the penis; a side effect of surgical treatment for benign prostate enlargement and some medications used to treat lower urinary tract symptoms (e.g., alpha blockers).

retropubic open prostatectomy. An operation for benign prostatic enlargement (BPE). Used when the prostate is too large for transurethral prostatectomy (TURP). Involves moving aside the bladder so that the inner prostate tissue can be removed without entering the bladder.

retropubic prostatectomy. An operation to remove prostate tissue referred to as *radical* when the entire prostate is removed for cancer or *simple* when only the inner portion of the prostate is removed for urinary obstruction due to prostate enlargement.

robotic-assisted laparoscopic prostatectomy. The use of laparoscopic instruments moved by robotic arms to remove the entire prostate for cancer (radical prostatectomy) or only the inner portion of the prostate (simple prostatectomy) for urinary obstruction.

S

salvage therapy. A secondary treatment following an initial treatment that did not eradiate a cancer. For example, the use of radiation therapy after surgery, or cryotherapy after radiation therapy for prostate cancer.

semen. Fluid that is ejaculated at the time of orgasm containing sperm produced in the testicles and seminal fluid produced by the seminal vesicles and prostate.

seminal vesicles. Paired glands located behind the bladder and above the prostate that produce part of the seminal fluid containing substances that maintain normal sperm function.

scrotum. The external pouch containing the testicles.

simple prostatectomy. A surgery for the treatment of lower urinary tract symptoms (LUTS) due to benign prostatic enlargement (BPE) that involves removing the obstructing inner tissue of the prostate gland. The procedure can be performed through an incision in the lower abdomen (retropubic or suprapubic), laparoscopically through holes in the abdominal wall, or through the urethra (transurethral resection/ablation of the prostate).

smooth muscle. An involuntary muscle found throughout the body (intestines, blood vessels) including the prostate gland and bladder neck, where it is involved in propelling seminal fluid into the urethra and out through the penis during ejaculation.

stress incontinence. The most common type of incontinence; involves the leakage of urine during coughing, sneezing, laughing, lifting, exercising, and other events that increase the pressure inside the bladder.

suprapubic open prostatectomy. An operation to treat lower urinary tract symptoms or complications from benign prostatic enlargement (BPE) that is performed when the prostate is too large to allow for transurethral prostatectomy (TURP). This approach involves an incision in the lower abdomen, opening the bladder, and removing the inner portion of the prostate through the bladder.

surgical castration. Surgical removal of either the testicles (bilateral orchiectomy) or the contents of the testicles (subcapsular orchiectomy) for treatment of prostate cancer.

T

testicles. Paired egg-shaped glands located in the scrotum that produce sperm and sex hormones.

testosterone. The primary male sex hormone, or androgen, produced in the testicles.

thermotherapy. Heat treatment of the prostate used for lower urinary tract symptoms. Heat is thought to reduce symptoms through the ablation of tissues including nerves within the prostate.

three-dimensional conformal radiation therapy (3D-CRT). A means of targeting external beam radiation more precisely to the prostate with image technology that results in delivery of high doses to the prostate with less exposure to surrounding tissue.

TNM system. A staging system based on the extent of the tumor (T), whether cancer cells have spread to nearby lymph nodes (N), and whether metastasis (M) has occurred.

total androgen blockade. A treatment for prostate cancer that interferes with the production and action of both testicular and adrenal androgens; involves combining an antiandrogen with a luteinizing hormone-releasing hormone (LHRH) agonist/analog or with surgical castration.

transition zone. The inner zone of the prostate that surrounds the urethra. The area where benign prostatic enlargement originates and, less often, prostate cancer.

transrectal ultrasound (TRUS). An imaging technique that involves placement of an ultrasound probe into the rectum. Ultrasound waves are used to create images of the entire prostate that are used to direct biopsy needles for diagnosing prostate cancer on prostate biopsy.

transurethral incision of the prostate (TUIP). A procedure performed through the urethra to relieve lower urinary tract symptoms; involves making small incisions in the prostate to relieve pressure caused by benign prostate growth.

transurethral microwave therapy (TUMT). A treatment for lower urinary tract symptoms caused by an enlarged prostate that utilizes microwave energy to heat and destroy prostate tissue. The energy is emitted from a catheter inserted in the urethra.

transurethral needle ablation (TUNA). A treatment for lower urinary tract symptoms caused by an enlarged prostate that uses radio frequency to generate heat within the prostate. Needles inserted into the prostate through the urethra deliver the energy.

transurethral resection of the prostate (TURP). A treatment for an enlarged prostate gland that involves the use of a special instrument (a resectoscope) inserted through the urethra and into the prostate to remove noncancerous prostate tissue. Also called TUR.

U

ureter. The tube that carries urine from each kidney to the bladder.

urethra. The tube through which urine is carried from the bladder, through the prostate, and out of the body during urination. In men, the urethra also carries semen that is released during ejaculation.

urethral stricture. Narrowing of the urethra.

urge incontinence. Leakage of urine accompanied by a sudden strong desire to urinate that cannot be suppressed.

urinalysis. The examination of urine under the microscope.

urinary incontinence. Uncontrolled loss of urine.

urinary tract infection. An infection of any part of the urinary system including the kidney, bladder, prostate, or urethra; often caused by bacteria such as *Escherichia coli*.

uroflowmetry. A noninvasive test in which a person urinates into a device that measures the rate of urine flow in milliliters per second. A reduced flow can be caused by a weak bladder or obstruction from a stricture or prostate enlargement.

urologist. A doctor who specializes in diagnosing and treating disorders of the genitorurinary system in males and females

V

vas deferens. The tube that transports sperm from the testicles to the urethra where it mixes with seminal fluid at the time of ejaculation.

vasectomy. A reversible surgical birth control procedure that prevents sperm transport through the vas deferens by removing a small section of the vas deferens on both sides within the scrotum.

W

watchful waiting. An approach to managing benign prostatic enlargement (BPE) or prostate cancer in which no treatment is initiated until symptoms appear. In men with prostate cancer, once treatment is initiated, it's palliative rather than curative.

The list below contains various public or private organizations that provide information and services related to prostate disorders.

The Brady Urological Institute
The Johns Hopkins Hospital
600 North Wolfe Street
Baltimore, MD 21287
410-955-6707
http://urology.jhu.edu/

From the leading urology center in America, this well-organized site provides the latest information on urological disease, including material on every major prostate disorder, interviews with leading urology experts, and links to clinical trials of experimental prostate therapies.

American Cancer Society
250 Williams Street NW
Atlanta, GA 30303
800-227-2345
www.cancer.org

The ACS, which sponsors the Man to Man support group, is a national community-based organization that answers questions about prostate cancer and other cancers, provides information on specific cancer topics, and provides referral information on treatment centers and self-help organizations.

AUA Foundation
1000 Corporate Boulevard
Suite 410
Linthicum, MD 21090
800-828-7866/410-689-3990
www.urologyhealth.org

The AUA Foundation is the world's leading nonprofit urological health foundation, and the official foundation of the American Urological Association. The foundation partners with physicians, researchers, health care professionals, patients, caregivers, families, and the public to support and improve the prevention, detection, and treatment of all urological diseases.

Cancer*Care*
275 Seventh Avenue
Floor 22
New York, NY 10001
800-813-4673
www.cancercare.org

Cancer*Care* is a national nonprofit organization that provides free, professional support services for anyone affected by cancer.

Cancer Information Service/National Cancer Institute
Public Inquiries Office
6116 Executive Boulevard
Suite 300
Bethesda, MD 20892-8322
800-4-CANCER (800-422-6237)
www.cancer.gov/cancertopics/types/prostate?
www.cancer.gov/aboutnci/cis

This federally funded service, established in 1975, provides scientifically based, unbiased information about all aspects of cancer, including research, clinical trials, prevention, and living with the disease. A service of the National Cancer Institute, this site also provides the latest information about prostate cancer screening, diagnosis, and treatments.

Malecare
125 Second Avenue
New York NY 10003
212-673-4920
www.malecare.org

This all-volunteer nonprofit men's prostate cancer support and advocacy group produces comprehensive men's cancer support programs, internationally and on the Internet. The group has a particular focus on gay and bisexual men and men with advanced disease.

National Association for Continence (NAFC)
PO Box 1019
Charleston, SC 29402-1019
800-BLADDER (800-252-3337)
www.nafc.org

This advocacy organization is dedicated to improving the quality of life of people with incontinence, voiding dysfunction, and related pelvic floor disorders.

National Kidney and Urologic Diseases Information Clearinghouse (NKUDIC)
3 Information Way
Bethesda, MD 20892
800-891-5390
www.kidney.niddk.nih.gov

This national service provides access to health information about all prostate disorders and links to patient organizations.

Prostate Cancer Foundation (PCF)
1250 Fourth Street
Santa Monica, CA 90401
800-757-2873/310-570-4700
www.prostatecancerfoundation.org

Founded in 1993 by Michael Milken, American financier and philanthropist, the PCF has been the driving force behind finding a cure for prostate cancer by supporting research that can translate into treatment and cure. The PCF has had a particular focus on supporting young investigators with novel ideas that might not be funded by traditional sources. Its informative Web site has background information on prostate cancer, from diagnosis to treatment.

Us TOO International
5003 Fairview Avenue
Downers Grove, IL 60515
800-808-7866/630-795-1002
www.ustoo.org

Founded in 1990 by five men who had been treated for prostate cancer, this nonprofit prostate cancer education and support network has 325 support group chapters worldwide. Us TOO provides men and their families with free information, materials, and peer-to-peer support so that they can make informed choices on detection, treatment options, and coping with ongoing survivorship.

ACKNOWLEDGMENTS

While writing a book can be a solitary endeavor, it is not accomplished without the direct or indirect input of so many. There are numerous friends and colleagues we would like to recognize for their assistance in helping us bring this book to you.

Thanks first and foremost to Stephen Hanselman from LevelFiveMedia, literary agent extraordinaire, who guided us through the publishing process. His faith in us from day one, and his dedication to this project has been extremely valuable and important. Without his keen instincts and direction, this book would not have found the widest audience possible.

Many thanks to Dominick Anfuso, our talented editor in chief at Free Press (Simon & Schuster), for understanding the importance of this book from its inception, and for all the work he did to move this from manuscript to published work.

We would like to thank Grace Young, award-winning cookbook author, who provided her insights and tasty recipes. A tip of the hat to Rob Duckwall of Dragonfly Media Group for his detailed medical illustrations that appear throughout the book. It's his talent that helps get our message across to you in the clearest manner possible.

A book like this makes extensive use of clinical studies. For every clinical trial or laboratory experiment discussed within these pages, there were dedicated researchers around the country behind them who had worked tirelessly in the cause of advancing science. We are grateful for the willingness of medical experts to take the time to discuss their work, including Wendy Demark-Wahnefried, PhD, from the University of Alabama at Birmingham Comprehensive Cancer Center for her insights about flaxseed and prostate cancer. Dr. Daniel A. Shoskes, the Cleveland Clinic urologist who is one of the leading experts on chronic pelvic pain syndrome and its diagnosis, and Mary McVearry, an extraordinary physical therapist who understands the burden of CPPS, offered their special treatment recommendations for this misunderstood disorder. For their approach to diagnosing and treating overactive bladder, Dr. Patricia Goode, medical director of the Continence Clinic at the University of Alabama at Birmingham, and Dr. Roger Dmochowski, from the Vanderbilt University Medical Center, were very helpful. For information on exercise and its effects on the prostate, Dr. J. Kellogg Parsons of the Moores Cancer Center at the University of California, San Diego, was quick to describe his latest research.

The urology faculty at the James Buchanan Brady Urological Institute at Johns Hopkins have provided invaluable insights through the years and have contributed to this book in many ways.

We would like especially to thank Dr. Patrick C. Walsh and Donald S. Coffey, PhD, for their mentorship that began in 1987 and continues today. Their leadership and teaching of so many has been felt throughout the world in the field of urology and is truly unprecedented.

To each and every one of you, thank you.

—H. Ballentine Carter, MD
Gerald Secor Couzens
May 2012

Page numbers in *italics* refer to illustrations and charts.

H. Ballentine Carter, MD, professor of urology and oncology and the director of adult urology at the Johns Hopkins University School of Medicine, is an international leader in research on the diagnosis and management of prostate cancer. He pioneered the concept of targeted prostate cancer screening with PSA, rather than a one-size-fits-all approach, through early publications with colleagues from the Baltimore Longitudinal Study of Aging. He continues to direct one of the largest active surveillance programs in the United States for monitoring carefully selected men with prostate cancer who have chosen no immediate treatment for their disease. He has published studies in the *Journal of the American Medical Association,* the *Journal of the National Cancer Institute, Cancer Research,* the *Journal of Urology,* and other major scientific publications, newspapers, and magazines. He lives in Baltimore, Maryland.

Gerald Secor Couzens, a medical writer who has written and coauthored more than twenty health, medical, fitness, and sports books, is the managing editor of the *Johns Hopkins Prostate Disorders Bulletin.* He lives with his family in New York City.